Internet of Things

Technology, Communications and Computing

The series Internet of Things - Technologies, Communications and Computing publishes new developments and advances in the various areas of the different facets of the Internet of Things.

The intent is to cover technology (smart devices, wireless sensors, systems), communications (networks and protocols) and computing (theory, middleware and applications) of the Internet of Things, as embedded in the fields of engineering, computer science, life sciences, as well as the methodologies behind them. The series contains monographs, lecture notes and edited volumes in the Internet of Things research and development area, spanning the areas of wireless sensor networks, autonomic networking, network protocol, agent-based computing, artificial intelligence, self organizing systems, multi-sensor data fusion, smart objects, and hybrid intelligent systems.

** Indexing: *Internet of Things* is covered by Scopus and Ei-Compendex **

More information about this series at http://www.springer.com/series/11636

Patrick Siarry • M. A. Jabbar
Rajanikanth Aluvalu • Ajith Abraham
Ana Madureira
Editors

The Fusion of Internet of Things, Artificial Intelligence, and Cloud Computing in Health Care

Springer

Editors
Patrick Siarry
Université Paris-Est Créteil
Créteil, France

M. A. Jabbar
Vardhaman College of Engineering
Hyderabad, Telangana, India

Rajanikanth Aluvalu
Vardhaman College of Engineering
Hyderabad, Telangana, India

Ajith Abraham
Machine Intelligence Research Labs
Auburn, Washington, USA

Ana Madureira
School of Engineering
Instituto Superior de Engenharia
Porto, Portugal

ISSN 2199-1073 ISSN 2199-1081 (electronic)
Internet of Things
ISBN 978-3-030-75219-4 ISBN 978-3-030-75220-0 (eBook)
https://doi.org/10.1007/978-3-030-75220-0

This Springer imprint is published by the registered company Springer Nature Switzerland AG
The registered company address is: Gewerbestrasse 11, 6330 Cham, Switzerland

Introduction

The healthcare industry is one of the most advanced in implementing and adopting emerging technology in some form. AI and cloud computing techniques, along with IoT, are useful in analyzing imaging and genetic data to extract information from clinical data. In many cases, IoT integrated with the cloud and AI will open new paths to innovation and insight in the medical domain. The fusion of AI, IoT, and cloud computing-based diagnostic systems will help doctors and medical practitioners predict various diseases by improving the speed of diagnosis and accuracy.

This book is a collective reference that provides a collection of research on the applications of IoT, cloud computing, and artificial intelligence in health care. This book is ideally designed for medical professionals, researchers, academicians, developers, and postgraduate students. The chapters presented in this book are unique to this book and explore the applications of emerging technologies in the healthcare domain.

The content is structured into 12 chapters, which are further classified into Part I and Part II. Part I discusses the foundational concepts of IoT, cloud, and artificial intelligence in health care. Part II covers the applications of IoT, cloud, and artificial intelligence in tackling COVID-19 and other pandemic diseases.

Chapter 1 provides an Overview of the Medical Internet of Things, Artificial Intelligence, and Cloud Computing Employed in Health Care from a Modern Panorama. The connected IoMT device provides objective reports of the patient's actual activity, helping to monitor their behavior and activities outside the office, allowing physicians to have real data of patient compliance and therapy recommendations.

The authors highlight Healthcare Data Storage Options Using the Cloud in Chap. 2. In this chapter, the healthcare data storage options on the cloud as well as the security of healthcare data are described.

A Review on Classification and Retrieval of Biomedical Images Using Artificial Intelligence is provided in Chap. 3. This chapter reviews the existing content-based medical image retrieval systems and techniques used for feature extraction and image classification.

The Diagnosis of Breast Cancer by Malignant Changes in Buccal Epithelium Using Artificial Intelligence, the Internet of Things, and Cloud Storage is discussed in Chap. 4. The authors proposed a model to detect tumor-associated changes in the fractal structure of chromatin in people with fibroadenomatosis and breast cancer.

Chapter 5 focuses on the Smart IoT Treatment: Making Medical Care More Intelligent. This chapter explores a conceptual model for understanding the factors determining patient satisfaction with the use of artificial intelligence in health care.

Chapter 6 highlights the Privacy and Security Concerns in IoT-Based Healthcare Systems. This chapter proposes a framework for securing healthcare information on the IoT-based platform. This chapter also demonstrates the architecture of the extensive healthcare system based on IoT, the technological problems, and some standard implementations relevant to comprehensive health care. Data safety, privacy, and confidentiality are looked into IoT-based security and privacy in healthcare systems.

Chapter 7 explores IoT Healthcare Applications. With the use of IoT technology, treatment and monitoring will be more precise and in proper order. This chapter concludes with IoT applications that enable patients to access data and personalized care and reduce visits to the hospital.

In Chap. 8 the authors examine a Tele Health Monitoring System in Rural Areas through Primary Health Centers using IOT for COVID-19. The project was successfully implemented in Abdullapurmet village in Telangana State. A small handbook was also created in the local language, Telugu, with a proper explanation of the operation of all the devices.

Chapter 9 discusses the applications of Artificial Intelligence for Disease Identification and Diagnosis. The chapter highlights the challenges of medical data processing for detecting and diagnosing diseases. The challenges include small datasets, missing data, and unbalanced datasets.

In Chap. 10 the authors propose a model for predicting epidemic outbreaks using IOT, Artificial Intelligence, and the Cloud. These emerging technologies will play an important role in fighting pandemic diseases.

Chapter 11 reviews Computational Intelligence Technologies for Tackling the COVID-19 Pandemic. This chapter talks about the symptoms and prevention of COVID-19. It also highlights the emerging technologies used to fight COVID-19. IoT technology is used to integrate medical equipment with the internet and provide remote treatment to infected patients, and many more technologies are highlighted.

Chapter 12 provides guidance on the role of artificial intelligence in healthcare management and the challenge of the Coronavirus pandemic. A review of the literature was conducted on the applications of artificial intelligence to tackle pandemic diseases like COVID-19.

Contents

Part I
Internet of Things, Artificial Intelligence, and Cloud Computing in Health Care

Chapter 1
An Overview of Medical Internet of Things, Artificial Intelligence, and Cloud Computing Employed in Health Care from a Modern Panorama

Ana Carolina Borges Monteiro, Reinaldo Padilha França, Rangel Arthur, and Yuzo Iano

1.1 Introduction

Cloud-based telemedicine for health care focuses on identifying important medical needs, how to integrate patients with telemedicine, facilitate collaboration between multidisciplinary health teams, and improve operational efficiency, with strict safety measures [1].

Innovation is needed mainly during the pandemic of the new coronavirus (SARS-CoV-2), which is drastically impacting the lives of people around the world and transforming health systems in the same way. After all, social isolation measures mainly affected the patient's access to medical care in elective consultations (when there is no risk of death), requiring increasingly personalized care and demanding daily updates on the latest protocols in the treatment of COVID-19 that is forcing new solutions to come up or for old ones to be rethought [2].

An important element for the health area is the remote monitoring of patients, such as after hospital discharge or in cases that do not require hospitalization. For this work to be effective, professionals must check the situation of patients daily, except that most of the tools available for this purpose are generally limited to phone calls and e-mails, in addition to the restricted technologies for secure videoconferencing [3].

A. C. B. Monteiro · R. P. França (✉) · Y. Iano
School of Electrical and Computer Engineering (FEEC), University of Campinas – UNICAMP, Barão Geraldo, Brazil
e-mail: monteiro@decom.fee.unicamsp.br; padilha@decom.fee.unicamp.br; yuzo@decom.fee.unicamp.br

R. Arthur
Faculty of Technology (FT), University of Campinas – UNICAMP, Jardim Nova Italia, Brazil
e-mail: rangel@ft.unicamp.br

P. Siarry et al. (eds.), *The Fusion of Internet of Things, Artificial Intelligence, and Cloud Computing in Health Care*, Internet of Things,
https://doi.org/10.1007/978-3-030-75220-0_1

Also related that digital health applications make it possible to monitor the health of patients by recording health data (or synchronizing the application with the connected medical devices (IoMT, ie, medical Internet of things), following their health conditions evolution through graphics, or even accessing central digital health. Also consider the possibility of carrying out monitoring of patient conditions, i.e., monitoring the health data of patients, or even keeping the record of clinical data in electronic medical records. By means of connected medical devices (IoMT) through cloud platforms, it is possible to be used synchronized with specific applications, making the data inclusion process simpler, ensuring reliable data [4].

With telemedicine through cloud for healthcare, healthcare organizations can create individualized care plans for patients or groups of patients. It is also possible to implement secure virtual consultations, initial screenings with chatbots, and remote monitoring, which enhance the online experience, and even using this service in self-assessment tools for infection, and, thus, seek to reduce the number of requests on their emergency lines [5].

Still considering that telemedicine solutions may involve telemedicine solutions based on teleconsultation, through a real-time video consultation platform, conducting online screenings, or even telemedicine sessions between doctors, nurses, and patients. Also consider the possibility of sharing information and sharing screens by video or chat, since medical devices can be integrated, and systems based on cloud and IoT technology (Internet of Things). This allows simultaneous connection of different communication points and the sending of medical images (via streaming) in real-time at the time of consultation [6].

Another important point is the continuous monitoring of patients through the IoT, enabling the monitoring of data coming from remote medical devices and allowing more efficient monitoring of patients, both inside and outside hospital facilities. With this information collected in real time, service teams can act before an emergency or fatality, reducing the chances of readmission of patients, among others [5, 6], resulting in telediagnosis through a platform for reports and management of medical information (exams and histories), organizing specific clinical protocols by specialties, still being able to attach exams in PDF, DOCX, PPT, images, and even videos formats, and emphasizing that such systems allow images to be attached to medical records and remote access to records via notebooks, tablets and smartphones, and other devices [7].

In this sense, cloud-based telemedicine ecosystem technologies using IoMT, cloud computing, and artificial intelligence (AI) offered a portfolio of complete solutions in eHealth with a focus on telemedicine and digital health through cloud infrastructure (cloud-based) assisting health institutions to act in a more agile, assertive, and sustainable way, representing that this technological performance helps in conducting teleconsultations and teleconsultations, monitoring patients with electronic medical records with prescription, teletriage and telediagnosis, scheduling appointments, and exams, managing service queues, among others, in various medical specialties [8].

In digital health, a range of monitoring solutions is offered that includes mobile health applications for patients, connected devices (IoMT), and compatibility for synchronization and personalized alerts in real time, registration of clinical data in electronic medical records, and clinical monitoring [9].

Therefore, this chapter aims to provide an updated overview of the cloud-based telemedicine ecosystem and adopting IoT, IoMT, cloud computing, and AI, addressing its branch of application, approaching with a concise bibliographic background, synthesizing the potential of the technologies.

1.2 IoMT Concept

The Internet of things (IoT) can be characterized in that several devices are connected to communication networks for the exchange and collection of information, generally involving the use of smart sensors in an environment (Fig. 1.1). Evaluating that obtaining more data and information about internal processes can increase the efficiency of operations by combining IoT technology with Big Data and AI tools, generating the possibility to identify patterns or internal areas that need improvement [10–12].

Internet of medical things (IoMT) is derived from Internet of things (IoT), which is related and used to develop and define devices that are connected to the Internet, with communication power, highlighting one of its main characteristics of IoT in the exchange of information [13].

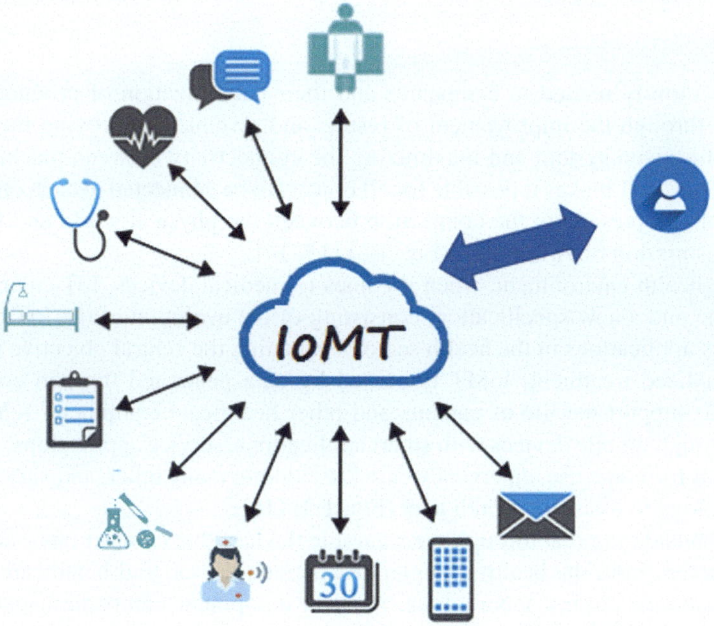

Fig. 1.1 Internet of medical things

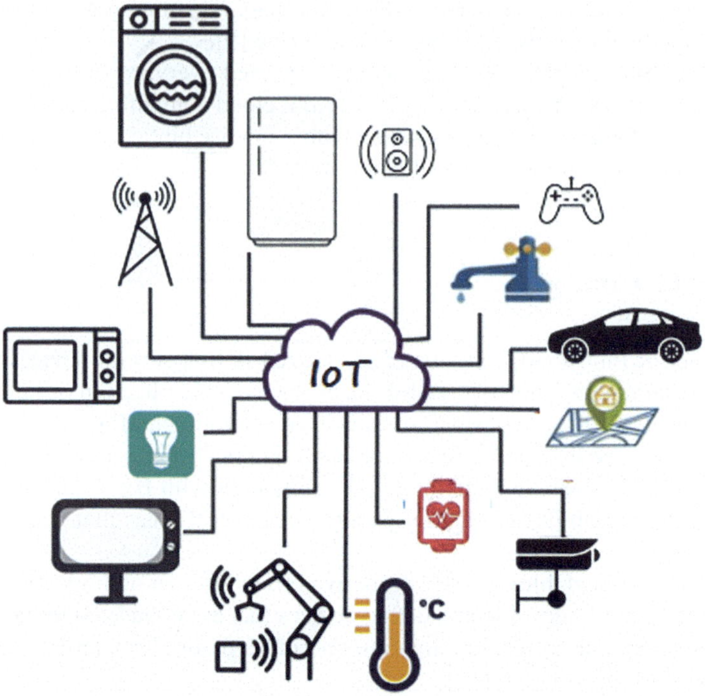

Fig. 1.2 Internet of things illustration

IoT is closely related to companies and their maximization of production and services, through the improvement of results and revenues, improving the performance of a given system and maximizing the connectivity between machines and people. Thus, IoT makes it possible for all objects to be connected to each other over the Internet, representing the connection between the physical world and the constant transmission of virtual data (Fig. 1.2) [13, 14].

In the health environment, when it comes to medical devices, IoT emerges as a new name and a new specification, consisting of the evolution of the IoT concept, having its applications in the health sector, evaluating the central objective in offering specialized treatment. IoMT is guided by data generated through connected devices to support the life of patients and other healthcare equipment. IoMT uses either through mobile devices with smart applications, service applications, medical equipment for home use, emergency care kits, among many other, and varied forms of technology to assist the health area (Fig. 1.3) [15].

Also considering that through the wearable devices that connect more and more diverse actors form the health triangle, i.e., patient, doctor, and healthcare institutions (hospitals, clinics, laboratories, medical equipment companies, medication companies, health insurance companies, and even preventive medicine clinics), which interconnect form an ecosystem [16].

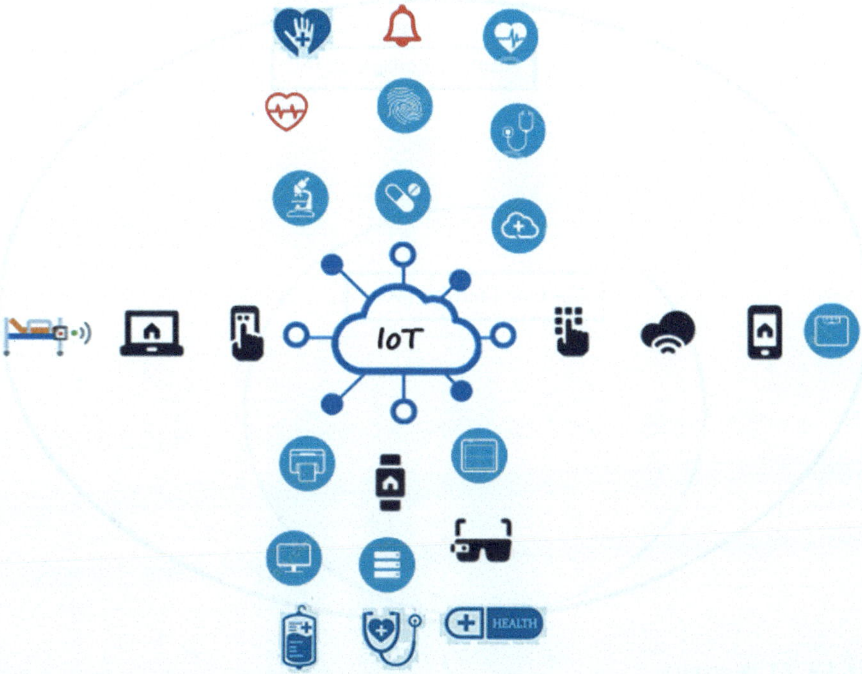

Fig. 1.3 Devices Internet of medical things

It is a fact that in modern times, IoT technology and medicine are increasingly closer, in a symbiosis in which health professionals use machines and devices connected to the Web to perfect exams, diagnoses, and even treatments, i.e., IoMT, with a lot more potential for use, and there is still much to explore from IoMT. Also evaluating that far beyond a data connection, IoMT is consistent with the integration between essential information from the patient's reality and the availability of data for consultation with doctors and specialists. Through IoMT, medicine has properties to benefit from greater agility in the verification of hospital pictures and even the early preparation for possible failures of both patients and medical equipment [17].

1.2.1 AI Application in Health

Artificial intelligence (AI) is considered a research area that uses technological resources capable of generating mechanisms and/or devices, computer intelligence, or machine learning, which are able to reproduce the human being's ability to think and solve problems, that is, to be rational. Applied to health, it brings countless benefits, as is the case of telemedicine advancing with the resources of artificial

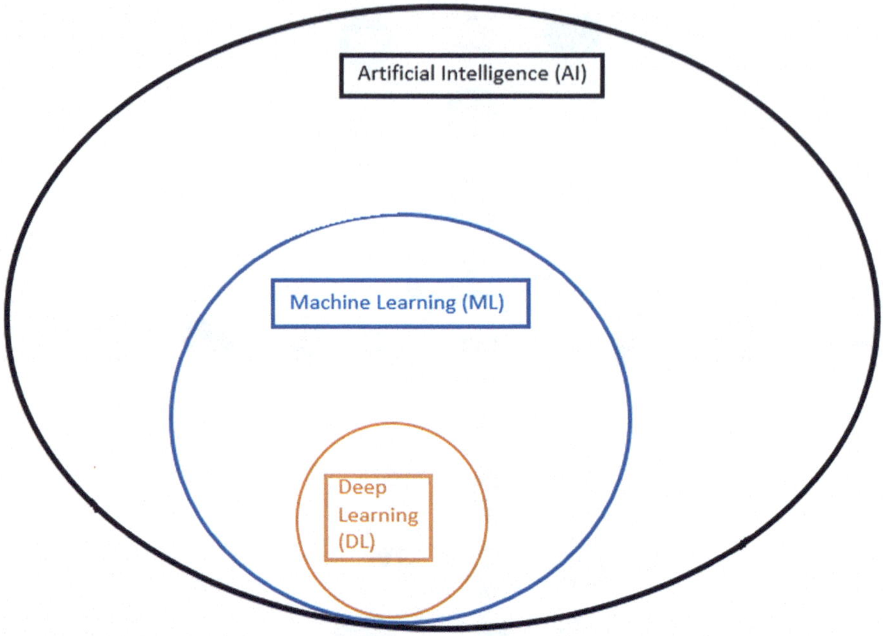

Fig. 1.4 AI illustration

intelligence, mainly related to automation and definition of medical priorities (emergency cases). AI-based solutions through imaging equipment are able to point out possible diseases, through machine learning and even deep learning (Fig. 1.4), and automatically forward notifications to the doctor, and even send the patient's vital signs directly to the medical records, among other features [18].

Health AI basically consists of automated statistics from a database and variables, consisting of computer systems capable of making decisions based on standards analyzed in a large amount of data, instead of a predefined fixed logic, such as those used in conventional systems. That is, it makes it possible to understand the scenario, model, and forecast demand, through an ideal cut and according to the type of activity or behavior being measured, still considering its property capable of "learning" and increasing its accuracy over time, contributing to diagnostic processes, identification of predispositions to diseases, and even treatment prescriptions [19].

With respect to telemedicine, inserted in a broader concept as to eHealth, it is the technology capable of storing and processing a huge repertoire of data, allowing the crossing of information and images digitally captured in exams and reports and transmitted via the telemedicine platform. This feature brings many benefits to doctors and patients in the definition of increasingly accurate diagnoses, relating the sum of this digital file to the patient's history, which is also stored digitally. Relating from the historical point of view, the call from before was telemedicine today; however, the technology has evolved to the point of the possibility of visualizing the image, still with limitations in terms of not being able to make a diagnosis without palpating the patient. However, this technology optimizes the doctor's time and provides an improvement in patients' routines, avoiding unnecessary travel [20].

Considering that eHealth is compatible with any Internet application, used in conjunction with other information technologies, such as AI techniques, i.e., machine learning and derivatives, it is focused on providing better conditions for clinical processes, patient treatment, and better costing conditions for the system of health. The concept includes many dimensions, ranging from the delivery of clinical information to actors and members of the healthcare chain, to the ease of interaction between them and reaching the availability of that same information in the most difficult and remote places. Including a set of tools and services capable of sustaining the service in an integrated way through the Web, allowing to mention Electronic Health Record (ePatient), mobile health (mHealth), Big Data, Cloud Computing, Personalized Medicine, Telemedicine among others [21].

Still relating employment together with Big Data technologies and machine learning algorithms (Fig. 1.5), information on patients will be more abundant, patterns are more easily identified, and new solutions to various health problems can be identified more easily, boosting the area of health entering a new era [11, 21].

Or even, it relates the collaboration between medical teams through cloud computing services and IoT gadgets making the medical routine safer and more effective, allowing the ability to diagnose patients more quickly. It uses technology creating personalized treatments and is more adapted to the unique profile of each patient [12].

The potential of IoT in health is related to the possibility of promoting greater integration between AI equipment and systems, in addition to feeding the database for AI. I see that through common medical devices connected to the Internet, they expand the data collection capacity and also expand the vision obtained through digital optics about symptoms and trends. This opens up the possibility of capturing data from multiparameter monitors, such as heart rate, respiratory rate, blood pressure, and patient temperature, among other types of digital data. Given that based on

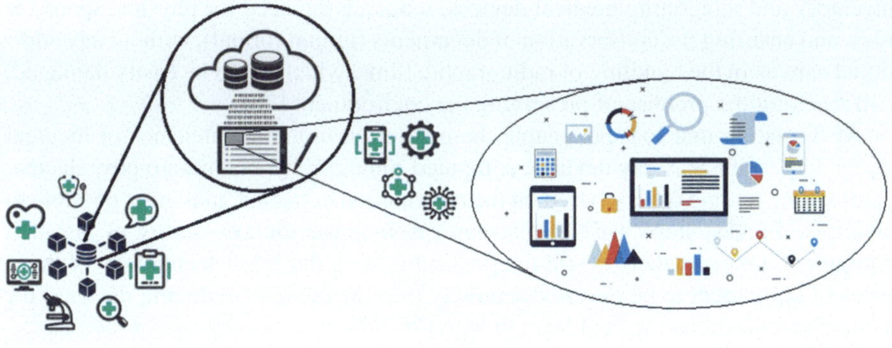

Fig. 1.5 Big data illustration

this information, AI tools can perform risk classification for patients, for example, optimizing care for the most vulnerable patients [22].

In hospitals, IoT is also present in equipment such as sensors that collect air quality data and incorporate AI, making autonomous robots used to disinfect facilities and allowing the development of applications for tracking infected people and creating security perimeters, very useful in the case of the COVID-19 pandemic, among many other applications [23].

Or the potential of IoT is that this technological concept makes possible some aspects of telemedicine, such as telemonitoring, contributing to making health more preventive, with regard to the possibility of measuring pressure and checking heartbeat in smartwatches, that is, via the Web, among many other possibilities of use. Regarding the monitoring of chronic diseases, IoMT can be used through smart apps, electronic medical records, sensors, and wearable devices, with smartwatches, collecting data related to symptoms, during their daily activities, and conditions of these patients. From this information, AI algorithms through machine learning are able to guide diagnostics and therapies at a distance and also monitor the evolution of the disease [24].

A useful utility in relation to IoMT is associated with oximetry sensors, widely used in hospitals and maternity hospitals, and used to measure the vital signs of inpatients and newborns. These oximeter sensors, through portable devices, can be placed on the wrist, finger, or ear, and with AI resources, they collect this event data, storing it in memory and still allowing remote or USB access [25].

1.2.2 IoT Technology

Currently, there are digital devices for performing diagnostic tests such as X-rays, computed tomography, and electrocardiogram, capable of generating and storing data digitally, eliminating the use of paper. Archiving digitally, these data and information allow greater simplicity in sharing between the entire medical chains. This characteristic of IoT in healthcare services helps in optimizing workflow, managing inventory and integrating medical devices, reducing the need for physical space for files, and ensuring the conservation of documents (digital format), without any additional care as in the handling of radiographic films, which could be easily damaged, still reaching the premise of preserving the environment [26].

Also relating that IoT can enable the prediction in the maintenance of medical equipment, such as X-ray devices, computed tomography, mammography, electrocardiogram, among others, based on the information collected, making it possible to anticipate breaks, stops and, in this sense, to increase the availability of installed equipment. Or even, there is still the possibility with the IoMT technology of these types of equipment to be operated remotely (remote control), reducing the need for a complete specialist medical team in loco [26, 27].

IoT technology is smart pacemakers facilitating the cardiac monitoring of thousands of people around the world. Consisting of the same modality as wearables, i.e., connected cardiac digital devices that can be implanted in the patient, they collect, store, and transmit data and information in real time about the patient's cardiovascular system. In this scenario, a cardiologist medical professional with the conditions to monitor the individual's health conditions from a distance, intervening when necessary, and having sufficient properties to be able to make decisions to improve the quality of life of this patient [28].

Another possibility of intelligent technology through IoT is devices with properties to monitor the glucose levels of diabetic patients, through continuous intelligent glucose monitoring (CGM) being able to register patterns and point out abnormalities in patients and even able to send data to another device, such as a smartphone, tablet, or medical device. These smart IoT devices allow diabetes, i.e., chronic disease that needs to be monitored daily, to be assessed using instant and accurate data through technology [29].

Or even mentioning the IoT technology applied through ingestible sensors (nanosensors), capturing and transmitting images of the gastrointestinal tract and the colon, replacing invasive procedures monitoring vital signs. And even, in specific cases, they allow the early detection of colorectal cancer, serving as an alternative to colonoscopy [30].

There are wearables with properties and characteristics to monitor symptoms and behaviors of people with depression and to follow through the application of tests and data collected through smartwatches with patients diagnosed with mild to moderate depression, mood assessments, and cognition effectively. Following through the usability of wearable devices, based on recorded information, i.e., patients who have their data collected while performing routine tasks, can be employed to monitor those patients with depression, or even following the evolution of Parkinson's symptoms. From there, it transmits this information to the physician and other specialists, analyzing this, and providing opting for more assertive treatments that improve the quality of life of those who suffer from this type of disease [31].

Or even with regard to those patients with serious diseases such as Alzheimer's disease, through the integration of IoT sensors with smartphones, it is possible to track hand tremors to the place where the user is. Through these data collected and transmitted on these devices, it is possible to identify the advances of Alzheimer's disease and the impact that this has on the patient's routine. From the patient's point of view, is obtained a better quality of life, since is acquired more security in your daily commutes and other situations in which Alzheimer's can affect your routine [32].

The deployment of IoT technology in hospitals and clinics can be achieved through the installation of smart hospital beds, through a differentiated approach assisting nurses and other professionals specialized in the accommodation and safety of patients at risk of falling from their beds. In addition, the beds have the properties of sending and informing messages about the best position to accommodate the patient, collaborating so that he is comfortable, in case they have not been repositioned properly after feeding or cleaning. Or even, the IoT technology applied in conjunction with artificial intelligence (AI) techniques allows identifying in advance, patients at risk, or in the circumstances of developing a generalized infection (sepsis) [33].

1.3 Telemedicine and Healthcare Concept

A series of IoT devices can be connected to the Wi-Fi network or other types of networks in a hospital, generating vast amounts of data and allowing the tracking of information, for professionals and medical teams, and even for patients, having their activities and monitoring health conditions. In this sense, it is possible to define health care as everything that encompasses the healthcare market, since this has become more and more specialized in the patient's demands, finding itself in the space of development of technologies and methodologies bringing a new approach in the provision and the promoting the health and well-being of the world population, developing an intelligent and sustainable health chain. Driven by people's life expectancy, it has increased over the years and in the same proportion the desire and interest in wanting to live with more quality and more independently. Thus, Health digital is the set of healthcare that aims to treat diseases and preserve health, encompassing all necessary medical, pharmaceutical, and diagnostic services [20, 33].

Telemedicine is attainable through a modern and intuitive platform, which records and stores information transmitted by connected devices, taking advantage of the potential of IoT by expanding the portfolio and reducing health costs. Through telemedicine, it is possible for clinics and hospitals to use digital equipment for diagnostic tests at a distance, which can be conducted by technicians in radiology or nursing [34].

IoT and telemedicine were born from the use of information and communication technologies; currently, the use of telemedicine is a provider of distance exam interpretation services. An example emphasizing how both technologies can work together is the sharing of data captured by digital devices during diagnostic tests, carried out via the telemedicine platform, enabling the issuance of distance reports with quality and efficiency, considering that this information is automatically added to the patient's medical record and is available for interpretation by specialists, enhancing the results for doctors, health units, and patients [35].

Through this type of platform, data from these exams are shared at one end and accessed at the other end by qualified specialists, responsible for interpreting the records. Also relating that with the support of the information available in the patient's record, usually collected in the emergency room, which is the gateway for patients in clinics, hospitals, and other health institutions, the specialists evaluate the exams and produce the report at a distance and even digitally signing it [36].

The properties of telemedicine technology speed up and reduce the processing time of exam results, considering that urgent exam requests are released in real time, supporting the choice of the best treatment through adverse events, such as heart attack, stroke, and serious incidents [37].

Telemedicine can be inserted into eHealth, and it can be subdivided into Telecare, given that the focus of communication is on the patient and his well-being, in which he is monitored in his own home or at a local health center by a doctor or any other health professional who communicates with other professionals at a distance. Teleconsultation is carried out among doctors, when a general practitioner seeks assistance from a specialist, such as a second opinion in the diagnosis, a more suitable medication, live guidance on how to perform a procedure, or even with the online consultation, made directly between doctors and patients. Tele-education is applied in medicine with a focus on training health professionals who are far from major centers, seeking to update and prepare them for various medical practice situations, using videoconferences, classes, lectures, e-learning, and recycling programs [38].

From a modern and current perspective, in combating the COVID-19 pandemic, which intensified the use of IoT and stimulated health tech that automates devices in the ICU (Intensive Care Unit) integrating management systems of electronic medical records and medical equipment. In an ICU environment, IoMT technology allows to connect data from devices that monitor the heart and lungs of patients with COVID-19, gathering all the information in a digital interface allowing doctors to be able to follow the evolution of the disease from a distance, either through a telemedicine platform even by smartphone, without risk of contamination [39].

Or even reflecting on the aspect of social distance, in view of the reality of the pandemic of COVID-19, telemedicine allows remote medical care making the routine in hospitals more agile and safer, since this technology allows the practice of consultations, diagnosis, and exams remote [40].

Thus, telemedicine covers all medical practice performed at a distance, regardless of the instrument used for this relationship; with the use of information technologies adding quality and speed in the exchange of knowledge, specialists and doctors can make decisions with greater agility and precision, being able to access exams from anywhere in the country, using computers and mobile devices, such as smartphones and tablets connected to the Internet.

1.3.1 Cloud-Related to Health Care

Over the past few years, the healthcare market has undergone a technological change, verifying the insertion of digital technologies in order to improve the clinical, operational, and financial aspects of the health business model, whether private or public, allied to the focus on generating benefits to the population as a whole, expanding the population's access to the provision of smarter healthcare services, within a smart and sustainable health chain [41].

The set of technologies such as IoT, Big Data, cloud computing, analytics, and AI allows a new perspective, completely changing the management of processes in the medical field. Through data on individual and even collective health, collected through smart devices, which represents, in addition to patients receiving personalized preventive treatments (more assertive), vital signs monitored remotely, resulting in a reduction in costs with hospital admissions, i.e., from the digital transformation in health care as key aspects influencing the global healthcare segment, financial sustainability in healthcare services is achieved [1, 3, 42].

With cloud computing, it was possible to accelerate the creation of new solutions and make them available to anyone, anywhere and anytime, making data storage infinite and anyone's access to cutting-edge solutions at a cost accessible. This technology has been an important protagonist in the response of the world society to the pandemic of COVID-19, with respect to telemedicine allowing the expansion of the number of people served, providing agility and security for all involved, collaborating even with online therapy, made through applications, online platforms, and even video conferencing [42, 43].

Due to measures of social distance to contain the spread of the disease, hospitals and clinics had to adapt to provide remote care. Cloud computing in the telemedicine background has made it more practical to access reports and test results and decrease spending by all institutions, doctors, patients, and greater reach to laboratories and offices. These measures have been consolidated as a "new normal" in the last months, adopted in an emergency way, offering a more efficient work model, and can be used as a complement to traditional care [43].

Still reflecting on COVID-19, deep learning techniques used in the learning of functions (neural network) are very specific imitating the functioning of the human brain, with supervised learning (Fig. 1.6), combined with computer vision to identify patterns in imaging exams, given how quickly technology adjusts to demands. This union is capable of detecting disease at an early stage, often imperceptible in the eyes of a doctor, representing a disruptive fact in favor of human life, exemplifying the potential of AI employed in cloud computing in favor of medicine, is the analysis of chest X-ray images of patients, based on a neural network analyzing examinations of healthy patients and patients with a positive diagnosis COVID-19, establishing analysis standards and becoming able to classify as low or high risk for complications pulmonary. The solution can be used in the cloud, given the high processing power of the technology, which is necessary for training neural networks and analyzing a digital image with the database [44].

Deep learning through the processing of molecular assays in order to carry out simulations for vaccines, against the new coronavirus, allows complex calculations and simulations with high demand for computational processing power to be performed, something that would be impossible to do without computer computing a cloud [45].

Technology should also be responsible for keeping the healthcare segment in a good cost-benefit ratio through modernization with the adoption of technologies such as cloud computing, AI, robotics, and IoT. In a connected world, health care is turning into digital; however, it is worth considering that the interconnection of data and information increases the cybersecurity concern, with the preservation of this data for health institutions to remain proactive protection and integrity of your systems against virtual attacks [36, 45].

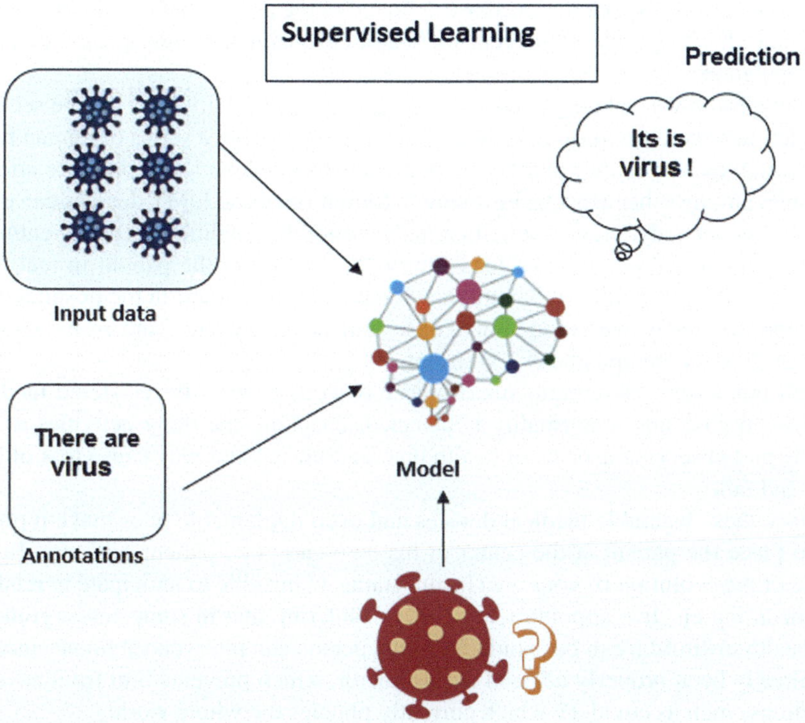

Fig. 1.6 Internet of things

Also correlating this factor with Cloud Computing technology, which allows data in the cloud to have greater digital security, agility, and cost reduction. In terms of cybersecurity, end-to-end encryption, secure authentication, and restricted server access in the cloud are barriers against system intrusions, considering that with respect to cloud computing it is to guarantee the integration and mobility of data, facilitating the sharing of them between managers and clinical staff of a hospital, whether on a tablet, smartphone, or even personal computer [46].

1.4 Discussion

The evolution of IoT and its extension in the health area through IoMT have been revolutionizing by means of disruptive technologies, through diagnoses occurring in real time and with increasingly efficient treatments, in addition to the revolutionary aspect representing health, proving that technology in the field of health has generated a lot of interest in life care, in patient care, and in improving diagnoses.

IoMT can be the great differentiator for communities to approach an overburdened health system that will only be under more stress as the population continues to age, i.e., as life expectancy increases, related to the aspect that the elderly tend to have more health problems, increasing health costs aimed at this specific niche of the population.

Examples IoMT is being used and changing people's daily lives can be seen on bracelets and watches fits, consisting of gadgets monitoring a series of human body items, such as movement, number of steps, heartbeat, sleep level, pressure arterial pressure, among other aspects. From this information, these IoMT devices can evaluate the human body, suggest activities, and monitor the condition of the patient/user.

The benefit and potential of IoMT through monitoring the patient in real time come from the possibility of having the vital data of the patient in the hospital beds in a centralized way, with reduction of costs with adverse events, and even considering that the data are updated every instant.

Still pondering that certain smart bracelets wore previously registered medical services in case any abnormality is detected, checking the daily activities of the elderly and observing aspects of health that are unusual and may cause loss of balance and fall.

Since these wearable medical devices and even implantable ones make it possible to place the patient at the center of his own care, i.e., patient self-care. Being aware of the evolution of your own health status, being able to anticipate in relation to scheduling elective appointments. Still considering that in some cases, going to any health institution can be avoided, and the person can intervene at home since he has already been properly advised by his doctor, which prevents him from adverse infections, such as covid-19 which currently plagues the whole world.

These IoMT gadgets range from the clock and can even be used to measure tremors related to disorders of the nervous system, such as Parkinson's disease, pills with a tiny sensor transmitting information and relaying to a cellphone monitored by the doctor, ensuring that the medication is being taken in time and the correct dosage, or even a contact lens for diabetics measuring blood sugar through the tear of the eyes, offering continuous data on blood sugar fluctuations, informing the patient to avoid complications and risk of life. Other related examples can still be considered in relation to the probes that can be swallowed facilitating the tracking of intestinal diseases or even voice assistants in medical clinics, among other IoMT applications.

The greater use and impact of IoMT in addition to helping in the diagnosis of patients, ensuring adherence to doctor's orders, providing data collected from IoMT devices for better diagnostics and treatment plans, in addition to reducing inefficiencies and waste in the health system. Relating that part of the waste in health is related to the wrong dispensing of medicines or even their poor packaging. Through the IoMT technology, it is possible to control the temperature and humidity of these drugs in hospital pharmacies and even in medical clinics, as well as checking the bedside before these drugs are administered to the patient.

The advantages of IoT in medicine through connected IoMT devices and gadgets are related to the autonomous registration of information, continuous monitoring of the patient, greater access to health information, and even ease of data sharing, together with automatic storage in cloud structures, providing a more complete medical history, with support for assertive diagnoses, generating patient empowerment as well as strengthening preventive and self-care actions.

With regard to the challenges of IoMT, digital security of data can be considered, both during transmission and during storage and sharing, highlighting that the information on the health of patients is confidential and sensitive. Assessing that in order to guarantee its digital protection, it requires a series of measures, establishing limits, which are often linked through regulation and legislation. The integration of intelligent digital systems is another barrier that prevents the popularization of IoMT in health, since it is necessary that different devices and gadgets be able to exchange information with each other.

In this context, it is understandable how it is possible to use IoMT sensors, for data collection and to generate information from it on a large scale to improve health services, considering that the options available to the patient have a level of customization never seen before. At the same time as it was seen using IoT technology in cars, watches, refrigerators, TVs, and even smartphones as a source of digital records about the life of each user (Fig. 1.7). In the same focus that IoMT will be

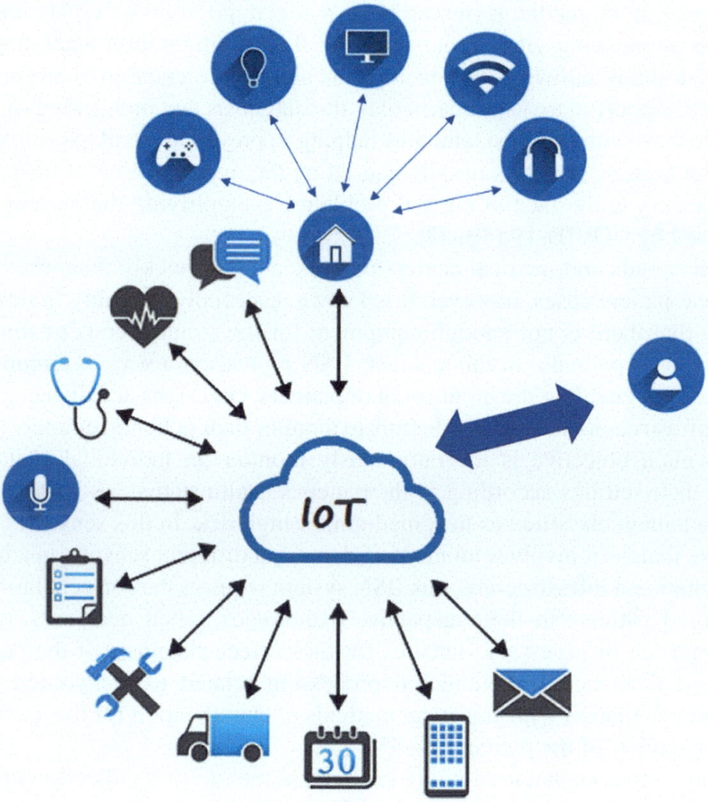

Fig. 1.7 Internet of things—body sensor network (BSN)

responsible for new models of health management, where doctors, specialists, and health institutions, and even the patient can better monitor the state of the body in search of more assertive treatments and healthier routines.

Related to advances in electronics, it has enabled the development of miniaturized and intelligent biomedical sensors, consisting of a group of sensors that form a network, body sensor network (BSN), and are attached to a patient's body in order to acquire physiological data and even be used to monitor the functioning of the human body. BSN employs the use of wireless communication as a suitable alternative, which provides less discomfort to patients and greater cost-benefit; however, technical and even social challenges must be addressed to allow its full practical adoption, relating the operational requirements for network wireless as energy efficiency, the heterogeneous composition of the network, and even the few computational resources. Therefore, the BSN infrastructure must be robust enough to assist its patients reliably and continuously [47–49].

BSN through wireless communications technology and sensors has enabled the creation of truly pervasive wireless sensor networks; this has the potential to enable monitoring of patients' vital signs from a distance through a robust infrastructure that allows doctors to monitor their patients remotely. By associating BSN with the advancement in biomedicine research, it made it possible to create integrated devices for monitoring vital signs, adjusting their configuration according to the patient's risk status, allowing the development and implementation of an application with sensor support to assist, in particular, the diagnosis and monitoring of patients in a simple way, with low cost, and thus helping to prevent the collapse of the medical hospital system, which is usually caused by the overcrowding of hospitals and medical centers in the face of current problems, exemplifying the current modern crisis caused by COVID-19 [49–52].

Since hospitals and medical centers must be able to quickly diagnose and efficiently treat patient cases, however, it is known, especially in reality in developing countries, that there is not enough equipment for the simultaneous treatment of a large number of patients. In this context, BSN represents a way of circumventing this problem by enabling the monitoring of patients' vital signs at a distance through a robust infrastructure that allows doctors to monitor their patients remotely [52–55].

BSN's main objective is to continuously monitor an individual's vital signs, adjusting their settings according to the patient's health status, associating the risk status of a patient classified as low, medium, or high risk. In this sense, it is important to note that, as it involves monitoring data from different sensors, in addition to the computational infrastructure, this BSN system requires the correct classification of monitored patients in their respective pathologies, when necessary, requiring solid knowledge in necessary statistics for the correct diagnosis of the pathology, and high-performance computational processing related to the volume of data required in association with statistical methods of classification for the accurate and efficient diagnosis of the patient [49–55].

BSN are networks that commonly encompass the use of a collection of devices and even BSN systems that belong to M-IoT supporting health care, whose main characteristics are low energy consumption, small size and weight, and ability to communicate wirelessly close to the body. These IoMT devices can be implanted on, in, or around the human body, commonly derived from sensors and actuators monitoring body functions and characteristics of the healthcare environment around them that influence the patient's health [47–55].

Still considering that this has some different characteristics of the sensor networks (WSN—wireless sensor network), since both need sensors of small dimensions and highly efficient in terms of energy consumption, relating that BSN, the sensors can be placed externally or internally to the human body or it can be placed in special garments and are generally placed in places that are difficult to access and the batteries are difficult to change because it can use the human body as means of transmission. Regarding the manipulation of collected data, reliability of the data obtained is necessary since it is private and confidential data requiring some type of encryption and access controls to the medium [52–55]

Thus, BSN also represents solutions for monitoring vital signs of patients at a distance, mainly in the homes of the monitored patients, mainly elderly people in the context of systems focused on assisted living environment, reified by means of integrated IoMT sensor devices for monitoring vital signs, thereby helping to bypass hospital contingency [52–55].

1.5 Trends

IoT applications require enhanced digital security due to sensors and integrated devices transmitting information between themselves and over the Internet. In this context, Blockchain technology guarantees the protection of these communications, by offering a standardized method to accelerate the exchange of data, allowing the execution of processes between IoT devices without intermediaries and securely, preventing the IoT devices from being compromised by cyberattacks and standards users' behaviors are revealed [56].

The principles of blockchain that allow the exchange of information, without a central server validating requests, making the IoT more secure are related to the possibility of anonymity; enhanced cybersecurity resources; and decentralization of transactions carried out through the blockchain. In an IoT network with distributed blockchain technology, it allows the users themselves to participate in the validation of all transactions on the network, still evaluating that the devices can be in a point-to-point mesh network, authenticating transactions and executing it based on predetermined rules [57].

AIoT comes from the union of AI with IoT based on the premise of creating systems that use the potential of these two innovations to have more efficient operations, improving the interaction between man and machine, and gaining more robustness in data analysis. On the one hand, IoT provides connectivity and data generation, and on the other, AI stands for intelligent systems with advanced machine learning techniques. AIoT combines the need for IoT data and analysis with the optimization and treatment of AI, creating solutions capable of offering customization, analyzing habits, patterns, and preferences of almost anything within the context of health, and making quick and assertive decisions [58].

Based on medical automation obtained by IoT through wearable devices and gadgets, edge computing technology is considered a counterpart for cloud computing, allowing digital connection and analysis closer to the edges of the network. Edge computing technology before the IoT, and the universe of devices connected via the Internet, deals with devices with the property to perform advanced processing and analysis, particularly for those that depend on cognitive computing for tasks such as face recognition, detection, language processing, and even preventing obstacles [59].

Fog computing is the technology that stands out as a great differential when applied in partnership with the IoT, since the storage services in cloud computing do not present the adequate speed that solutions offered in IoT will require in the near future. This is based on the premise of the growing volume of IoT devices that will be in use, in the context of health care, and currently, cloud computing systems will not be able to handle all of the virtual data traffic and data load [60].

Thus, computing in fog aims to expand the capacity of the computing device and cloud storage across the network, essentially consisting of the application of an intermediate layer (fog) between the cloud and the hardware allowing for processing, analysis, and storage digitalization of these data more quickly, giving faster answers to certain questions. In other words, fog computing establishes a process that precedes cloud computing, managing, and analyzing the digital environment to store what is really needed [61].

1.6 Conclusions

IoT is an innovating society, given that its potential is enormous, given its characteristics of bringing smart connections to millions of devices, exponentially expanding the number of records available for various sectors, connecting simple everyday devices, such as coffee makers, toasters, refrigerators, TVs, and even other diverse devices for focused use, such as temperature, humidity sensors, and thermostats, collecting information from that.

In the health context, IoT expands innovation in patient monitoring, making the prevention of health problems more effectively with a real-time collection of information from the human body, at the same time as enabling more accurate diagnoses, allowing the creation of a patient profile with long-term records, resulting in a gain in a better quality of life, with fewer diseases and more time to deal with diagnoses and treatments.

The connected IoMT device provides objective reports of the patient's actual activity, helping to monitor their behavior and activities outside the office, allowing physicians to have real data for patient compliance and therapy recommendations.

IoMT technology allows internal surveillance of a patient; this feature helps the medical team to monitor the progression of a disease, for example, and to learn things that can impact guidelines and patients. In this sense, IoMT opens the door to more personalized health care for each individual, from creating personalized diagnoses to determining care guidelines based on a particular patient's unique biological systems.

In addition to IoMT solutions provide continuous improvement of medical care with more accurate diagnostic results and more assertive treatments, increasing its efficiency, i.e., IoMT technology is the next frontier in patient care, both inside and outside the hospital. Considering that through these solutions, whether in the hospital, in the office, or at home, they allow the best decision making of the doctor, in the way of treating health problems, chronic or not.

In this same scenario, it is possible to highlight IoMT as a trend that allows the creation of new treatments, more accurate and with a greater wealth of information, based on reality with information obtained in real time, ranging from the blood pressure of patients to the number of steps taken.

References

1. França, R. P., et al. (2020). Potential proposal to improve data transmission in healthcare systems. Deep Learning Techniques for Biomedical and Health Informatics. Academic Press, 267–283.
2. Cucinotta, D., & Vanelli, M. (2020). WHO declares COVID-19 a pandemic. *Acta Bio-Medica: Atenei Parmensis, 91*(1), 157–160.
3. França, R. P., et al. (2021). A methodology for improving efficiency in data transmission in healthcare systems. In *Internet of things for healthcare technologies* (pp. 49–70). Springer.
4. Mavrogiorgou, A., et al. (2019). IoT in healthcare: Achieving interoperability of high-quality data acquired by IoT medical devices. *Sensors, 19*(9), 1978.
5. Jin, Z., & Yu, C. (2015). Telemedicine in the cloud era: Prospects and challenges. *IEEE Pervasive Computing, 14*(1), 54–61.
6. Wootton, R., Craig, J., & Patterson, V. (2017). *Introduction to telemedicine*. CRC Press.
7. Ozkan, H. (2016). A comparison of classification methods for telediagnosis of Parkinson's disease. *Entropy, 18*(4), 115.
8. Jayaraman, P. P., et al. (2020). Healthcare 4.0: A review of frontiers in digital health. *Wiley Interdisciplinary Reviews: Data Mining and Knowledge Discovery, 10*(2), e1350.
9. Adarsha, A. S., Reader, K., & Erban, S. (2019). User experience, IoMT, and healthcare. *AIS Transactions on Human-Computer Interaction, 11*(4), 264–273.
10. França, R. P., et al. (2021). An overview of internet of things technology applied on precision agriculture concept. In *Precision agriculture technologies for food security and sustainability* (pp. 47–70).
11. França, R. P., et al. (2021). Big data and cloud computing: A technological and literary background. In *Advanced deep learning applications in big data analytics* (pp. 29–50). IGI Global.
12. Franca, R. P., et al. (2020). Better transmission of information focused on green computing through data transmission channels in cloud environments with rayleigh fading. In *Green computing in smart cities: Simulation and techniques* (pp. 71–93). Springer.
13. Gatouillat, A., et al. (2018). Internet of medical things: A review of recent contributions dealing with cyber-physical systems in medicine. *IEEE Internet of Things Journal, 5*(5), 3810–3822.
14. Tran, C., & Misra, S. (2019). The technical foundations of IoT. *IEEE Wireless Communications, 26*(3), 8–8.

15. Zanjal, S. V., & Talmale, G. R. (2016). Medicine reminder and monitoring system for secure health using IoT. *Procedia Computer Science, 78*(3), 471–476.
16. Jayanth, S., et al. (2017). Wearable device to measure heartbeat using IoT. 2017 international conference on inventive systems and control (ICISC). IEEE.
17. Manoj, A. S., Hussain, M. A., & Teja, P. S. (2019). Patient health monitoring using IoT. In *Mobile health applications for quality healthcare delivery* (pp. 30–45). IGI Global.
18. Joshi, P. (2017). *Artificial intelligence with python.* Packt Publishing Ltd.
19. Wahl, B., et al. (2018). Artificial intelligence (AI) and global health: How can AI contribute to health in resource-poor settings? *BMJ Global Health, 3*(4), e000798.
20. França, R. P., et al. (2019). Potential model for improvement of the data transmission in healthcare systems.
21. Nelson, R., & Staggers, N. (2016). *Health informatics-E-book: An Interprofessional approach.* Elsevier Health Sciences.
22. Butt, S. A., et al. (2019). IoT smart health security threats. 2019 19th international conference on computational science and its applications (ICCSA). IEEE.
23. Kanase, P., & Gaikwad, S. (2016). Smart hospitals using internet of things (IoT). *International Research Journal of Engineering and Technology (IRJET), 3*(3).
24. Purri, S., et al. (2017). Specialization of IoT applications in health care industries. 2017 international conference on big data analytics and computational intelligence (ICBDAC). IEEE.
25. Nayyar, A., Puri, V., & Nguyen, N. G. (2019). Biosenhealth 1.0: A novel internet of medical things (iomt)-based patient health monitoring system. In *International conference on innovative computing and communications.* Springer.
26. Popereshnyak, S., et al. (2018). IoT application testing features based on the modelling network. 2018 XIVth international conference on perspective technologies and methods in MEMS design (MEMSTECH). IEEE.
27. Monteiro, A. C. B., et al. (2018). Health 4.0: Applications, management, technologies and review. *Personalized Medicine, 5*, 6.
28. Park, K. H., Park, J., & Lee, J. W. (2017). An IoT system for remote monitoring of patients at home. *Applied Sciences, 7*(3), 260.
29. Deshkar, S., Thanseeh, R. A., & Menon, V. G. (2017). A review on IoT based m-health systems for diabetes. *International Journal of Computer Science and Telecommunications, 8*(1), 13–18.
30. Singh, K. (2020). Nanosensors for food safety and environmental monitoring. In *Nanotechnology for food, agriculture, and environment* (pp. 63–84). Springer.
31. Deepika Mathuvanthi, P., Suresh, V., & Pradeep, C. (2019). IoT powered wearable to assist individuals facing depression symptoms.
32. Varatharajan, R., et al. (2018). Wearable sensor devices for early detection of Alzheimer disease using dynamic time warping algorithm. *Cluster Computing, 21*(1), 681–690.
33. Nguyen, H. H. (2016). Advanced assistive control strategies for smart hospital beds. Diss.
34. Cruz-Cunha, M. M., ed. (2016). Encyclopedia of E-health and telemedicine. IGI Global.
35. Albahri, A. S., et al. (2020). IoT-based telemedicine for disease prevention and health promotion: State-of-the-art. *Journal of Network and Computer Applications, 173*, 102873.
36. Monteiro, A. C. B. (2019). Proposta de uma metodologia de segmentação de imagens para detecção e contagem de hemácias e leucócitos através do algoritmo WT-MO.
37. Monteiro, A. C. B., et al. (2018). Methodology of high accuracy, sensitivity and specificity in the counts of erythrocytes and leukocytes in blood smear images. In *Brazilian technology symposium.* Springer.
38. Jordanova, M., & Lievens, F. (2011). Global telemedicine and eHealth (a synopsis). 2011 e-health and bioengineering conference (EHB). IEEE.
39. Azizy, A., Fayaz, M., & Agirbasli, M. (2020). Do not forget Afghanistan in times of COVID-19: Telemedicine and the internet of things to strengthen planetary health systems. *OMICS: A Journal of Integrative Biology.*

40. Munir, M. S., Kim, S. F. A. D. H., & Hong, C. S. (2020). A risk-sensitive social distance recommendation system via bluetooth towards the COVID-19 private safety. *Korean Computer Congress (KCC)*.
41. Obinikpo, A. A., & Kantarci, B. (2017). Big sensed data meets deep learning for smarter health care in smart cities. *Journal of Sensor and Actuator Networks, 6*(4), 26.
42. França, R. P, et al. (2020). Lower memory consumption for data transmission in smart cloud environments with CBEDE methodology. In *Smart systems design, applications, and challenges*. (pp. 216–237). IGI Global.
43. Tuli, S., et al. (2020). Predicting the growth and trend of COVID-19 pandemic using machine learning and cloud computing. *Internet of Things, 11*, 100222.
44. Huang, L., et al. (2020). Serial quantitative chest ct assessment of covid-19: Deep-learning approach. *Radiology: Cardiothoracic Imaging, 2*(2), e200075.
45. Beznik, T., et al. (2020). Deep learning to detect bacterial colonies for the production of vaccines. arXiv preprint arXiv:2009.00926.
46. França, R. P., et al. Applying a methodology in data transmission of discrete events from the perspective of cyber-physical systems environments. In *Artificial intelligence paradigms for smart cyber-physical systems* (pp. 278–300). IGI Global.
47. Fortino, G., et al. (2012). Enabling effective programming and flexible management of efficient body sensor network applications. *IEEE Transactions on Human-Machine Systems, 43*(1), 115–133.
48. Zheng, M., et al. (2018). An emerging wearable world: New gadgetry produces a rising tide of changes and challenges. *IEEE Systems, Man, and Cybernetics Magazine, 4*(4), 6–14.
49. Fortino, G., et al. (2014). BodyCloud: A SaaS approach for community body sensor networks. *Future Generation Computer Systems, 35*, 62–79.
50. Chen, M., et al. (2011). Body area networks: A survey. *Mobile Networks and Applications, 16*(2), 171–193.
51. Fortino, G., et al. (2009). SPINE2: Developing BSN applications on heterogeneous sensor nodes. 2009 IEEE international symposium on industrial embedded systems. IEEE.
52. Iyengar, S., et al. (2008). A framework for creating healthcare monitoring applications using wireless body sensor networks. Proceedings of the ICST 3rd international conference on Body area networks.
53. Yang, G. (2006). In G.-Z. Yang (Ed.), *Body sensor networks* (Vol. 1). Springer.
54. Fortino, G., et al. (2009). Platform-independent development of collaborative wireless body sensor network applications: SPINE2. 2009 IEEE international conference on systems, man and cybernetics. IEEE.
55. Aloi, G., et al. (2016). A mobile multi-technology gateway to enable IoT interoperability. 2016 IEEE first international conference on internet-of-things design and implementation (IoTDI). IEEE.
56. França, R. P., et al. (2020). A review on the technological and literary background of multimedia compression. In *Handbook of research on multimedia cyber security* (pp. 1–20). IGI Global.
57. Drescher, D. (2017). *Blockchain basics* (Vol. 276). Apress.
58. Hsu, C.-S., et al. Challenges and prospects of AIoT application in hospitality and tourism marketing.
59. Shi, W., et al. (2016). Edge computing: Vision and challenges. *IEEE Internet of Things Journal, 3*(5), 637–646.
60. Bonomi, F., et al. (2012). Fog computing and its role in the internet of things. Proceedings of the first edition of the MCC workshop on mobile cloud computing.
61. Yousefpour, A., et al. (2019). All one needs to know about fog computing and related edge computing paradigms: A complete survey. *Journal of Systems Architecture, 98*, 289–330.

Chapter 2
Healthcare Data Storage Options Using Cloud

Sandhya Armoogum and Patricia Khonje

2.1 Introduction

In this era of digitalization, information and communication technologies (ICT) are widely adopted and form part of our daily life. Likewise, the healthcare system is embracing ICT to improve healthcare access, the quality of healthcare, and to be more cost-effective. Such smart healthcare system uses technologies such as wearable devices and the Internet of things (IoT), mobile Internet, big data analytics, cloud computing, and artificial intelligence (AI) to provide better diagnostics, better treatment, and intelligent tools and devices (e.g., for ambient assisted living) that improve the quality of life for patients [1]. As the global population is aging, chronic diseases are increasing. With the emergence of new viruses such as the COVID-19 coronavirus, which is causing a worldwide pandemic, smart healthcare solutions are fundamental to improve the efficiency of medical care, enhance the health service experience of citizens, and decrease the operational cost.

Wearable devices or medical devices which are integrated in an IoT network or connected to a smartphone mobile application can now monitor and collect patient information which enables remote real-time alerting, tracking, and monitoring of patients which permits personalized treatments, better accuracy, and more apt intervention by doctors. Such real-time monitoring via connected devices can save lives in event of a medical emergency like heart failure, diabetes, and asthma attacks. Body sensor networks (BSN), which consist of wireless sensor networks designed for monitoring human physiological signals, are rapidly emerging as human-centric cyber–physical systems. Fortino et al. [2] proposed the BodyCloud, which allows BSNs to be integrated on the cloud and supports the development and deployment

S. Armoogum (✉) · P. Khonje
University of Technology Mauritius, La Tour Koenig, Pointe-aux-Sables, Mauritius
e-mail: sandhya.armoogum@umail.utm.ac.mu

P. Siarry et al. (eds.), *The Fusion of Internet of Things, Artificial Intelligence, and Cloud Computing in Health Care*, Internet of Things,
https://doi.org/10.1007/978-3-030-75220-0_2

of cloud-assisted BSN applications. Furthermore, Gravina et al. [3] proposed a cloud-based activity as a service cyber–physical framework for human activity monitoring in mobility built atop the BodyCloud platform. Healthcare IoT devices are interconnected through wireless communication protocols like COAP, MQTT, Zigbee, and Bluetooth [4]. Big data analytics on medical data provide much insight into diseases and treatments [5]. Similarly, AI enables to interpret complex data and act intelligently to achieve a goal. AI and machine learning are commonly used to analyze patient data and medical imaging to make recommendations that can help doctors in their diagnostics, evaluate diseases, and perform epidemiological analysis.

Large amount of data is generated by smart healthcare system, which is referred to as healthcare big data. Such data include traditional data from electronic medical records (EMRs) or electronic health record (EHR) systems (e.g., patient's medical history, physician notes, clinical reports, laboratory reports, medications, insurance information, medical imaging such as CT scans, MRIs, X-ray reports, PET scans, tomography), and data related to computerized provider order entry (CPOE) systems. Moreover, high volume of real-time IoT-based health care and wearable devices as well as mobile applications data is also recorded such as blood pressure, oxygen and blood sugar levels monitoring, pulse oximeter readings, pacemaker readings, and stress level [6]. Research in medical field also involves omics data such as genomics (genome sequence data) and proteomics (proteome is a set of proteins produced in an organism). The size of a single sequenced human genome is approximately 200 GB [7].

Current estimates suggest a single patient generates close to 80 MB each year only in imaging and electronic medical record (EMR) data [8]. It has been estimated that up to 30% of the entire world's stored data is health-related (on the yottabyte scale) [9]. Data from the U.S. healthcare system alone reached 150 exabytes in 2011 [10]. The Global Healthcare Data Storage market is expected to reach $8.11 billion by 2026 growing at a CAGR of 16.4% from 2019 to 2026 [11]. Healthcare data are projected to grow faster than manufacturing data, financial services data, or media. Thus, the amount of healthcare data is increasing exponentially, and the need to effectively store and manage healthcare big data is crucial.

This chapter delves into the storage of healthcare big data. In Sect. 2.2, the healthcare big data management challenges are discussed. Section 2.3 presents the cloud option of storing healthcare data. Section 2.4 introduces the different types of storage that are available for storing data, as well as the different storage systems on the cloud. The storage security aspect on the cloud is described in Sect. 2.5. Finally, Sect. 2.6 summarizes and concludes the chapter by discussing the future directions.

2.2 Healthcare Big Data Management Requirements and Challenges

When storing healthcare data, the healthcare data management requirements need to be considered. Figure 2.1 depicts the main requirements of healthcare data management.

Healthcare systems have gone though the digitalization phase and have increasingly adopted IoT technology to enhance their services and improve their efficiency. This has resulted in increasing amount of data generated which has to be stored. Big data can be primarily defined as having three V characteristics, i.e., volume, variety, velocity. Healthcare data, apart from the sheer volume, are also of a disparate nature i.e., it consists of structured, semi-structured, and unstructured data as the data can be in different forms such as a table, email, image, video, and sensor feeds. Sensor monitoring often produces real-time data that need to be recorded; this depicts the velocity characteristics of healthcare big data. Similarly, with the improving

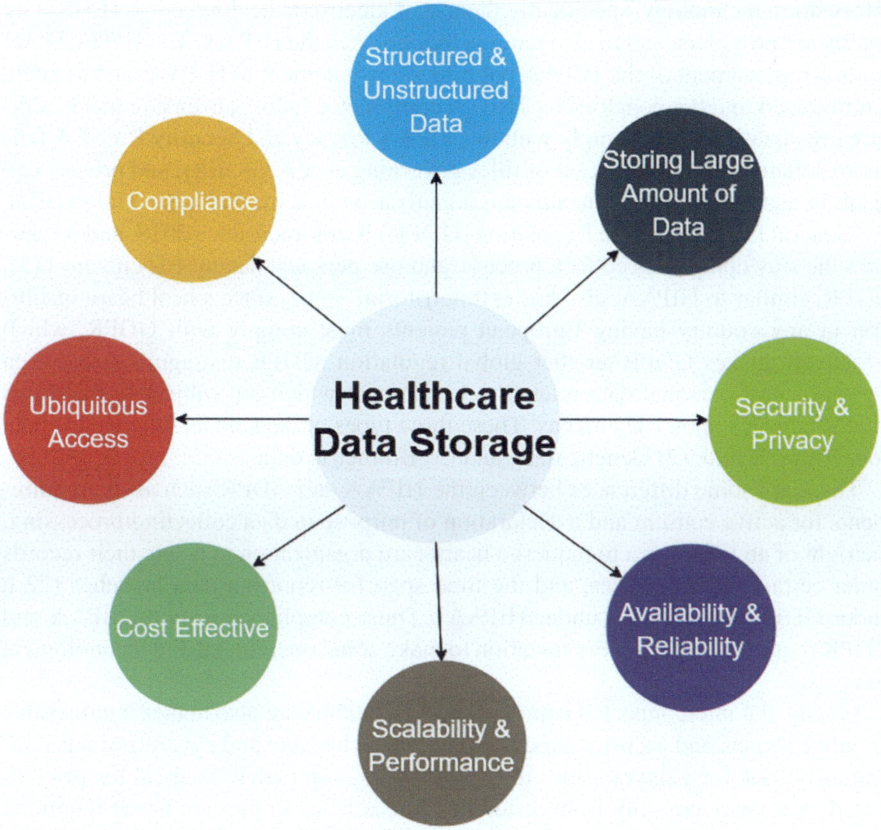

Fig. 2.1 Healthcare data management requirements

medical devices now available, the quality and size of medical imaging data have also increased. There is thus the need to adopt a scalable architecture for storing the increasingly amount of healthcare big data [12]. Moreover, for large healthcare institutions, which have care centers in different geographical locations, the data are also distributed across different servers in different locations. Often though, such data need to be accessible to different users from different locations. Healthcare data storage should be accessible 24/7, which means that the storage system has to be reliable and available.

The healthcare industry has to invest largely on upgrading and increasing their storage capacity such that it is more flexible and scalable, which can be costly. It can also be challenging to manage the different variety of clinical data generated from EMR, IoT, medical imaging, genome sequencing, etc.

Another important requirement for the data storage system is compliance, as the healthcare industry is highly regulated. In the USA, most of the regulations are represented in the Health Insurance Portability and Accountability Act (HIPAA) of 1996. In 2009, the HITECH Act (Health Information Technology for Economic and Clinical Health Act) was created to promote and expand the adoption of health information technology, specifically the use of electronic health records (EHRs) by healthcare providers, and to also remove loopholes in the HIPAA. The HITECH Act is not a replacement of the HIPAA but rather a supplement to HIPAA, and as such, it introduced tougher penalties for HIPAA compliance failures to ensure that healthcare organizations duly comply with the HIPAA Privacy and Security Rules. A failure to adhere to the complex set of rules governing access, security, and privacy can result in heavy fines for the healthcare organization. For the European Union (EU), the General Data Protection Regulation (GDPR) is enforced since 2018, and it regulates the way companies collect, process, and use personal data of EU citizens [13]. GDPR, similar to HIPAA, also has extraterritorial scope, since a healthcare institution in any country having European patients must comply with GDPR, which effectively makes GDPR another global regulation. GDPR distinguishes between three types of personal data related to health care which are subject to the rights GDPR conveys upon EU citizens. These three types of data are as follows: (1) data concerning health, (2) Genetic data, and (3) Biometric data.

There are some differences between the HIPAA and GDPR such as the requirements for active consent and a declaration of purpose in data collecting/processing, the right of an EU citizen to request a healthcare organization to delete their records under certain circumstances, and the time span for reporting data breaches (72 h under GDPR and 60 days under HIPAA). Thus, compliance to both HIPAA and GDPR requires healthcare organization to make some operational and technological changes.

Finally, the interconnected nature of modern health care also makes it vulnerable to online threats and security attacks in general as hackers and cybercriminals continuously look for vulnerabilities to exploit. Accessing patient medical history collected over years possibly from different sources helps to provide better treatment but also puts at risk the healthcare network. The healthcare industry is plagued by a myriad of cybersecurity attacks such as distributed denial-of-service attacks (DDoS) which can disrupt an organizations ability to provide patient care, theft of data, medical insurance fraud, identity theft, insider misuse and unintentional actions, and ransomware attacks. According to Millard [14], ransomware incidents increased by 300% from 2015 to 2016. The UK's National Health System (NHS) hospitals were held hostage in May 2017 to the WannaCry ransomware which resulted in delayed treatment plans. Universal Health Services, one of the largest healthcare provider in the USA, was hit by the Ryuk ransomware in September 2020, whereby all of the 250 healthcare facilities' computer infrastructure were locked resulting in chaotic conditions which tremendously affected patient treatment [15]. In September 2020, due to a ransomware attack at the Duesseldorf University Hospital, a woman who needed urgent medical care died after being rerouted to a hospital in the city of Wuppertal, more than 30 km away [16]. This incident marked the first reported human death indirectly caused by a ransomware attack.

Going forward, the healthcare industry has to improve its data management capabilities in order to keep pace in a digital landscape and ensure security of data.

2.3 Cloud for Healthcare Big Data Storage

Traditionally, healthcare institutions have been storing their data on-premise as this allows them to have full control over the in-house data, where they minimize risks associated with data breach and maintain their own backup and recovery systems. However, today with the growing complexity of healthcare big data, which includes different geographically located healthcare facilities and the increasing number of smart health applications, there is no "one-size-fit-all" solution. It is becoming more challenging to handle big data storage, the evolving real-time data from IoT devices, Bring Your Own Devices (BYOD) practices, to enforce security, compliance, availability, and to provide ubiquitous access for on-premise healthcare data storage.

On-premise storage is often not very agile. It is required that the storage solution is scalable such that more storage capacity can be added without requiring a complete upgrade and conversion, which may not always be the case. Increasing on-premise storage capacity also implies increasing physical space within the premises which might not be easy to accommodate. Apart from the costs of additional storage solutions, there is also the operational cost incurred such as power supply, cooling of server rooms, IT staff, which makes on-premise data storage a rather costly option. Depending on the backup strategy in place, on-premise storage may also have more latency in recovery from an attack or failure. Healthcare data being critical, longer downtime can significantly impact on the quality of care given to patients when patient data is not readily available.

The cloud has emerged as a most convenient and viable, more global and holistic data storage solution for the healthcare industry [17–22]. Cloud storage is definitely more scalable and more cost-effective in terms of capital expenditure and operational expenditures as well as secure. In Sect. 2.5, the security mechanisms proposed for securing healthcare applications and data are described. More smart health applications are being deployed on the cloud today and consequently using cloud storage for the related data [23–29]. Aileni et al. [30] propose the use of cloud for storing and processing big data from biosensors. The authors, Kolodner et al. [31], proposed an architecture of a scalable and flexible cloud environment for data-intensive storage cloud services for health care, which enable data mobility across providers and allow computational and content-centric access to storage and deploy new data-oriented mechanisms for QoS and security guarantees. The use of cloud computing has also been proposed for healthcare underground wireless sensor network [32]. Mobile cloud computing (MCC) is also popularly proposed for mobile healthcare (m-healthcare) applications [33–35]. This results in more accessibility, improved performance, better disaster recovery, and more efficiently managed systems which positively impacts the quality of medical care provided to patients ultimately. For healthcare institutions that already have on-premise storage, it is also possible to extend their storage and ICT infrastructure requirements by using the cloud platform, i.e., a hybrid solution.

The NIST [36] defines the cloud as follows "Cloud computing is a model for enabling ubiquitous, convenient, on-demand network access to a shared pool of configurable computing resources (e.g., networks, servers, storage, applications, and services) that can be rapidly provisioned and released with minimal management effort or service provider interaction." There are four cloud deployment models, namely public cloud, private cloud, hybrid cloud, and community cloud. Public cloud is cloud infrastructure owned and operated by a third-party cloud service provider (CSP), delivered over the Internet. The public cloud resources can be used by anyone who subscribes to the cloud offerings. The private cloud is exclusively for the use of a single organization. Often, it is owned and built on the organizations premises, but it could also be outsourced from a third-party organization. Hybrid cloud is the result, when companies partly use their own private cloud and partly use resources from one or several public cloud. In such scenario, usually all sensitive and confidential data are kept on the private cloud. The community cloud is set up from a collaborative effort, for the specific needs of an industry, and shared by the partners. The three-service delivery model of the cloud includes the Software as a Service (SaaS) where software is consumed by users, Platform as a Service (PaaS) which allows developers to build applications, and Infrastructure as a Service (IaaS) which mainly allows to get access to a compute node on the cloud in the form of a virtual machine (VM) with its own virtual disk or even a virtual network of VMs. Cloud customers can use one or more of the service delivery model. The term Storage as a Service mainly refers to the storage of data in the form of files such as document, images, and videos. Common Storage as a Service offering on the cloud includes Google Drive, Microsoft One Drive, Apple's iCloud, and Dropbox. Such storage mechanisms are mainly for storing data or data backups as well as for sharing data among users.

Rajabion et al. [37] state that "Cloud computing is one of the main choices for handling and processing of this type of data (healthcare)." Smart healthcare applications and m-healthcare applications can easily and quickly be deployed on the cloud today where all the required resources are provisioned for the applications including storage, whether it is in the form of relational databases, NoSQL databases, file storage, or object store.

2.4 Cloud Storage

For the healthcare industry to deliver patient care and coordinate medical information, there is the need for storage that is both reliable and secure. The suitable data storage solution is the cloud storage and the hybrid storage; i.e., healthcare facilities can migrate all their ICT services and storage on the cloud, or they can use both their on-premise systems and storage and extend their storage onto the cloud for more storage capacity.

According to Gartner [38], the leaders for Public Cloud Storage Services are Amazon Web Services (AWS), Microsoft Azure, and Google. All three major cloud providers are proposing new cloud services including cloud storage for hospitals and other healthcare facilities [39]. Recently, Microsoft has launched its new cloud service, Cloud for Healthcare, specifically designed for health care. The new services include scheduling telehealth visits, allowing virtual care via virtual visits, and support the Fast Healthcare Interoperability Resources (FHIR), which is a common data standard for health care, and a tool called Patient 360 which allows health providers to get the full information about the patient [40]. Mayo Clinic has signed a 10-year strategic partnership with Google to accelerate innovation in AI and analytics through digital technologies [41]. Amazon is also proposing solutions to store, protect, and optimize healthcare data in AWS. Cerner, a major company that supplies health information technology services, devices, and hardware, is working with AWS for developing innovative healthcare solutions using AI and machine learning (ML) [42].

2.4.1 Cloud Storage Type

Similar to the on-premise infrastructure, the cloud storage consists of magnetic storage (hard disks) and solid-state storage (flash disks).

Magnetic Storage: Hard Disk Drive (HDD)

HDD are magnetic storage media whereby data is stored in a magnetized medium. They are mechanical hard drives as they have moving parts, namely the central spindle that allows the disk platters of the HDD to rotate and the actuator that allows the read/write head to move. The speed at which the disk spins affects the time taken to read/write data from/to the HDD among others. The higher the revolutions per minute (RPM), the faster data can be read. Magnetic tapes are also another type of magnetic storage, which is popularly used to store old patient records, and clinical data. Magnetic tapes are also suitable for storing backups as they can store data reliably for a long period of time, but data stored on magnetic tapes cannot be accessed fast online.

HDD can store very large amount of data (high capacity) at relatively cheap price and have better data access times compared to magnetic tapes. Traditionally in the healthcare industry, most data are stored on HDD and backup data on magnetic tapes. Magnetic tapes are preferred despite that they are slow and prove to be expensive when it comes to managing and maintaining them, as they are more secure given that they may not be directly accessible via the network.

Cloud data storage options also include HDD. The cloud is equipped with a large number of HDD storage arrays which are mounted on racks. The popular vendors of storage arrays include NetApp, Dell EMC, Hewlett Packard Enterprise (HPE), IBM, Huawei, and Hitachi Vantara [43]. Three different kinds of HDD are typically used: Serial ATA (SATA), Serial Attached SCSI (SAS), and Near Line SAS (NL-SAS). SATA drives typically have RPM of 5400 RPM and 7200 RPM; thus, their performance is the lowest among the three types of HDD. However, they are reliable and have large storage capacity and are relatively cheap. SAS drives typically have 10,000 and 15,000 RPM and provide the best performance and low latency, and are typically used to store data for mission critical application as they are also more reliable. The SAS drives have additional commands that control the disks, which contribute to make SAS drives more efficient than SATA. They are also more expensive than SATA drives. NL-SAS disk consists of spinning SATA platters but with the native command set of SAS drives. Due to their low rotational speed, their performance is lower than SAS drives, but overall, they are more efficient than SATA drives. The cloud data centers have all three types of HDD as well as SSD storage. Storage on SAS drives and SSD drives on the cloud provides better performance but are also more expensive. Cloud providers offer storage tiering to allow customers to optimize the use of storage. Thereby, backup data can be stored on SATA drives, for instance, while production data is stored on SAS drives instead of both being stored on SAS drives. This allows the customer to save on the cost storage by making the best use of the storage type for the different kind of data to be stored. Typically, Tier 1 could represent storage which has best performance and reliability, while also being the most expensive. Tier 2 could represent the storage which is slower and less efficient, but which is also usually cheaper. In this regards, SAS drives can be considered as being Tier 1 storage, while SATA drives could be offered as Tier 2 storage on the cloud. Tiering is further addressed in Sect. 2.4.2.

Flash Storage: Solid-State Drive (SSD)

Flash storage is a nonmechanical and nonmagnetic storage whereby data is stored using electronic circuits, i.e., NAND-based flash memory. Given that SSD drives do not have mechanical parts, they are less susceptible to physical shock, are silent, and have overall better performance than HDD and are also much smaller in size for the same capacity HDD. However, they are also more expensive. Overtime, the cost of flash memory is becoming more affordable and SSD of larger capacity is increasingly available. SSD is the storage of choice for healthcare data that need to be readily accessible especially in cases of emergency. For instance, it would take over 15 s to read an MRI image of the size 1.8 GB stored on a HDD as compared to just 0.15 s from SSD flash storage [44]. Flash storage can also offer built-in encryption which can be particularly useful for securing healthcare data for HIPAA compliance.

Traditional Flash storage uses the SATA III interface, primarily used by HDD, which is not designed to support SSD. SATA III can support 6 GB/s of peak bandwidth theoretically, but due to overhead associated with the interface, the effective bandwidth peaks at about the 555 MB/s. This limits the access speed to the SSD storage. PCIe is one of the fastest storage communication protocols. Nonvolatile memory express (NVMe) is a new storage access and transport protocol that uses PCIe. NVMe flash storage is the next-generation SSD that delivers high bandwidth and low latency for all types of complex workloads. NVMe SSD drives are up to six times faster than the typical SATA SSD. NVMe Over Fabric (NVMe-oF) is a storage networking protocol for NVMe-enabled storage disk arrays. It enables faster and more efficient connectivity between storage disk arrays and the servers. Cloud storage providers are heavily using All-Flash NVMe arrays to provide low latency and high-throughput storage. Facebook uses NVMe cloud storage technology in their data centers around the clock to address the hyperscale issues regarding the data of their 2.5 Billion users [45].

2.4.2 Cloud Storage Tiering

Storage tiering distinguishes between more important or frequently accessed data, which should ideally be stored on the fastest type of storage (but also more costly) with less important and rarely accessed data (e.g., backup data) that can be stored on the slowest and cheapest storage type. The simplest tiering system has two tiers: Tier 1 (also known as hot storage)—provides high performance, usually expensive; and Tier 2 (also known as cold storage)—characterized by lower performance, but is cheaper. Most of the popular public cloud offers more than two tiers of storage, thus offering more choice and granularity for classifying and storing data accordingly onto the different storage tiers.

A four-tier model could involve Tier 0,1,2,3 or mission critical, hot, warm, cold tiers. Here, the tier 3/cold would be used to store rarely accessed data, e.g., old patient health records; tier 2/warm would be used for data which are not constantly accessed, e.g., outpatient health records; tier 1/hot would be data constantly used, e.g., in-patient records; and tier 0/mission critical could be data which is used constantly and which needs to be speedily accessible, e.g., medical imaging data of patient during surgery. Tiering thus allows storage resources to be used more efficiently and is also more cost-effective while at the same time providing good performance access for each class of data.

Because data classification can change over time or in certain situation, e.g., emergency health crisis of a patient, data can be moved from a lower tier to a higher tier as required or vice versa i.e. old patient data can be moved from higher tier to lower tier. Automated storage tiering is also supported whereby data can be moved across storage tiers dynamically, e.g., based on the frequency with which some records are being accessed; they can be moved to a higher tier automatically by the storage system, while data that have been less frequently used from a higher tier can be shifted to a lower tier accordingly.

Typically, the cloud providers offer more storage tier levels for their object storage offerings. Object storage is described in Sect. 2.4.3.3. An object can be stored in one storage class i.e. tier level. Users can configure policies (i.e., object life cycle management) to set up rules describing actions to be taken on objects, e.g., downgrade data not accessed for more than 30 days from the current tier to a lower tier with the aim to reduce long-term storage costs. Google object storage tiering are as follows: (1) *Standard*: Hot data or short storage periods; (2) *Nearline*: Lower cost, good for data accessed once a month or less; (3) *Coldline*: Very low cost, better for data read or modified once per quarter; (4) *Archive*: Lowest cost, for data accessed less than once a year but still with millisecond access times. Microsoft Azure offers three tiering levels for the Azure Blob Storage as follows: (1) *Hot*: Data in active use or expected to be accessed frequently; (2) *Cool*: Lower cost, monthly access or less; (3) *Archive:* Lowest cost, access time is several hours. Typically, data stored in Archive access tier is considered offline, and it takes longer to get the data online and accessible. AWS storage tiering is provided for the object storage Amazon Simple Storage Service (S3) where it has the following storage classes—(1) *Standard*: Low latency and high throughput, used for frequently accessed data and more expensive; (2) *Standard-Infrequent Access (IA)*: Same performance, lower storage charges, with retrieval charges, which is ideal for long-term storage; (3) *Glacier*: Ideal for data archiving and has low cost with a retrieval range from 1 min up to 12 h; (4) *Glacier Deep Archive*: Lowest cost storage but data is restored within 12 h. AWS S3 also supports the object life cycle management allowing users to define policies regarding the shifting of data from one tier to another. However, AWS also has another storage class called ***S3 Intelligent Tiering***, which is a two-tiered storage in a single class (frequent access/hot tier, and infrequent access/cold tier). It is ideal for long-lived data with unknown or unpredictable access patterns. Data objects in this tier are initially placed in the hot tier, and AWS automatically downgrade objects which have not been accessed for 30 consecutive days to the cold tier, and shift them back to the hot tier if they are accessed.

2.4.3 Cloud Storage: File, Block, and Object Storage

Data can be stored on the cloud as files, blocks, or objects.

File Storage

File Storage is one of the old styles of storage that are file system-based methods of storing and retrieving data. File storage organizes and represents data as files. These files are, in turn, organized in folders, and these folders are then arranged into directories and subdirectories in a hierarchical fashion. To access a file, computers need the path from directory to subdirectory to folder to file. Limited amount of metadata is stored for each file such as the name of the file and size of the file. The files can be stored locally on a directly attached storage (DAS) or remotely on network-attached storage (NAS). The NAS storage uses a network file system (e.g., NFS, CIFS, SMB) to expose data stored. AWS's Elastic File System is an NFS file system-based storage, while Azure also offers cloud-based file storage access via SMB. Google Cloud Filestore is the network file storage solution of the Google Cloud. File storage is scalable as using scale-out NAS devices such as the Dell EMC Isilon; the storage capacity can be increased. Data can be easily shared between users in cloud file storage for collaboration. Administrators can also easily set access rights of files, while security and version control are easily managed. However, file storage is suitable for small organizations. The tree-like file system hierarchy can handle millions of files quite easily, but when the number of files increases further, the file access start to slow down due to the overhead of the underlying file system lookup to find the file location. File storage on cloud can be used to store some type of healthcare data, but it is not the ideal solution for large healthcare facilities. It is also not suitable for storing all the different variety of healthcare data and especially the large volume of real-time healthcare big data generated by health IoT networks.

Block Storage

Block storage chunks data into arbitrarily organized, evenly sized volumes. Each block of data is given a unique identifier, which allows a storage system to store the block of data anywhere on the storage area. No metadata are stored for the block of data. When data are requested, the storage system retrieves and reassembles the blocks of data. Block storage is usually deployed in storage area network (SAN) environments and must be tied to a functioning server (controller). A SAN is a specialized high-speed network that provides block-level network access to storage devices which are typically all-flash disk arrays. SAN environments typically have high performance, consistent low latency, high availability, and resilience. Due to their centralized architecture, consistent methodologies, and tools for security, data protection and disaster recovery can be applied to the SAN. Data can be replicated for reliability and/or stored in a RAID configuration. Block storage and SAN are often used for performance-hungry applications like databases, email servers, virtual disks associated to virtual machines, and large virtual desktop infrastructures (VDIs). Block storage is suited for structured data and is costly as SAN consists often of a bunch of SSD disks arrays. It can be used for storing structured healthcare data.

AWS offers the Amazon Elastic Block Store (EBS) which is an easy-to-use, high-performance block storage service designed for use with Amazon Elastic Compute Cloud (EC2). It is most suitable for transaction-intensive applications and workloads requiring high throughput at any scale. On EBS, users can store data on five types of storage to optimize storage performance and cost for a broad range of applications, namely three types of SSD (io2, io1, and gp2) and two types of HDD (st1 and sc1) [46, 47]. The Microsoft block storage offering is the Azure Managed Disk where data can be stored on different types of storage media for different performance levels: Premium SSD, Standard SSD, Standard HDD, and Ultra Disk. Google Cloud Persistent Disk provides block storage which is reliable and has high performance; it is used by all virtual machines in Google Cloud (Google Cloud Compute Engine). Data can be stored on three storage types: standard persistent disks, balanced persistent disks, and SSD persistent disks; the latter are designed for enterprise applications and high-performance database needs that require lower latency and more IOPS. SSD persistent disk storage option is also the most expensive. Google also allows choosing where the storage is located (i.e., which region) and the type of availability. Regional persistent disks are replicated in different zones within a region and offer high availability, whereas zonal disks (cheaper option) also provide high availability but with disks replicated only within a single zone [48, 49].

Object Storage

With object storage, data items are not stored in blocks or files but rather in flexibly sized containers called "objects" or "blobs." The object size can vary from a few kilobytes to multiterabytes. Object stores can hold any type of data (e.g., text, image, video, and sensor data) as the object is essentially stored as binary data. Object storage is thus suitable for storing a large volume of unstructured data. Each object is uniquely identified by means of an objectID; they are stored in a flat address space, whereby it is easier to locate and retrieve them, even if they are stored in geographically distributed storage clusters. Each object is linked to associated metadata. With object storage, lots of metadata can be stored about the object, and the objects can be accessed directly through REST APIs or HTTP/HTTPs requests using their identifier. Object storage is potentially good for analytics/searching due to its rich metadata. But it is not convenient for transactional data, e.g., databases. Object storage is cost-efficient and extremely scalable as it can be scaled out and managed simply by adding additional nodes to the storage cluster. Object storage is also very robust and resilient. To protect data stored in an object store from both disk failure (i.e., one node fails, data can still be accessed) and data corruption, replication or erasure coding (EC) or both are applied. Object store is most convenient for hospitals which with the growth in digitalization are required to store large amounts of unstructured data more efficiently and securely.

Traditionally, object storage, due to their highly scalable and reliable storage mechanism for storing large volumes of data, is also suitable for storing archived data, backup data, large datasets of unstructured data for analytics, and Web applications that require large storage capacity which can be accessed via REST APIs. Cloud providers offer different storage tiers based on performance, cost, and frequency of access for object storage which makes it more and more suitable for IoT applications, Web applications, and data analytics. Thus, today, the cloud object storage can be used for storing and accessing a wide variety of applications data. According to Symonds [50], "Modern object storage is cloud-native and suited for containerization and orchestration, making it truly elastic."

Microsoft Azure has Blob storage which is the object storage solution where large amount of unstructured data can be stored. The storage service offers three types of blobs: block blobs, append blobs, and page blobs. They are all geared toward providing better read/write access. Block blobs are optimized for uploading large amounts of data efficiently. Page blobs are a collection of 512-byte pages optimized for random read and write operations. An append blob is comprised of blocks and is optimized for append operations. For cost-effective data storage, Azure block storage supports two performance tiers: (1) Premium: optimized for high transaction rates and single-digit consistent storage latency where data is stored on SSD; and (2) Standard: optimized for high capacity and high throughput [51]. Google object storage solution is the "Google Cloud Storage." Tiering is supported as described in Sect. 2.4.2. Similarly, Amazon offers the Simple Storage Service (Amazon S3) as an object storage service which provides scalability, data availability, security, and performance.

Healthcare Cloud Storage

Healthcare big data consist of large volumes of structured as well as unstructured data. File storage is not scalable enough to be able to store healthcare big data. Block storage is suitable for storing structured transactional healthcare data such as appointment scheduling, invoicing, and insurance data, but it cannot easily scale up and is also a more costly option. Thus, for storing and accessing unstructured clinical data in the healthcare industry such as patients' health records, prescriptions, medical imaging, IoT data, genome data for research, bioinformatics datasets, object storage is most suitable as it is easily scalable, reliable and secure, has good performance, and is extremely cost-effective compared to block storage solutions [52]. Modern healthcare applications communicate through RESTful APIs which is inherently compatible with cloud object storage solutions such as AWS S3. The FHIR (Fast Healthcare Interoperability Resources) Specification, which is a standard for exchanging healthcare information electronically, is also based on RESTful APIs. Cloud healthcare applications can also easily access IoT data stored at the edge of the cloud. The Broad Institute has adopted the Google Cloud Platform for storage and processing of human genome sequence with the aim of finding patterns, which may reveal the origins of diseases. It was revealed that the cloud platform analyzes human genomes 400% faster, while also ensuring security and privacy of the data [53]. On-premise storage can also easily be leveraged to include cloud object storage.

2.4.4 Blockchain Technology for Storage of Data in Health Care

A blockchain is a digital distributed ledger; i.e., it consists of a time-stamped series of immutable records of data also known as "blocks" that are managed and stored in a network connected through peer-to-peer nodes. Each of these blocks of data is secured and bound to each other using cryptographic hashing mechanisms to constitute a "chain." Blockchain is inherently reliable due to its distributed nature and is also highly secure. Access to the blockchain is based on authentication; new blocks are authorized and secured by means of digital signatures. Furthermore, blocks in the blockchain are safeguarded from tampering, thus providing integrity, by means of cryptographic hashing and chaining principles. The use of blockchain was first introduced in the context of cryptocurrency for the Bitcoin protocol. However, today, blockchain technology is being explored and used in various industries such as business, finance, retail, agriculture, manufacturing, real estate, and the IoT. Blockchain technology is also being increasingly adopted in the healthcare industry for a wide range of applications and data storage.

Blockchain technology can effectively be used as a distributed storage mechanism [54]. The authors propose the use of the Interplanetary File System (IPFS) and blockchain for storing patient diagnostic reports in healthcare facilities [54]. Blockchain technology can improve healthcare data sharing and storing due to its decentralized nature, immutability of data stored in the blockchain, and the transparency and traceability features of the blockchain [55, 56]. Shahnaz et al. [57] proposed to implement a scalable EHR using blockchain technology where granular access control is provided to secure the storage of patient data. Similarly, Mayer et al. [58] looked into the use of blockchain for storing and sharing EHR data and which can facilitate trust between healthcare providers for sharing data, EHR interoperability, auditability, and privacy. Usman and Qamar [59] used the permissioned Hyperledger blockchain platform for implementing a prototype of EMR Management System. Zheng et al. [60] proposed the use of blockchain technology for users to securely store and share such personal health data in a GDPR compliant manner using cloud storage. Wearable/fitness devices (e.g., Apple Watch, Fitbit Charge 4, Samsung Galaxy Fit, Garmin Vivosmart 4, Whoop Strap 3.0) and mobile applications also store large amount of personal health-related data in databases. Such data can be useful for research or commercial project and can be shared via a blockchain. Kassab et al. [61], in a review article, suggest that blockchain technology has lots of potential in the sphere of health care. It can not only securely store and manage patient data (the most popular use case scenario for blockchain) but also track the entire supply chain of medicines and medical equipment such that it facilitates accountability and transparency as well as providing reliable data for clinical research and insurance claims. The four key benefits of using blockchain technology were (1) improved availability of data; (2) improved transparency; (3) improved security; and (4) improved performance. The following challenges were also identified: (1) Scalability and performance; (2) Usability; (3) Secure identification of patients; and (4) Lack of Incentives and willingness to adopt blockchain technology. Tariq et al. [62] recommend that the use of blockchain technology for IoT-enabled smart healthcare systems, which are particularly vulnerable to security breaches, can be beneficial but there are also challenges regarding the deployment of large scale blockchain. Esposito et al. [63] in their paper title "Blockchain: A Panacea for Healthcare Cloud-Based Data Security and Privacy?" discuss the potential of using the Blockchain technology to protect healthcare data hosted within the cloud.

2.5 Cloud Storage Security

Deploying healthcare applications and big data storage on public or hybrid cloud is vulnerable to threats posed by attackers, cloud employees, or vendors subcontracted by the cloud service provider. Healthcare providers have to adhere to storing and sharing data securely whether the data are stored on-premise or on the cloud. For HIPAA and GDPR compliance, healthcare data security and privacy are even more important. Protected Health Information (PHI) relates to identifiable health information that is stored in electronic form such as EHR/EMRs health records, laboratory test results, health histories, diagnoses, treatment information, insurance information, and lists of allergies. Basic security mechanisms such as firewall protection, AES data encryption at rest, SSL security for data in transit, secure key management, strong authentication, policy-based data loss protection (DLP) controls for storage have to be implemented [64]. Some of the security and privacy concerns that are thought to come with the use of the cloud include abuse of privileges, poor encryption, identity theft, data loss, and theft because of the shared and open environment [65]. Issues to do with trust, security attacks, and confidentiality are some of the concerns causing reluctance in embracing cloud storage [66–68]. Zhang and Liu [69] presented the important security concepts related to data sharing in EHR system deployed on the cloud and analyzed the arising security and privacy issues in the access and management of the cloud-based EHR systems. Carter [70] emphasizes the considerations and importance for genomic data privacy and security when working in the cloud to ensure compliance. Much research is being conducted to propose novel ways of securing healthcare data and applications deployed on the cloud to address the security shortcomings.

Khattak et al. [71] present the analysis of security concerns of cloud-based healthcare systems such as availability, trust, confidentiality, compliance, integrity, and audit and concludes that a single-cloud solution is more vulnerable to attack from malicious cloud employees and denial-of-service attacks due to some component failure. While most focus has been on the security related to single cloud, the authors propose a multi-cloud model also known as cloud-of-clouds, as a more secure cloud computing and storage environment for e-healthcare. Similarly, Ziglari and Negini [72] propose the use of several cloud service providers collaborating to offer security in EHR systems; for instance, the EHR application can be deployed on one cloud provider, while the data storage is implemented on another cloud provider for more resilience and security of the overall EHR system. Likewise, a backup of the data could be stored with a third cloud provider. Tunneled communication (cryptographically secured) is used for communication between cloud providers for the purpose of the application.

Hombal and Dayananda [73] address the security issue of accessing and sharing data among the medical practitioners of different healthcare facilities in an efficient manner, i.e., sharing data among a group. The proposed system involves the group members to perform a key agreement protocol, whereby they obtain a common group key that allows sharing of data securely while also detecting malicious users during the group data sharing.

Tupakula and Varadharajan [74] proposed techniques to establish trust on the tenant virtual machine (VM) by performing attestation using the Trusted Platform Module (TPM) chip as well as securing the tenant communication in the context of healthcare facilities (customer/tenant) using the IaaS on the cloud. Attestation allows the customer to ensure integrity of the VM.

Dean et al. [75] depict the design and implementation of a scalable and secure multitenant cloud environment for storage and processing of PHI data in a compliant manner. Alexander and Sathyalakshmi [76] proposed a privacy-aware system and anonymization techniques for data publishing on cloud for PHI based on k-anonymity algorithm and the Advanced Encryption Standard (AES). Shakil et al. [77] focus on the authentication of users accessing and managing the cloud-based BAMHealthCloud system. A behavioral biometric signature-based authentication is proposed for secure data access and retrieval. Al Hamid et al. [78] proposed a key agreement protocol based on a bilinear pairing cryptography for generating a session key to be used to secure medical big data to be shared among the users with whom the session key is shared. Attackers attempting to access the secure data are redirected to decoy data gallery, while only verified users are allowed access to the medical data. Roy et al. [79] propose a fine-grained data access control over multiple cloud servers in a mobile cloud computing-based healthcare applications.

Moreover, cloud storage providers also provide security for data. AWS S3 provides access control mechanisms to block the public in general from accessing the data stored on the cloud as well as configuring the bucket access control lists to set access rights for users based on the principle of least privilege [47]. Users must be authenticated to get access to the storage. AWS typically uses SSL/TLS for securing data in transit from the cloud to the user. Server-side encryption (SSE) can be opted for the encryption of the data stored. Three SSE options are available as follows: (1) Server-side encryption with Amazon S3-managed keys (SSE-S3); (2) Server-side encryption with customer master keys stored in AWS Key Management Service

(SSE-KMS); and (3) Server-side encryption with customer-provided keys (SSE-C). If data stored on the S3 cloud storage are data which do not require modification, e.g., X-Ray image, by using the "Object Lock" feature of S3, they can be stored using a "Write Once Read Many" (WORM) storage. The Object Lock feature prevents accidental or malicious deletion of data. For data that can be modified, the versioning feature can be used to preserve, retrieve, and restore the different versions of the object. Likewise, versioning builds resilience in the storage system. To provide high availability, data can be replicated in multi regions. Finally, AWS S3 also has features that allow the user to monitor and log access to the data.

Microsoft Azure also supports several security features for the cloud storage [80]. Azure role-based access control (Azure RBAC) allows setting up access rights to users. Only authenticated and authorized users are allowed access to the data. Azure Defender, if enabled, detects unusual and potentially harmful attempts to access or exploit storage accounts and trigger security alerts to inform the administrator. The administrator can lock users so that they cannot intentionally or unintentionally modify or delete data. Azure storage can also store blob as WORM state whereby the data are immutable. Azure storage soft delete feature allows recovering blob data after it has been deleted. Blobs can also be encrypted and stored at rest as well as in transit (256-bit AES encryption). Similar security features are also provided by Google Cloud Object Storage [49].

2.6 Conclusion

In this chapter, the healthcare data storage options on the cloud as well as the security of healthcare data are described. The healthcare industry is rapidly evolving and turning into smart healthcare systems with the adoption of new technologies such as cloud computing, mobile computing, IoT, AI and machine learning, and data analytics. New challenges will be faced as the smart healthcare systems mature and become more agile, reliable, secure, and robust. The use of blockchain technology for storing healthcare data in the cloud is also promising due to the security provided by the blockchain technology. The demand for storage capacity for healthcare data will only increase with time. For offloading archived healthcare data from cloud storage, new storage may be adopted such as DNA storage, which involves the use of synthetic DNA for storing data. DNA has very high storage density, has potentially low maintenance cost, is energy efficient, and can store data reliably for a longer period of time as compared to both HDD and SDD. Currently, DNA storage is expensive and not being used on a large scale.

References

1. Aceto, G., Valerio, P., & Antonio, P. (2020). Industry 4.0 and health: Internet of things, big data, and cloud computing for healthcare 4.0. *Journal of Industrial Information Integration, 18*, 100129. ISSN: 2452-414X.
2. Fortino, G., Parisi, D., Pirrone, V., & Di Fatta, G. (2014). BodyCloud: A SaaS approach for community body sensor networks. *Future Generation Computer Systems, 35*, 62–79., ISSN 0167-739X.. https://doi.org/10.1016/j.future.2013.12.015
3. Gravina, R., Ma, C., Pace, P., Aloi, G., Russo, W., Li, W., & Fortino, G. (2017). Cloud-based activity-aaService cyber–physical framework for human activity monitoring in mobility. *Future Generation Computer Systems, 75*, 158–171., ISSN 0167-739X.. https://doi.org/10.1016/j.future.2016.09.006
4. Zeadally, S., Siddiqui, F., Baig, Z., & Ibrahim, A. (2019). Smart healthcare: Challenges and potential solutions using internet of things (IoT) and big data analytics. *PSU Research Review, 4*(2), 149–168. https://doi.org/10.1108/PRR-08-2019-0027
5. Rath, M. (2018). Real time analysis based on intelligent applications of big data and IoT in smart health care systems. *International Journal of Big Data and Analytics in Healthcare, 3*(2), 45–61.
6. Suter-Crazzolara, C. (2018). Better patient outcomes through mining of biomedical big data. *Journal of Frontiers in ICT, 5*, 30.
7. Robison, R. J. (2014). How big is the human genome? *Precision Medicine*. https://medium.com/precision-medicine/how-big-is-the-human-genome-e90caa3409b0. Accessed 24 October 2020.
8. Huesch, D., & Mosher, T. J. (2017). Using it or losing it? The case for data scientists inside health care. *Journal of NeJM Catalyst Innovations in Care Delivery*. https://catalyst.nejm.org/case-data-scientists-inside-health-care/
9. Faggella, D. (2019). Where Healthcare's big data actually comes from. https://www.techemergence.com/where-healthcares-bigdata-actually-comes-from. Accessed 20 June 2018.
10. Raghupathi, W., & Raghupathi, V. (2014). Big data analytics in healthcare: Promise and potential. *Health Information Science System, 2*, 3. https://doi.org/10.1186/2047-2501-2-3
11. Syngene Research. 2020. Global healthcare data storage market analysis 2020. https://www.researchandmarkets.com/reports/5136822/global-healthcare-data-storage-market-analysis. Accessed 24 November 2020.
12. Dash, S., Shakyawar, S. K., Sharma, M., et al. (2019). Big data in healthcare: management, analysis and future prospects. *Journal of Big Data, 6*. https://doi.org/10.1186/s40537-019-0217-0. Article no. 54.
13. Argaw, S. T., Troncoso-Pastoriza, J. R., Lacey, D., et al. (2020). Cybersecurity of hospitals: Discussing the challenges and working towards mitigating the risks. *BMC Medical Informatics and Decision Making, 20*, 146. https://doi.org/10.1186/s12911-020-01161-7
14. Millard, W. B. (2017). Where bits and bytes meet flesh and blood. *Annals of Emergency Medicine, 70*(3), A17–A21. https://doi.org/10.1016/j.annemergmed.2017.07.008
15. Guardian. (2020). US hospital systems facing 'imminent' threat of cyber attacks, FBI warns. https://www.theguardian.com/society/2020/oct/28/us-healthcare-system-cyber-attacks-fbi. Accessed 29 October 2020.
16. Cimpanu, C., (2020). First death reported following a ransomware attack on a German hospital, September 17, 2020. https://www.zdnet.com/article/first-death-reported-following-a-ransomware-attack-on-a-german-hospital/. Accessed 30 October 2020.
17. Ali, O., Shrestha, A., Soar, J., & Wamba, S. F. (2018). Cloud computing-enabled healthcare opportunities, issues, and applications: A systematic review. *International Journal of Information Management* . ISSN: 0268-4012., *43*, 146–158. https://doi.org/10.1016/j.ijinfomgt.2018.07.009

18. Casola, V., Castiglione, A., Choo, K. R., & Esposito, C. (2016, November-December). Healthcare-related data in the cloud: Challenges and opportunities. *IEEE Cloud Computing, 3*(6), 10–14. https://doi.org/10.1109/MCC.2016.139
19. Kumari, A., Tanwar, S., Tyagi, S., & Kumar, N. (2018). Fog computing for healthcare 4.0 environment: Opportunities and challenges journal of. *Computers and Electrical Engineering, 72*, 1–13.
20. Shanmugam, M., & Singh, M. (2017). A comparitive study on traditional healthcare system and present healthcare system using cloud computing and big data. 2017 international conference on signal processing and communication (ICSPC) (pp. 269–273). Coimbatore. https://doi.org/10.1109/CSPC.2017.8305852
21. Yu, W. D., Kollipara, M., Penmetsa, R., & Elliadka, S. (2013). A distributed storage solution for cloud based e-healthcare information system. 2013 IEEE 15th international conference on e-health networking, applications and services (Healthcom 2013) (pp. 476–480). Lisbon. https://doi.org/10.1109/HealthCom.2013.6720723
22. Zhan, H., & Zhang, W. (2014). Cloud storage-based medical data integration technology. In H. Jeong, S. M. Obaidat, N. Yen, & J. Park (Eds.), *Advances in computer science and its applications. Lecture notes in electrical engineering* (Vol. 279). Springer. https://doi.org/10.1007/978-3-642-41674-3_152
23. Candela-Mendoza, E., Cruz-Ipanaque, L., & Armas-Aguirre, J. (2018). Mobile technology model to ambulatory healthcare information online using cloud platform. In *2018 IEEE XXV international conference on electronics* (pp. 1–4). Electrical Engineering and Computing (INTERCON). https://doi.org/10.1109/INTERCON.2018.8526466
24. Hameed, R. T., Mohamad, O. A., Hamid, O. T., & Tapus, N. (2015). Design of e-Healthcare management system based on cloud and service oriented architecture. 2015 E-health and bioengineering conference (EHB) (pp. 1–4). Iasi. https://doi.org/10.1109/EHB.2015.7391393
25. Ibrahim, L. F., Sadek, S., Hakeem, S., Al-Sabban, L., Ibrahim Mohammed Ahmed, A., & Hassan Al-Sayed, A. (2014). Enhanced hospital information system by cloud computing: SHEFA'A. In A. Marcus (Ed.), *Design, user experience, and usability. User experience design for everyday life applications and services. DUXU 2014. Lecture notes in computer science* (Vol. 8519). Springer. https://doi.org/10.1007/978-3-319-07635-5_6
26. Liu, W., & Park, E. K. (2013). e-healthcare cloud computing application solutions: Cloud-enabling characteristics, challenges and adaptations. 2013 international conference on computing, networking and communications (ICNC) (pp. 437–443). San Diego, CA. https://doi.org/10.1109/ICCNC.2013.6504124
27. Mourya, A. K., Shafqat-Ul-Ahsaan, & Idrees, S. M. (2020). Cloud computing-based approach for accessing electronic health record for healthcare sector. In A. Chaudhary, C. Choudhary, M. Gupta, C. Lal, & T. Badal (Eds.), *Microservices in big data analytics*. Springer. https://doi.org/10.1007/978-981-15-0128-9_16
28. Reddy C.T., Sirisha, G., & Reddy, A. M. (2018). Smart healthcare analysis and therapy for voice disorder using cloud and edge computing. 2018 4th international conference on applied and theoretical computing and communication technology (iCATccT) (pp. 103–106). Mangalore, India. https://doi.org/10.1109/iCATccT44854.2018.9001280
29. Tawalbeh, L. A., & Habeeb, S. (2018). An integrated cloud based healthcare system. 2018 fifth international conference on internet of things: systems, management and security (pp. 268–273). Valencia. https://doi.org/10.1109/IoTSMS.2018.8554648
30. Aileni, R. M., Pasca, S., & Valderrama, C. (2015). Cloud computing for big data from biomedical sensors monitoring, storage and analyze. 2015 conference grid, cloud & high performance computing in science (ROLCG), Cluj-Napoca (pp. 1–4). https://doi.org/10.1109/ROLCG.2015.7367419
31. Kolodner, E. K., et al. (2011). A cloud environment for data-intensive storage services. 2011 IEEE third international conference on cloud computing technology and science (pp. 357–366). Athens. https://doi.org/10.1109/CloudCom.2011.55

32. Zungeru, A. M., Gorata, M., Mangwala, M., & Chuma, J. (2017). Healthcare cloud computing for underground wireless sensor networks. 2017 2nd international conference on frontiers of sensors technologies (ICFST) (pp. 136–140). Shenzhen. https://doi.org/10.1109/ICFST.2017.8210490
33. Hanen, J., Kechaou, Z., & Ayed, M. B. (2016). An enhanced healthcare system in mobile cloud computing environment. *Vietnam Journal of Computer Science, 3*, 267–277. https://doi.org/10.1007/s40595-016-0076-y
34. Jemal, H., Kechaou, Z., Ayed, M. B., & Alimi, A. M. (2015). Mobile cloud computing in healthcare system. In M. Núñez, N. Nguyen, D. Camacho, & B. Trawiński (Eds.), *Computational collective intelligence. Lecture notes in computer science* (Vol. 9330). Springer. https://doi.org/10.1007/978-3-319-24306-1_40
35. Karaca, Y., Moonis, M., Zhang, Y.-D., & Gezgez, C. (2019). Mobile cloud computing based stroke healthcare system. *International Journal of Information Management.*, ISSN: 0268-4012.*, 45*, 250–261. https://doi.org/10.1016/j.ijinfomgt.2018.09.012
36. NIST, Mell, P., & Grance, T. 2011, September. The NIST definition of cloud computing. NIST Special Publication 800–145. Computer Security Resource Center. https://csrc.nist.gov/publications/detail/sp/800-145/final. Accessed 1 November 2020.
37. Rajabion, L., Shaltooki, A. A., Taghikhah, M., Ghasemi, A., & Badfar, A. (2019). Healthcare big data processing mechanisms: The role of cloud computing. *International Journal of Information Management.*, ISSN: 0268–4012.*, 49*, 271–289.
38. Gartner. (2018). Gartner magic quadrant for public cloud storage services, worldwide. ID: G00340206. https://www.gartner.com/en/documents/3884480/magic-quadrant-for-public-cloud-storage-services-worldwi
39. Evans, M. (2019). Google, Amazon and Microsoft in battle to store health data in the Cloud. Wall Street Journal. https://www.wsj.com/articles/google-amazon-and-microsoft-in-battle-to-store-health-data-in-the-cloud-11568122202. Accessed 5 November 2020.
40. Landi, H. (2020a, September). Microsoft makes big play for healthcare cloud business in competition with Google, Amazon, Fierce healthcare. https://www.fiercehealthcare.com/tech/microsoft-makes-big-play-for-healthcare-cloud-business-competition-google-amazon. Accessed 5 November 2020.
41. Landi, H. (2020b, September). Mayo Clinic taps Google cloud as strategic partner to accelerate innovation in AI, analytics and digital tools, Fierce healthcare. https://www.fiercehealthcare.com/tech/mayo-clinic-taps-google-cloud-as-strategic-partner-to-accelerate-innovation-ai-digital. Accessed 5 November 2020.
42. Miliard, M. (2019, December). Cerner expands AWS relationship with new machine learning initiatives. https://www.healthcareitnews.com/news/cerner-expands-aws-relationship-new-machine-learning-initiatives. Accessed 6 November 2020.
43. Hernandez P. (2020). 20 top enterprise data storage vendors: An overview of leading data storage vendors, based on a variety of enterprise storage needs. https://www.enterprisestorageforum.com/products/20-top-enterprise-data-storage-vendors.html. Accessed 5 November 2020.
44. Delkin Industrial. (2020, July). Delkin blog: Medical hardware flash storage: factors to consider. https://www.delkin.com/blog/medical-hardware-flash-storage-factors-to-consider/. Accessed 5 November 2020.
45. Stenfort R. (2019, December). How Facebook leverages NVMe™ cloud storage in the datacenter, NVM express. https://nvmexpress.org/how-facebook-leverages-nvme-cloud-storage-in-the-datacenter/. Accessed 24 October 2020.
46. Amazon (2020a). Amazon EBS volume types. https://aws.amazon.com/ebs/volume-types/. Accessed 6 November 2020.
47. Amazon (2020b). Data protection in Amazon S3. https://docs.aws.amazon.com/AmazonS3/latest/dev/DataDurability.html. Accessed 4 November 2020.
48. Google. (2020a). Block storage performance. https://cloud.google.com/compute/docs/disks/performance. Accessed 29 October 2020.

49. Google. (2020b, June). 5 ways to enhance your cloud storage security and data protection. https://cloud.google.com/blog/products/storage-data-transfer/5-ways-to-enhance-your-cloud-storage-security-and-data-protection
50. Symonds J. (2020, February). Why the healthcare industry is adopting high performance object storage. https://blog.min.io/why-the-healthcare-industry-is-adopting-high-performance-object-storage/. Accessed 24 October 2020.
51. Microsoft. (2019). Performance tiers for block blob storage. https://docs.microsoft.com/en-us/azure/storage/blobs/storage-blob-performance-tiers. Accessed 6 November 2020.
52. Tso, M. (2018). Forbes Technology Council, May 2018, health care information and the object storage VNA. https://www.forbes.com/sites/forbestechcouncil/2018/05/17/health-care-information-and-the-object-storage-vna/?sh=43e9453a6744. Accessed 24 October 2020.
53. Broad Institute. (2020). Broad Institute and Google Genomics. https://www.broadinstitute.org/google. Accessed 30 October 2020.
54. Kumar, R., & Tripathi, R. (2020) Chapter 2 -Blockchain-based framework for data storage in peer-to-peer scheme using interplanetary file system. Handbook of research on blockchain technology (pp. 35–59). https://doi.org/10.1016/B978-0-12-819816-2.00002-2
55. Shah, B., Shah, N., Shakhla, S., & Sawant, V. (2018). Remodeling the healthcare industry by employing blockchain technology. 2018 international conference on circuits and systems in digital enterprise technology (ICCSDET) (pp. 1–5). Kottayam, India. https://doi.org/10.1109/ICCSDET.2018.8821113
56. Shi, S., He, D., Li, L., Kumar, N., Khan, M. K., & Choo, K.-K. R. (2020). Applications of blockchain in ensuring the security and privacy of electronic health record systems: A survey. *Journal of Computers & Security*., ISSN: 0167-4048., *97*, 101966. https://doi.org/10.1016/j.cose.2020.101966
57. Shahnaz, A., Qamar, U., & Khalid, A. (2019). Using Blockchain for electronic health records. *IEEE Access, 7*, 147782–147795. https://doi.org/10.1109/ACCESS.2019.2946373
58. Mayer, A. H., da Costa, C. A., & Righi, R. d. R. (2020). Electronic health records in a Blockchain: A systematic review. *Health Informatics Journal, 26*(2), 1273–1288. https://doi.org/10.1177/1460458219866350
59. Usman, M., & Qamar, U. (2019). Secure electronic medical records storage and sharing using blockchain technology. *Procedia Computer Science*., ISSN: 1877–0509., *174*, 321–327. https://doi.org/10.1016/j.procs.2020.06.093
60. Zheng, X., Mukkamala, R. R., Vatrapu, R., & Ordieres-Mere, J. (2018). Blockchain-based personal health data sharing system using cloud storage. 2018 IEEE 20th international conference on e-health networking, applications and services (Healthcom) (pp. 1-6). Ostrava. https://doi.org/10.1109/HealthCom.2018.8531125
61. Kassab, M. H., DeFranco, J., Malas, T., Laplante, P., Destefanis, G., & Graciano Neto, V. V. (2019). Exploring research in blockchain for healthcare and a roadmap for the future. In IEEE transactions on emerging topics in computing. https://doi.org/10.1109/TETC.2019.2936881
62. Tariq, N., Qamar, A., Asim, M., & Khan, F. A. (2020). Blockchain and smart healthcare security: A survey. *Procedia Computer Science, 175*(2020), 615–620. https://doi.org/10.1016/j.procs.2020.07.089
63. Esposito, C., De Santis, A., Tortora, G., Chang, H., & Choo, K. R. (2018, January/February). Blockchain: A panacea for healthcare cloud-based data security and privacy? *IEEE Cloud Computing, 5*(1), 31–37. https://doi.org/10.1109/MCC.2018.011791712
64. Michelson, S. (2019). Key considerations for securing your digital healthcare cloud. https://www.idigitalhealth.com/news/. Accessed 6 November 2020.
65. AbuKhousa, E., Mohamed, N., & Al-Jaroodi, J. (2012). E-health cloud: Opportunities and challenges. *Future Internet, 4*(3), 621–645.
66. Dong, N., Jonker, H., & Pang, J. (2011). Challenges in eHealth: From enabling to enforcing privacy, in foundations of health informatics engineering and systems. In Z. Liu & A. Wassyng (Eds.), *FHIES 2011. Lecture notes in computer science* (pp. 195–206). Springer.

67. ENISA, European Network Information Security Agency. (2009). *An SME perspective on cloud computing*. European Network Information Security Agency.
68. Kuo, A. M.-H. (2011). Opportunities and challenges of cloud computing to improve health care services. *Journal of Medical Internet Research, 13*(3), e67.
69. Zhang, R, & Liu, L. (2010). Security models and requirements for healthcare application clouds. In Proceedings of the 2010 IEEE 3rd international conference on cloud computing (pp. 268–275). Miami, FL.
70. Carter, A. B. (2019, July). Considerations for genomic data privacy and security when working in the cloud. *The Journal of Molecular Diagnostics, 21*(4), 542–552. https://doi.org/10.1016/j.jmoldx.2018.07.009
71. Khattak, H. A. K., Abbass, H., Naeem, A., Saleem, K., & Iqbal, W. (2015). Security concerns of cloud-based healthcare systems: A perspective of moving from single-cloud to a multi-cloud infrastructure. 2015 17th international conference on E-health networking, application & services (HealthCom) (pp. 61–67). Boston, MA. https://doi.org/10.1109/HealthCom.2015.7454474
72. Ziglari, H., & Negini, A. (2017). Evaluating cloud deployment models based on security in EHR system. 2017 international conference on engineering and technology (ICET) (pp. 1–6). Antalya. https://doi.org/10.1109/ICEngTechnol.2017.8308142
73. Hombal, U., & Dayananda, R. B. (2019). An effective security protocol for GDS (group data sharing) in healthcare cloud environment. 2019 international conference on communication and electronics systems (ICCES) (pp. 488–492). Coimbatore, India. https:/doi.org/10.1109/ICCES45898.2019.9002033
74. Tupakula, U., & Varadharajan, V. (2014). Trust enhanced cloud security for healthcare services. 2014 IEEE 13th international conference on trust, security and privacy in computing and communications (pp. 344–351). Beijing. https://doi.org/10.1109/TrustCom.2014.46
75. Dean, D. J. et al. (2017). Engineering scalable, secure, multi-tenant cloud for healthcare data. 2017 IEEE world congress on SERVICES (SERVICES) (pp. 21–29). Honolulu, HI. https://doi.org/10.1109/SERVICES.2017.13
76. Alexander, E., & Sathyalakshmi. (2017). Privacy-aware set-valued data publishing on cloud for personal healthcare records. In *Artificial intelligence and evolutionary computations in engineering systems* (pp. 323–334). Springer.
77. Shakil, K. A., Zareen, F. J., Alam, M., & Jabin, S. (2020, January). BAMHealthCloud: A biometric authentication and data management system for healthcare data in cloud. *Journal of King Saud University - Computer and Information Sciences, 32*(1), 57–64. https://doi.org/10.1016/j.jksuci.2017.07.001
78. Al Hamid, H. A., Rahman, S. M. M., Hossain, M. S., Almogren, A., & Alamri, A. (2017). A security model for preserving the privacy of medical big data in a healthcare cloud using a fog computing facility with pairing-based cryptography. *IEEE Access, 5*, 22313–22328. https://doi.org/10.1109/ACCESS.2017.2757844
79. Roy, S., Das, A. K., Chatterjee, S., Kumar, N., Chattopadhyay, S., & Rodrigues, J. J. P. C. (2019, January). Provably secure fine-grained data access control over multiple cloud servers in mobile cloud computing based healthcare applications. *IEEE Transactions on Industrial Informatics, 15*(1), 457–468. https://doi.org/10.1109/TII.2018.2824815
80. Microsoft. (2020, June). Security recommendations for Blob storage. https://docs.microsoft.com/en-us/azure/storage/blobs/security-recommendations

Chapter 3
A Review on Classification and Retrieval of Biomedical Images Using Artificial Intelligence

K. V. Greeshma and J. Viji Gripsy

Abbreviations

AI	Artificial intelligence
BoVW	Bag of visual words
CBIR	Content-based image retrieval
CBMIR	Content-based medical image retrieval
CMBs	Cerebral microbleeds
CNN	Convolutional neural network
ConvNet	Convolutional neural networks
CT	Computed tomography
DL	Deep Learning
DoG	Difference of Gaussian
DR	Diabetic retinopathy
HOG	Histogram of oriented gradient
ILD	Interstitial lung diseases
IoMT	Internet of medical things
IOT	Internet of things
LBP	Local binary patterns
MIRS	Medical image retrieval systems
ML	Machine learning
MR	Magnetic resonance
MRI	Magnetic resonance imaging
NN	Neural networks
OPT	Optical projection tomography
PACS	Picture archiving and communication system

K. V. Greeshma (✉) · J. Viji Gripsy
Department of Computer Science (UG), PSGR Krishnammal College for Women, Coimbatore, India
e-mail: gripsy@psgrkcw.ac.in

P. Siarry et al. (eds.), *The Fusion of Internet of Things, Artificial Intelligence, and Cloud Computing in Health Care*, Internet of Things,
https://doi.org/10.1007/978-3-030-75220-0_3

PET	Positron emission tomography
PFN	Perifissural nodules
RBMs	Restricted Boltzmann machines
ReLU	Rectified linear unit
RFRM	Relevance feedback retrieval method
SIFT	Scale-invariant feature transform
SURF	Speeded-up robust features
SVM	Support vector machine

3.1 Introduction

Nowadays, IOT plays a vital role in healthcare industry for collecting, visualizing, and transmitting data to provide decision making and proper diagnosis and treatment. Using artificial intelligence, machine learning and deep learning-based approaches help to collect and process the data captured by the IOT devices. To implement these technologies, high computational power and services are needed which are often available by means of cloud. For better medical treatment, various computer-aided diagnosis tools and techniques have been adopted. These tools provide visual information using various medical image modalities for the diagnosis and treatment in medical science.

Medical image analysis is a very complex task for medical experts to interpret the information from the visual data that contains complex structure of human body organs. A medical expert can take better decisions and treatment for serious medical problems by analyzing similar past relevant cases. However, due to the availability of many types of medical image modalities in medical science, bounteous number of medical visual records is generated daily. This is a very challenging and time-consuming task to handle this big data of medical records and retrieve relevant information by medical professionals. In healthcare industry to handle such a problem in an effective and efficient way, we can use the fusion of IOT, artificial intelligence, and cloud computing technologies.

Internet of medical things (IoMT) devices and architectures [1], content-based medical image retrieval (CBMIR) [2] systems, and computer-based medical image retrieval systems (MIRS) help the medical experts to retrieve relevant cases similar to a medical condition from this huge amount of data. Content-based image retrieval (CBIR) [3] and image classification are the most important area in image processing and computer vision. CBIR is an image search and retrieval techniques based on the visual content within the large amount of data. To develop a better medical image retrieval system, image classification is the key challenge. Machine learning and artificial including deep learning algorithms and methods can provide a better classification and high retrieval performance in medical images.

Deep learning has a great impact in medical image analysis and has shown remarkable performance in general CBIR approaches. Deep learning models have made many contributions in healthcare industry such as diabetic retinopathy (DR), brain tumor detection, retinal fundus images, brain MRI, heart disease diagnosis, and many cancer detection problems [4]. Medical imaging technology is growing rapidly, but the content-based image retrieval tasks are in the developmental phase. This paper reviews the major deep learning and machine learning models used in the medical image classification and retrieval [5–17].

Content-based image retrieval classification is an active area of research with considerable applications in medical education, training, clinical diagnosis, and medical research areas. CBMIR [18] systems or picture archiving and communication system (PACS) [19] can store many solved patient treatment records of different diseases. PACS helps the medical experts to consider a patient's image records by allowing them to finds all similar images related to that particular patient. CBMIR systems have been proposed by many researchers to assist physicians in healthcare for better treatment and diagnosis.

We have surveyed various research papers describing machine learning and deep learning models using convolutional neural networks (ConvNet) for single modal-based and multimodal-based image classification and retrieval of medical images. The performances of these architectures are compared with various conventional feature extraction techniques and state-of-the-art methods used in CBIR [20–22].

The rest of the chapter is organized as follows: Section 3.2 describes the state-of-the-art methods and approaches. Sect. 3.3 presents an overview of medical image retrieval techniques—content-based image retrieval (CBIR) and content-based medical image retrieval (CBMIR). Image classification techniques are presented in Sect. 3.4. We have reviewed different machine learning and deep learning algorithms used in medical CBIR in Sect. 3.5. Section 3.6 provides various feature descriptors used in medical image classification and retrieval systems, and finally, we draw a conclusion in Sect. 3.7.

3.2 State of the Art

Researchers have presented many methods for the improvement in classification and retrieval of biomedical images. In the recent studies, a significant breakthrough has done in medical field, and they are classified as single modality and multiple modalities of medical images. As the single modality method, Ciompi et al. [23] have proposed an approach for the automatic classification of perifissural nodules (PFN). They presented a pretrained convolutional neural network for feature extraction and have high relevance on the subject of lung cancer screening. In the paper of Setio et al. [24], they presented a novel CAD system for pulmonary nodule detection from lung CT scans using multiview convolutional networks (ConvNets). Van Tulder et al. [25] proposed a convolutional classification restricted Boltzmann machines (RBMs) by combining the generative and discriminative learning objectives for lung CT analysis.

Anthimopoulos et al. [26] presented a deep convolutional neural network (CNN)-based system for the classification of interstitial lung diseases (ILD) patterns by extracting the features of ILD from the ILD CT scan image dataset. Yan et al. [27] proposed a novel multistage deep learning framework for image classification and applied it on recognition of different body organs. In the pretrained stage, they have trained a CNN on local patches to separate discriminative and noninformative patches from the training data. Then, the network is further fine-tuned by these local patches for the classification task. In a research paper, Dou et al. [28] presented a novel automatic approach to detect cerebral microbleeds (CMBs) from magnetic resonance (MR) images. In this work, they proposed a two-stage framework under 3D convolutional neural networks for the task of CMB detection. In the work of Chowdhury et al. [29], an efficient CBMIR system using convolutional neural network is presented for the automatic retrieval of radiographic images. In the first stage, a set of images are retrieved by using CNN-based feature comparisons, and in the second stage, outlier images are filtered out with the help of edge histogram feature descriptor.

In the research papers that discussed about multiple-based modalities, Qayyum et al. [30] presented a deep learning-based framework for content-based medical image retrieval by training a deep convolutional neural network for the classification task. Two strategies have been proposed for the retrieval of biomedical images, one is by getting prediction about the class of query image by the trained network, and other is to search relevant images in that specific class. Owais et al. [2] proposed a medical image classification framework for retrieving heterogeneous medical images by utilizing recent deep learning techniques. The proposed deep learning-based framework bridges the semantic gap by exploring the discriminative features (i.e., all low-level and high-level features) directly from the images. These extracted features are used to perform class prediction-based image retrieval tasks. The performance of the proposed system is evaluated on various multimodal databases for all possible real-world configuration modes (i.e., closed-world, open-world, and mixed-world) (Table 3.1).

3.3 Medical Imaging and Image Retrieval

In just 1 year, a leading medical facility in Texas generated more than half a million medical images in their fight against cancer. With there being so many images to analyze, harnessing the power of IoT was a must in early diagnosis to present the correct treatments.

The facility installed a smart CT scanner that uses something known as computer vision. The scanner sends data directly to the cloud or a series of connected clouds and uses neural networks and deep learning algorithms to process that in a split second. The application is able to interpret the image from everything it has learnt in the past and identify the indicators of cancer that could have potentially gone unnoticed. This is not a slight against healthcare professionals, but there are some

Table 3.1 State-of-the-art methods for medical image classification and retrieval

Imaging modalities		Study	No of classes	Methodology
Single modality	CT	Ciompi et al. [23]	2	Pretrained convolutional neural networks
	CT	Setio et al. [24]	2	Multiview convolutional neural networks
	CT	van Tulder et al. [27]	5	Restricted Boltzmann machines
	CT	Anthimopoulos et al. [26]	7	Deep CNN
	CT	Yan et al. [31]	12	Multistage deep learning framework
	MRI	Dou et al. [28]	2	3D CNN
	X-ray	Chowdhury et al. [29]	31	CNN + edge histogram descriptor
Multiple modalities	MRI, CT, PET, OPT, fundus camera	Qayyum et al. [30]	24	CBMIR using CNN
	MRI, CT, PET, OPT, fundus camera, X-ray, ultrasound, endoscopy, visible light camera	Owais et al. [2]	50	Deep residual CNN

early stage symptoms that are virtually impossible to spot, and the AI was able to pinpoint those. Doctors are able to provide patients with an on-the-spot diagnosis and treatment plan.

Smart image processing connected technologies like the CT scanner will also allow medical device manufacturers to innovate. Integrating smart cloud platforms to medical devices, they bring to market and licensing cloud analytics capabilities to their customers as a premium service. Subscription-based cloud analytic services for medical diagnosis have the potential to drastically improve workflows by allowing for faster and more accurate diagnosis.

Medical image retrieval system is a tool for medical experts to retrieve similar images to query image in content. Nowadays, with the help of IOT and cloud, the healthcare industry can maintain large number of patient treatment records in an efficient manner. The medical experts can access the patients integrated reports stored in the database and process it for proper diagnosis and treatment. The medical image data are increasing day by day which exist in many formats, namely computed tomography, magnetic resonance imaging, ultrasound, and X-ray images. The medical images produced are large in number because of increasing tomographic images. Hence, managing and the getting grant use to these large image databases have become extremely complex. It has a great influence on the clinical factor in the medical field [32].

While image processing has the capability of changing how we perceive the healthcare industry, it is important to be aware of other developments that are already being use or coming soon. These are a few of the key ones.

- Managing beds and records: AI is being used to manage patient records and place them in the best room/bed based on their condition.
- Repetitive jobs: AI can automate previously manual jobs such as analyzing X-rays and scans.
- Treatment design: Create patient treatment plans based on data.
- Virtual doctors: AI applications are being used to offer 24/7 virtual doctor services and reduce waiting room times.
- Medication and inventory management: Track medication and inventory across multiple locations and stocks.

Other developments such as health monitoring (devices like Garmin and Fitbit) and drug creation through medicine analysis are also in their early stages but look set to revolutionize the industry.

3.3.1 Content-Based Image Retrieval (CBIR)

A block diagram of a generic content-based image retrieval system is illustrated in Fig. 3.1. In CBIR, based on the features extracted from the image content, the images are retrieved from the database. CBIR system contains two phases. One is offline phase, and other is online. During the offline phase, features are extracted from each image to establish a local features database. In the online processing phase, the same feature extraction is performed on the query image and the similarity measurement is calculated between the query image's features and features of database images. The measurements can then be used to find the high similarity, or

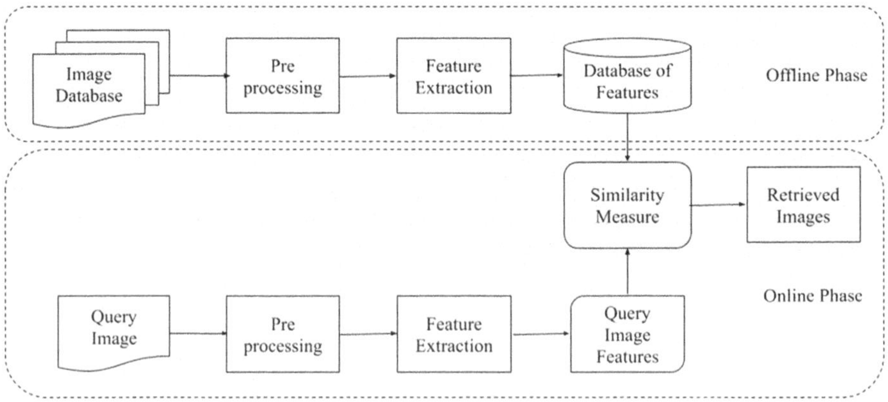

Fig. 3.1 Block diagram of a generic content-based image retrieval system

low distance is then displayed to users as retrieval results. The preprocessing and feature extraction procedures are same in both phases [33].

3.3.2 Content-Based Medical Image Retrieval (CBMIR)

Content-based medical image retrieval system is a method to search and retrieve similar images to query image from the medical image repository. With the widespread dissemination of picture archiving and communication systems (PACS) in hospitals, the sizes of medical image collections are increasing rapidly. Therefore, to manage such large medical databases, the development of effective medical image retrieval system is required. Apart from this task of managing database, a specific CBMIR system helps the doctors in making critical decisions about a specific disease or injury. By retrieving similar images and case histories, the doctors could make a more informed decision about the patient's disease stage and diagnosis [34]. For medical images, global feature extraction-based systems have failed to provide compact feature representations as clinically beneficial information is highly localized in small regions of the image [35–38].

Although a number of methods and approaches have been suggested, it remains one of the most challenging problems in current (CBMIR) studies, largely due to the well-known "semantic gap" issue that exists between machine-captured low-level image features and human-perceived high-level semantic concepts. There have been many techniques proposed to bridge this gap. Ahmed et al. proposed a novel relevance feedback retrieval method (RFRM) for CBMIR. The feedback implemented here is based on voting values performed by each class in the image repository.

3.4 Image Classification Techniques

Image classification plays a major role in various computer vision domains, like image retrieval, online shopping, driverless car, and surveillance. In image classification, the main aim is the feature extraction from the images and classifies it into right classes using any one of the classifiers or classification methods [39]. Soft computing approaches like neural networks and SVM [40] have made major breakthrough for the image classification tasks. For classifications of images or patterns, one of the best classification methods is multiclass support vector machine (SVM). Histogram of oriented gradient (HOG) [41] is an efficient gradient-based feature descriptor for data discrimination, and its performance is excellent comparing with other feature sets.

Nowadays, the most exciting technology revolution has been the rise of the deep learning. In the area of computer vision, convolutional neural networks (CNN or ConvNet) are default deep learning model used for image classification problems. In these deep network models, feature extraction is figured out by itself and these models tend to perform well with huge number of samples. Deep learning often refers to some hidden elements as hyperparameters as they are one of the most crucial components of any deep learning applications. Hyperparameters are the fine-tuning elements that live outside the model but that can heavily influence its behavior and the performance of the model immensely dependent on the selection of right hyperparameter.

Image classification is a supervised machine learning problem. The labeled training data are given, and the subset of this training data is used as validation data for training algorithm. And iterate through training until the model is good. And test the images using this model, and evaluate the accuracy [42] (Fig. 3.2).

3.5 Machine Learning and Deep Learning Algorithms

Machine learning is the study of algorithms that can extract or learn information's automatically. It is the application of artificial intelligence in which the system's ability to learn automatically or to make better decision for future and to make improvement from experiments without being explicitly programmed (Fig. 3.3).

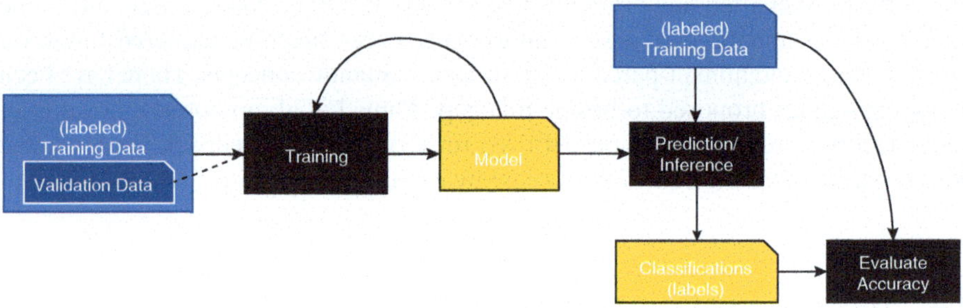

Fig. 3.2 Image classification using machine learning

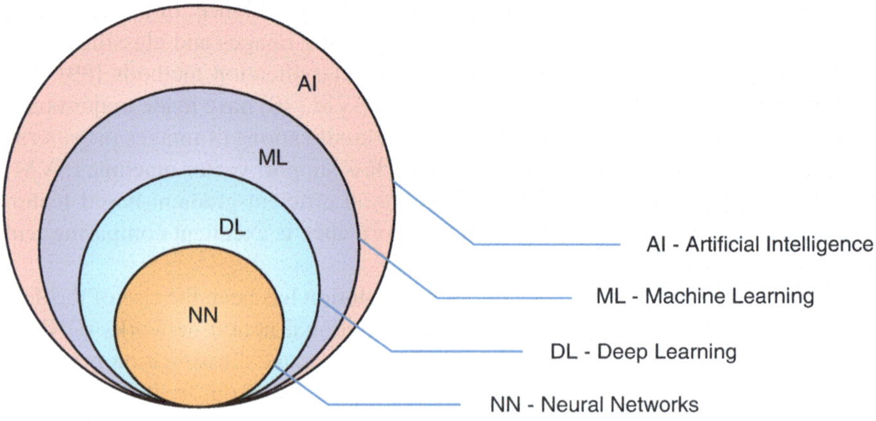

Fig. 3.3 Relationship between AI, ML, and DL

Deep learning is a subset of ML algorithms specifically all the various types of neural networks, and when applied to massive datasets and given massive computing power, these NN will outperform all other models. DL is the popular fields in AI (Fig. 3.4).

Machine learning is a field that is focused on the construction of algorithms that make predictions based on data. Machine learning algorithms can be largely classified into three categories by the type of datasets that are used as experience. These categories are as follows:

- Supervised learning.
- Unsupervised learning.

Supervised learning systems make use of labeled datasets. Unsupervised learning systems use unlabeled datasets to train the system (Fig. 3.5).

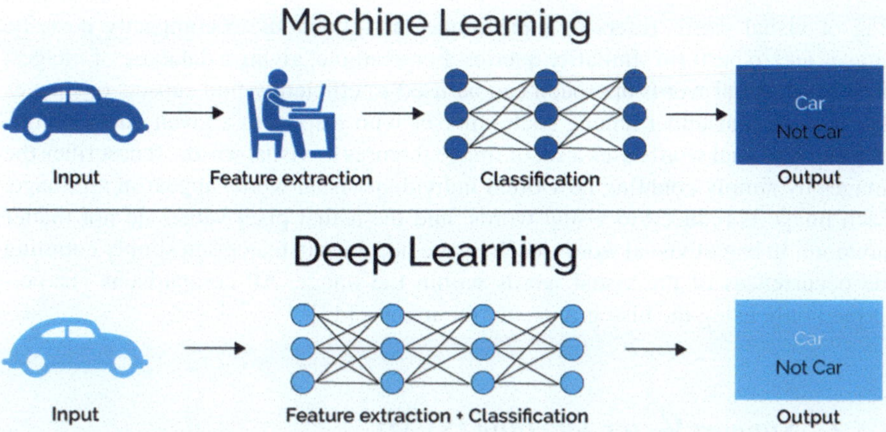

Fig. 3.4 Machine learning vs. deep learning

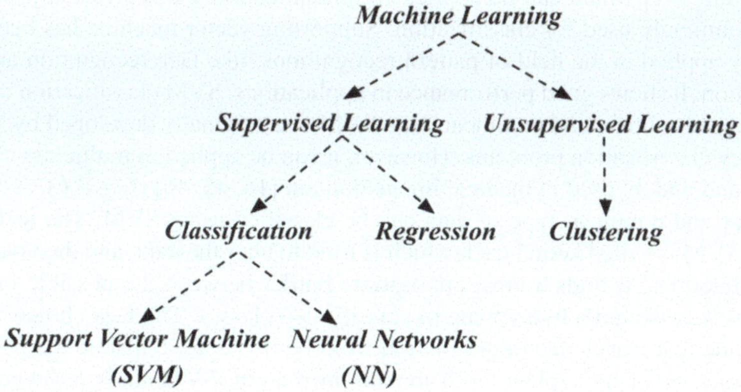

Fig. 3.5 Types of machine learning

ML and DL have various types of applications in medical domain. Some of them are as follows:

- Image recognition.
- Image retrieval.
- Image classification.

Image classification is a supervised machine learning problem. The labeled training data are given, and the subset of this training data is used as validation data for training algorithm. And iterate through training until the model is good. And test the images using this model, and evaluate the accuracy.

3.5.1 Bag of Visual Words (BoVW)

Bag of visual words refers to a technique that allows us to compactly describe images and to perform similarity queries. For example, giving a database of images, the bag of visual words approach can be used to efficiently find subsets of images that look similar either among each other or with respect to a given query image. The bag of visual words uses a set of image features as visual words. It describes the images by simply counting how often individual visual words appear in an image. Each image is reduced to visual words, and the actual pixel values do not matter anymore. In bag of visual words, each image becomes in histogram simply counting the occurrences of the visual words within the image. All comparisons are performed only using the histograms, not the images [43].

3.5.2 Support Vector Machine (SVM)

In ML, one kind of the most common and successful classifier in supervised learning is SVM [44] which can be applied for classification and regression problems. But it commonly used for classification. Supporting vector machine has been successfully applied in the field of pattern recognitions, like face recognition and text recognition. It shows good performance in applications. SVM classification method can be used for linear and nonlinear data. SVM was originally developed by Vapnik for binary classification problems. However, it can be applied in multiclass classifications and widely used in medical image domain [16, 45, 46] (Fig. 3.6).

Linear and nonlinear type of data can be classified using SVM. The technique used in SVM is called kernel trick which is used to alter the data, and then based on these alterations, it finds a most appropriate border between the possible outputs. The goal is to design a hyperplane to classify two classes. The best choice will be hyperplane that leaves maximum margin from both classes. Separate the points of two classes using hyperplane with maximum margin. SVM finds its hyperplane using support vectors and margins.

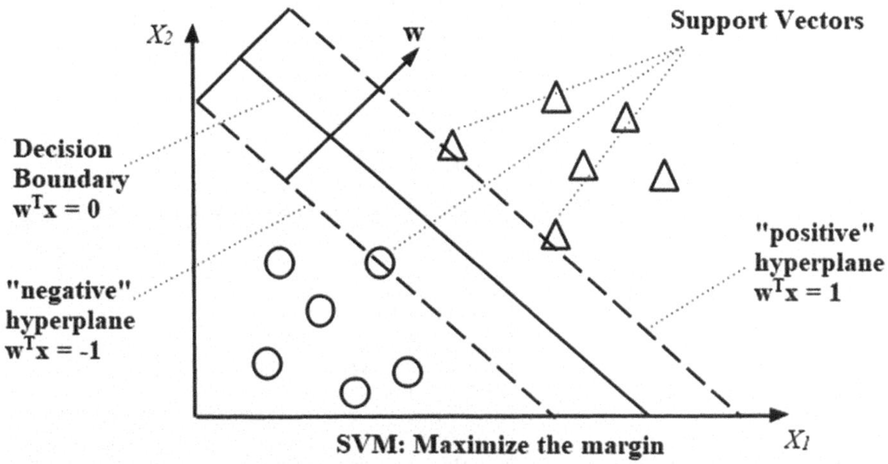

Fig. 3.6 Support vector machine

3.5.3 Convolutional Neural Networks

Convolutional neural networks (CNN or ConvNets) [42] is a type of deep neural network which made up of neurons. It is a specific class of feed-forward neural network in which the connectivity between the neurons inspired by the animal visual cortex. It is generally used to analyze the visual images by processing data with grid like topology. A CNN is also called as a "ConvNet." The first ConvNet called LeNet is built in 1988. It was used for character recognition tasks like reading zip codes and digits. This ConvNet was trained by the complex algorithm like backpropagation.

All CNN model consists of mainly four operations. These are the building blocks of ConvNets. These are:

1. Convolution.
2. Nonlinearity (ReLU).
3. Pooling or subsampling.
4. Fully connected layer.

Convolution

All color images have 3 channels—red, green, and blue. These channels have pixel values ranging from 0 to 255. But in the case of grayscale images, there is only one channel with values from 0 to 255. The values which are very close to 0 represent the black and values closer to 255 represent the black. To collect features from the images is the main purpose of the convolution operation.

Fig. 3.7 Image in matrix form

1	1	1	0	0
0	1	1	1	0
0	0	1	1	1
0	0	1	1	0
0	1	1	0	0

Fig. 3.8 Feature matrix

1	0	1
0	1	0
1	0	1

For example, by considering an image of 5 × 5 matrix with values 1 and 0 (Fig. 3.7).

Considering with a 3 × 3 matrix (Fig. 3.8),

Now, the convolution operation performed on the 5 × 5 image with a 3 × 3 feature matrix can be computed as (Fig. 3.9).

The 3 × 3 matrix which is slide over the image is known as a kernel or filter. The filter moves over the input image pixel by pixel, and in each cell of the pixel, an element-wise multiplication operation is performed. And all these outputs are summed up to get the value which is added to the resultant matrix. This resultant matrix is called as convolved feature or feature map which is shown in the above picture. By using different kernel matrices, it produces various types of feature maps for the same input. Different features of an image like color, patterns, and boundaries can be extracted using this several filters.

CNN model can learn the values of the filter by itself during the training process, but it has to specify the parameters like size and number of filters before the

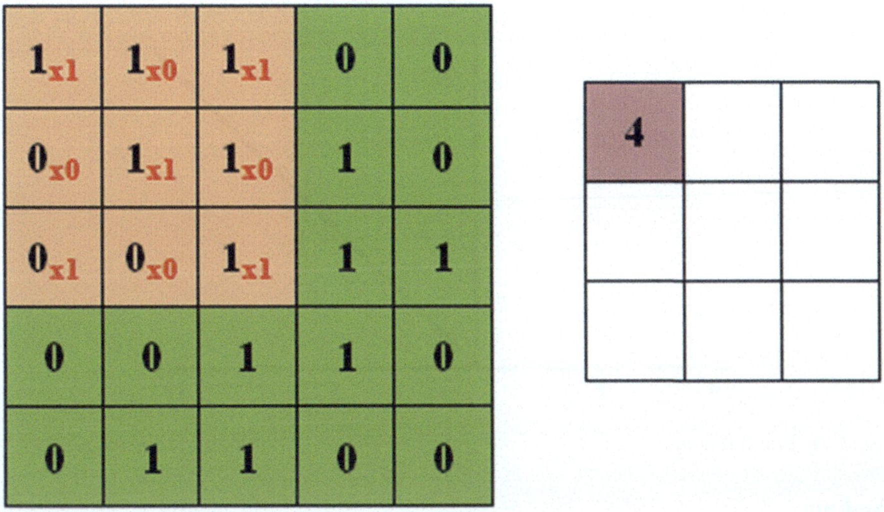

Fig. 3.9 Convolution operation on image

training. When the number of filters increased, more features of the images are retrieved and more efficient recognition of patterns can be achieved [47].

- Stride: The number of pixels on which we move the kernel over the given input image.
- Zero padding: It can change and modify the size of the filter. For applying filter to the bordering elements of the input matrix of the image, the border of the image matrix is padded with zeros.
- Depth: The number of filters needed for the convolution operation.

Nonlinearity (ReLU)

Rectified linear unit (ReLU) is a very popular activation function when it comes with deep learning and even normal neural networks. ReLU is just max (0, x) means; whenever the x is less than zero, it gives 0, and whenever it is greater than zero, it remains as it is.

Figure 3.10 depicts the graph of a ReLU function.

$$\text{Output} = \max\left(\text{zero}, \text{Input}\right)$$

Comparing with other nonlinear activation functions like tanh and sigmoid ReLU performs the best.

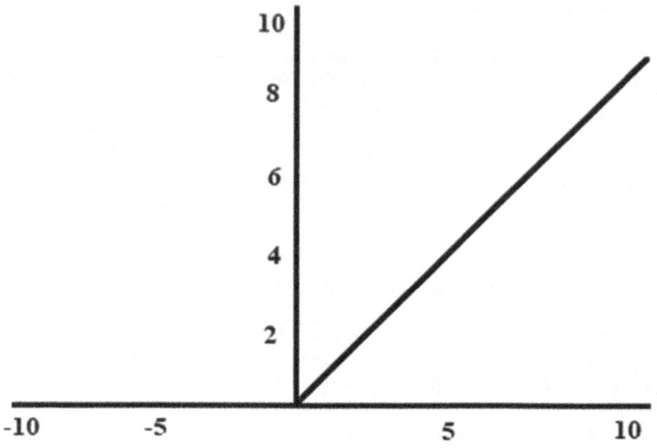

Fig. 3.10 ReLU function

Pooling

Pooling or subsampling reduces the dimension of the image, but it preserves the important information from the feature map. Several types of pooling operation are used in ConvNets. They are max pooling, sum pooling, and average pooling.

Figure 3.11 displays the pooling operation.

In max pooling function, the maximum value in the feature map is retrieved from the given region of elements. In average pooling, it takes the average of the all elements in the specified region. Like in sum pooling, it consider the sum of the elements in that region. Considering all pooling functions, the max pooling performs the best.

Figure 3.12 depicts a max pooling operation of an input image.

Fully Connected Layer

Fully connected layers are those where each node is connected to every previous and every next node. These layers can lead to overfitting (Fig. 3.13).

Even if the very large training set is given for classification, the ConvNets can perform well on the unseen images and classify them correctly into the relevant classes.

3.6 Feature Descriptors

Combining feature descriptors in content-based image retrieval (CBIR) systems plays a key role due to improve the retrieval performance and reduce semantic gap between the visual features and semantics concepts. Texture and shape are the two

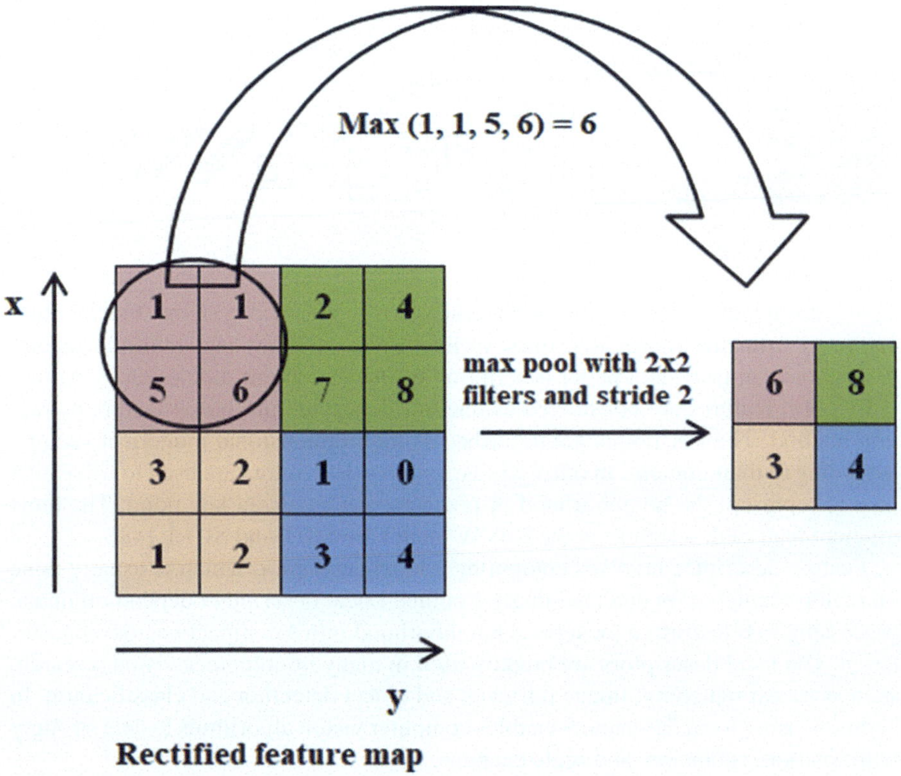

Fig. 3.11 Subsampling operation

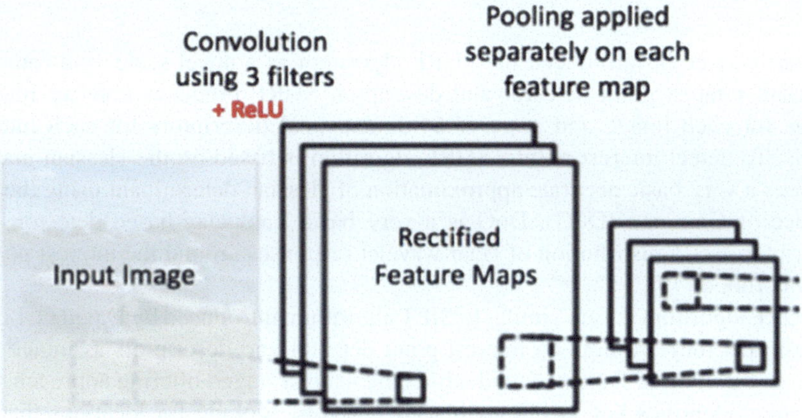

Fig. 3.12 Max pooling performed on an input image

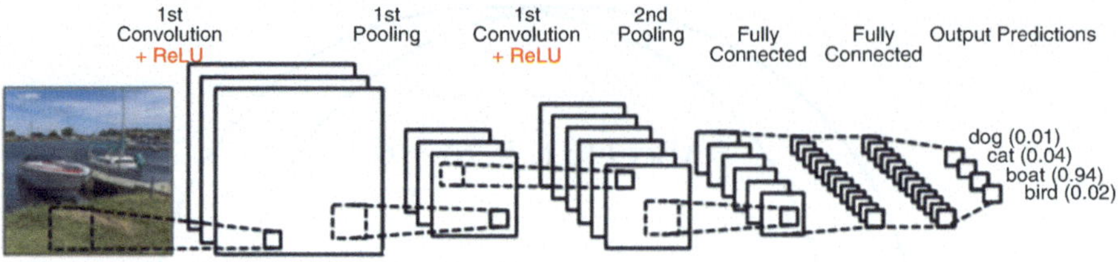

Fig. 3.13 CNN layers

significant features in content-based medical image retrieval systems. Each feature extracted from the image describes various point of view, and multiple feature descriptors can provide a better description of image content. Local binary pattern (LBP) [41] features are considered as one of the best texture-based feature extraction method. The key points are described as multidimensional numerical vectors, according to their content. In other words, features descriptors are used to determine how to represent the neighborhood of pixels near a localized key point. The most efficient feature descriptors in the BoVW model are SIFT and SURF [48].

Feature descriptor involves computing a local descriptor, which is usually done on regions centered on detected interest points. Local descriptors depend on image processing to transform a local pixel neighborhood into a compact vector representation. The local descriptors are broadly used in many of computer vision research, such as robust matching, image retrieval, and object detection and classification. In addition, using local descriptors enables computer vision algorithms to deal strongly with rotation, occlusion, and scale changes.

3.6.1 Speeded-Up Robust Features (SURF)

Herbert Bay et al. introduced the SURF algorithm as a novel scale- and rotation-invariant interest point detector and descriptor. SURF produces a set of interest points for each image and a set of 64-dimensional descriptors for each interest points. To detect interest points, SURF algorithm is based on the Hessian matrix, but uses a very basic accurate approximation of Hessian determinant using the difference of Gaussian (DoG). DoG is a very basic Laplacian-based detector. The descriptor uses a distribution of Haar wavelet responses around the interest point's neighborhood [49].

SURF algorithm is very similar to SIFT algorithm, introduced by David G. Lowe, in term that they are both an interest point detector and descriptors as image features. In SIFT, these features are identified by using a staged filtering approach. The first stage identifies key locations in scale space by looking for locations that are maxima or minima of a difference of Gaussian (DoG) function. Each point is used to generate a feature vector that describes the local image region sampled relative to its scale-space coordinate frame [50].

3.6.2 *Histogram of Oriented Gradients (HOG)*

One kind of simple and effective feature extraction methods is HOG feature descriptor. It is a fast and efficient feature descriptor in comparison to the SIFT and LBP due to the simple computations; it has been also shown that HOG features are successful descriptor for detection. Mainly, it is used for the purpose of object detection in image processing and CV. Using HOG, the shape and appearance of the image can be described. It divides the image into small cells like 4-by-4 which is used in this work and computes the edge directions [44]. For improving the accuracy, the histograms can be normalized. And it contains enough information to visualize the fashion image shape. For identifying the suitable parameter setting configuration of HOG parameters, more training and testing processes using the classifier have to be performed.

3.6.3 *Local Binary Patterns (LBP)*

Local binary patterns (LBPs) coverts a grayscale image at pixel level to a matrix of integer numbers. This matrix of labels describes the original image. It computes the local representation of the texture. It is a visual descriptor used in CV for classification. This model is proposed in 1990 and first described in 1994 [44]. When combining with the HOG feature descriptors, it significantly improves the performance. LBP feature descriptor is a powerful feature used for texture classification.

3.7 Conclusion

Digital images are generated increasingly with the help of IOT sensors and devices, and this big volume of data is stored in clouds so that they can be accessed by medical experts or radiologists for decision making and disease diagnosis. The early detection of diseases is possible in an efficient way with these smart computer systems. Artificial intelligence techniques like machine learning and deep learning algorithms are widely used in biomedical image domain. Content-based image retrieval systems provided state-of-the-art results with the help of different feature descriptors and classification algorithms. The deep learning technique, convolutional neural networks, machine learning algorithm, and support vector machine have been used in many research areas for feature classification. In this paper, we present the review of existing content-based medical image retrieval systems and techniques used for feature extraction and image classification. AI has a bright future in the healthcare industry, and this article only touches the surface on the possibilities. As new technology such as the connected cloud, edge computing, and 5G become commonplace, the capabilities of innovation will be pushed further to save time, lower costs, and ultimately improve accuracy.

References

1. Greco, L., Percannella, G., Ritrovato, P., Tortorella, F., & Vento, M. (2020). Trends in IoT based solutions for health care: Moving AI to the edge. *Pattern Recognition Letters, 135*, 346–353.
2. Owais, M., Arsalan, M., Choi, J., & Park, K. R. (2019). Effective diagnosis and treatment through content-based medical image retrieval (CBMIR) by using artificial intelligence. *Journal of Clinical Medicine, 8*(4), 462.
3. Carvalho, E. D., Antônio Filho, O. C., Silva, R. R., Araújo, F. H., Diniz, J. O., Silva, A. C., ... Gattass, M. (2020). Breast cancer diagnosis from histopathological images using textural features and CBIR. *Artificial Intelligence in Medicine, 105*, 101845.
4. Wong, K. K., Fortino, G., & Abbott, D. (2020). Deep learning-based cardiovascular image diagnosis: A promising challenge. *Future Generation Computer Systems, 110*, 802–811.
5. Haripriya, P., & Porkodi, R. (2021). Parallel deep convolutional neural network for content based medical image retrieval. *Journal of Ambient Intelligence and Humanized.*
6. Haq, N. F., Moradi, M., & Wang, Z. J. (2020). A deep community based approach for large scale content based X-ray image retrieval. *Medical Image Analysis, 68*, 101847.
7. Ismail, W. N., Hassan, M. M., Alsalamah, H. A., & Fortino, G. (2020). CNN-based health model for regular health factors analysis in internet-of-medical things environment. *IEEE Access, 8*, 52541–52549.
8. Karimi, D., Dou, H., Warfield, S. K., & Gholipour, A. (2020). Deep learning with noisy labels: Exploring techniques and remedies in medical image analysis. *Medical Image Analysis, 65*, 101759.
9. Kaur, P., & Singh, R. K. (2020, June). A panoramic view of content-based medical image retrieval system. In 2020 international conference on intelligent engineering and management (ICIEM) (pp. 187–192). IEEE.
10. Khan, S. R., Sikandar, M., Almogren, A., Din, I. U., Guerrieri, A., & Fortino, G. (2020). IoMT-based computational approach for detecting brain tumor. *Future Generation Computer Systems, 109*, 360–367.
11. Kumar, A., Kim, J., Cai, W., Fulham, M., & Feng, D. (2013). Content-based medical image retrieval: A survey of applications to multidimensional and multimodality data. *Journal of Digital Imaging, 26*(6), 1025–1039.
12. Kumar, M., & Singh, M. (2016). CBMIR: Content based medical image retrieval system using texture and intensity for eye images.
13. Litjens, G., Kooi, T., Bejnordi, B. E., Setio, A. A. A., Ciompi, F., Ghafoorian, M., ... Sánchez, C. I. (2017). A survey on deep learning in medical image analysis. *Medical Image Analysis, 42*, 60–88.
14. Lowe, D. G. (1999, September). Object recognition from local scale-invariant features. In proceedings of the seventh IEEE international conference on computer vision (Vol. 2, pp. 1150–1157). IEEE.
15. Muhammad, K., Khan, S., Del Ser, J., & de Albuquerque, V. H. C. (2020). Deep learning for multigrade brain tumor classification in smart healthcare systems: A prospective survey. IEEE transactions on neural networks and learning systems.
16. Nandpuru, H. B., Salankar, S. S., & Bora, V. R. (2014, March). MRI brain cancer classification using support vector machine. In 2014 IEEE Students' conference on electrical, electronics and computer science (pp. 1–6). IEEE.
17. Piccialli, F., Di Somma, V., Giampaolo, F., Cuomo, S., & Fortino, G. (2021). A survey on deep learning in medicine: Why, how and when? *Information Fusion, 66*, 111–137.
18. Pilevar, A. H. (2011). CBMIR: Content-based image retrieval algorithm for medical image databases. *Journal of Medical Signals and Sensors, 1*(1), 12.
19. Greenspan, H., & Pinhas, A. T. (2007). Medical image categorization and retrieval for PACS using the GMM-KL framework. *IEEE Transactions on Information Technology in Biomedicine, 11*(2), 190–202.

20. Alinsaif, S., & Lang, J. (2020). Texture features in the Shearlet domain for histopathological image classification. *BMC Medical Informatics and Decision Making, 20*(14), 1–19.
21. Alroobaea, R., Rubaiee, S., Bourouis, S., Bouguila, N., & Alsufyani, A. (2020). Bayesian inference framework for bounded generalized Gaussian-based mixture model and its application to biomedical images classification. *International Journal of Imaging Systems and Technology, 30*(1), 18–30.
22. Asnaoui, K. E., Chawki, Y., & Idri, A. (2020). Automated methods for detection and classification pneumonia based on x-ray images using deep learning. arXiv preprint arXiv:2003.14363.
23. Ciompi, F., de Hoop, B., van Riel, S. J., Chung, K., Scholten, E. T., Oudkerk, M., ... van Ginneken, B. (2015). Automatic classification of pulmonary peri-fissural nodules in computed tomography using an ensemble of 2D views and a convolutional neural network out-of-the-box. *Medical Image Analysis, 26*(1), 195–202.
24. Setio, A. A. A., Ciompi, F., Litjens, G., Gerke, P., Jacobs, C., Van Riel, S. J., ... van Ginneken, B. (2016). Pulmonary nodule detection in CT images: False positive reduction using multi-view convolutional networks. *IEEE Transactions on Medical Imaging, 35*(5), 1160–1169.
25. van Tulder, G., & de Bruijne, M. (2016). Combining generative and discriminative representation learning for lung CT analysis with convolutional restricted Boltzmann machines. *IEEE Transactions on Medical Imaging, 35*(5), 1262–1272.
26. Anthimopoulos, M., Christodoulidis, S., Ebner, L., Christe, A., & Mougiakakou, S. (2016). Lung pattern classification for interstitial lung diseases using a deep convolutional neural network. *IEEE Transactions on Medical Imaging, 35*(5), 1207–1216.
27. Yan, Z., Zhan, Y., Peng, Z., Liao, S., Shinagawa, Y., Zhang, S., ... Zhou, X. S. (2016). Multi-instance deep learning: Discover discriminative local anatomies for bodypart recognition. *IEEE Transactions on Medical Imaging, 35*(5), 1332–1343.
28. Dou, Q., Chen, H., Yu, L., Zhao, L., Qin, J., Wang, D., ... Heng, P. A. (2016). Automatic detection of cerebral microbleeds from MR images via 3D convolutional neural networks. *IEEE Transactions on Medical Imaging, 35*(5), 1182–1195.
29. Chowdhury, M., Bulo, S. R., Moreno, R., Kundu, M. K., & Smedby, Ö. (2016, December). An efficient radiographic image retrieval system using convolutional neural network. In 2016 23rd international conference on pattern recognition (ICPR) (pp. 3134–3139). IEEE.
30. Qayyum, A., Anwar, S. M., Awais, M., & Majid, M. (2017). Medical image retrieval using deep convolutional neural network. *Neurocomputing, 266*, 8–20.
31. Scherer, R., & Ditzinger, S. (2020). *Computer vision methods for fast image classification and retrieval*. Springer International Publishing.
32. Amini, A., Chen, W., Fortino, G., Li, Y., Pan, Y., & Wang, M. D. (2020). Editorial special issue on "AI-driven informatics, sensing, imaging and big data analytics for fighting the COVID-19 pandemic". *IEEE Journal of Biomedical and Health Informatics, 24*(10), 2731–2732.
33. Ahmed, A. (2020). Implementing relevance feedback for content-based medical image retrieval. *IEEE Access, 8*, 79969–79976.
34. Swapna, T., & Kunnan, S. Content-based image retrieval system for bio-medical images.
35. Behnam, M., & Pourghassem, H. (2013, December). Feature descriptor optimization in medical image retrieval based on genetic algorithm. In 2013 20th Iranian conference on biomedical engineering (ICBME) (pp. 280–285). IEEE.
36. Camalan, S., Niazi, M. K. K., Moberly, A. C., Teknos, T., Essig, G., Elmaraghy, C., ... Gurcan, M. N. (2020). OtoMatch: Content-based eardrum image retrieval using deep learning. *PLoS One, 15*(5), e0232776.
37. Fallahi, A. R., Pooyan, M., & Mohammadnejad, H. (2009, June). Application of morphological operations in human brain CT image with SVM. In 2009 3rd international conference on bioinformatics and biomedical engineering (pp. 1–4). IEEE.
38. Garg, M., & Dhiman, G. (2021). *A novel content based image retrieval approach for classification using glcm features and texture fused lbp variants*. Neural Computing and Applications (Vol. 33, pp. 1311–1328).

39. Quelhas, P., Monay, F., Odobez, J. M., Gatica-Perez, D., & Tuytelaars, T. (2007). A thousand words in a scene. *IEEE Transactions on Pattern Analysis and Machine Intelligence, 29*(9), 1575–1589.
40. Nithya, S., & ShineLet, G. (2012). Bio-medical image retrieval using SVM. *International Journal of Advanced Research in Computer Engineering & Technology (IJARCET), 1*(10), 14–18.
41. Alhindi, T. J., Kalra, S., Ng, K. H., Afrin, A., & Tizhoosh, H. R. (2018, July). Comparing LBP, HOG and deep features for classification of histopathology images. In 2018 international joint conference on neural networks (IJCNN) (pp. 1–7). IEEE.
42. Greeshma, K. V., & Sreekumar, K. (2019). Hyperparameter optimization and regularization on fashion-MNIST classification.
43. Bansal, D., Khanna, K., Chhikara, R., Dua, R. K., & Malhotra, R. (2020). Classification of magnetic resonance images using bag of features for detecting dementia. *Procedia Computer Science, 167*, 131–137.
44. Greeshma, K. V., & Gripsy, J. V. (2020). Image classification using HOG and LBP feature descriptors with SVM and CNN.
45. Othman, M. F. B., Abdullah, N. B., & Kamal, N. F. B. (2011, April). MRI brain classification using support vector machine. In 2011 fourth international conference on modeling, simulation and applied optimization (pp. 1–4). IEEE.
46. Wang, L. (Ed.). (2005). *Support vector machines: Theory and applications* (Vol. 177). Springer Science & Business Media.
47. Wang, Z., Wu, D., Gravina, R., Fortino, G., Jiang, Y., & Tang, K. (2017). Kernel fusion based extreme learning machine for cross-location activity recognition. *Information Fusion, 37*, 1–9.
48. Alfanindya, A., Hashim, N., & Eswaran, C. (2013, June). Content based image retrieval and classification using speeded-up robust features (SURF) and grouped bag-of-visual-words (GBoVW). In 2013 international conference on technology, informatics, management, engineering and environment (pp. 77–82). IEEE.
49. Bay, H., Tuytelaars, T., & Van Gool, L. (2006, May). Surf: Speeded up robust features. In *European conference on computer vision* (pp. 404–417). Springer.
50. Govindaraju, S., & Kumar, G. P. R. (2016). A novel content based medical image retrieval using SURF features. *Indian Journal of Science and Technology, 9*(20), 1–8.

Chapter 4
Diagnosis of Breast Cancer by Malignant Changes in Buccal Epithelium Using Artificial Intelligence, Internet of Things, and Cloud Storage

Dmitriy Klyushin, Kateryna Golubeva, Natalia Boroday, and Dmytro Shervarly

4.1 Introduction

The problem of early diagnosis of breast cancer against the background of increasing morbidity and mortality from this kind of cancer in the world is undoubtedly one of the most important. In order to diagnose cancer at an early stage, an automated mass examination of large groups of the population is needed in order to detect cancer at an early, asymptomatic stage. An effective screening test must be highly sensitive and specific, i.e., clearly separate healthy people from people at risk.

The standard diagnosis of breast cancer consisting of clinical examination, mammography, and aspiration biopsy (Breast Triple Assessment) guarantees high accuracy. However, it can be achieved only using quite dangerous invasive procedures involving radiation and trauma to the tumor, in addition provided that the malignant process has reached a stage where the tumor can be seen on an X-ray and get into it with a fine needle. The use of such methods for screening is not effective enough. Therefore, the second important property of an effective screening method should be non-invasive and harmless, i.e., it must guarantee the absence of tumor injury and other dangerous factors.

Some investigations [1] have directly demonstrated the emergence of tumor-associated changes that are manifested in DNA damage of far-tumor cells in mice

D. Klyushin (✉) · K. Golubeva
Taras Shevchenko National University of Kyiv, Kyiv, Ukraine

N. Boroday
Institute for Problems of Cryobiology and Cryomedicine of the National Academy of Sciences of Ukraine, Kharkiv, Ukraine

D. Shervarly
SourceMe, Stockholm, Sweden

P. Siarry et al. (eds.), *The Fusion of Internet of Things, Artificial Intelligence, and Cloud Computing in Health Care*, Internet of Things,
https://doi.org/10.1007/978-3-030-75220-0_4

with M05076 sarcoma, B16 melanoma, and COLON26 carcinoma. The most probable cause of tumor-associated changes in tissues distant from the tumor is considered as reaction of the immune system to the presence of a tumor.

On the other hand, in [2] the team of authors proved that the DNA in the cell nucleus is packed as a fractal globule, i.e., twisted along a three-dimensional Peano curve. Thus, we can hope that a combination of malignancy-associated changes in the buccal epithelium and fractal nature of DNA packaging in chromatin would be useful for breast cancer diagnosis and screening. Based on this idea, we developed a new classifier that would separate healthy people from patients with breast cancer or fibroadenomatosis by digital image processing of cell nucleus using new technologies: cloud storages, cloud platforms, and IoT.

Today, the fractal analysis is considered as one the most perspective field of investigation of cell heterogeneity. For example, the fractal dimension is used for defining heterogeneity of cells of complex endometrial hyperplasia and well-differentiated endometrioid carcinoma [3]. It is also used a prognostic factor for survival in melanoma [4], leucemia [5, 6], and other diseases [7–9]. The investigations of Nikolaou and Papamarkos [10], Ohri et al. [11], Losa and Castelli [12], Muniandy and Stanlas [13], etc. have shown the significant potential of fractal analysis in estimation of the morphological data. Meanwhile, the objects of these investigations were solely tumor cells but not normal cells with the malignancy-associated changes.

The malignancy-associated changes (MAC) in cells far from a tumor were investigated in papers of Susnik et al. [14], Us-Krasovec et al. [15], Andrushkiw et al. [16], Boroday et al. [17], etc. In these papers it was shown that the analysis of MAC in buccal epithelium is one of the perspective non-invasive methods for the effective screening of cancer. Such methods can be divided in two groups: methods involving the analysis of MAC in non-tumor cells located near a tumor [14, 15] and methods involving the analysis of MAC in non-tumor cells located far from a tumor, in particular, in buccal epithelium (oral mucosa) [16, 17].

Thus, the aim of the chapter is to describe the novel highly accurate AI system for screening of breast cancer based on investigation of fractal properties of chromatin in Feulgen-stained nuclei of buccal epithelium. The chapter is organized as follows. Section 4.1 contains the introduction and a short survey of papers on the malignancy-associated changes and fractal analysis in morphology. Section 4.2 describes the material and methods for analysis of MAC in buccal epithelium. In Sect. 4.3 the system for screening is described. Section 4.4 contains the results of analysis of control and test groups. Section 4.5 concludes the presentation and describes some open problems.

4.2 Materials and Methods

The subject of the study were three groups of people: a control group (29 people), a group of patients with breast cancer of the second stage (68 patients), a group of patients with fibroadenomatosis (33 patients), whose diagnosis was confirmed histologically. The dataset consists of 20,256 images of interphase nuclei of buccal epithelium (6752 nuclei scanned without filter, through a yellow filter, and through a violet filter).

The initial materials for the study were scrapings of epitheliocytes of the oral mucosa from the average depth of the spinous layer, obtained after drying at room temperature, fixation in a mixture of Nikiforov and histochemical reaction of Feulgen with cold hydrolysis in 5*n* HCl for 15 min at $t = 21–22$ °C. The DNA content stained by Feulgen was estimated using the Olympus computer analyzer, consisting of the Olympus BX microscope, Camedia C-5050 digital zoom camera, and a computer. We investigated 52 cells in average in every preparation. The DNA-fuchsine content in the nuclei of the epitheliocytes was defined as a product of the optical density on area. Thus under investigation of the interphase nucleus we obtained a scanogram of the DNA distribution which is rectangular table (matrix) 160×160 pixels.

One of the main requirements that must be met when fixing the parameters of digital photography of the nucleus is the invariance with respect to the rotation of the scan, because the orientation of the nucleus on a microscope slide can be completely random. In order to obtain the invariance with respect to rotation, we propose to use space-filling curves [18], i.e., to read the RGB values of the colors of the pixels of the scan not line by line, but along the Hilbert curve. In this way, we can use any orientation of the nucleus in the image and can consider our image as a vector, not as a matrix.

The digital images analyzed had a size of 128 by 128 pixels, which allows you to read all the pixels of the image, following the Hilbert curve of the seventh order. Thus, we analyzed three arrays of brightness of pixel corresponding to three color components (Red Green Blue) for each curve.

To apply the space-filling curves, we first binarized the image using as a threshold the median brightness of all the pixels (Fig. 4.1).

Next, we cleaned an image deleting background artifacts (Fig. 4.2).

Then, we cleaned the image by binarization and the mask from the previous stage (Fig. 4.3).

At the last stage, we overlaid the mask onto the initial image and obtained the image that further was used for analysis (Figs. 4.4 and 4.5).

However, these dependencies can be interpreted somewhat differently. We decided to consider the data sequences that occur during the walking along a curve as the values of the corresponding color component: red, blue, and green. Now you can use a mathematical apparatus designed for such data sequences (Fig. 4.6).

Given the hypothesis of the fractal nature of chromatin distribution, the Hurst exponent was chosen for data sequences analysis, which is related to the fractal

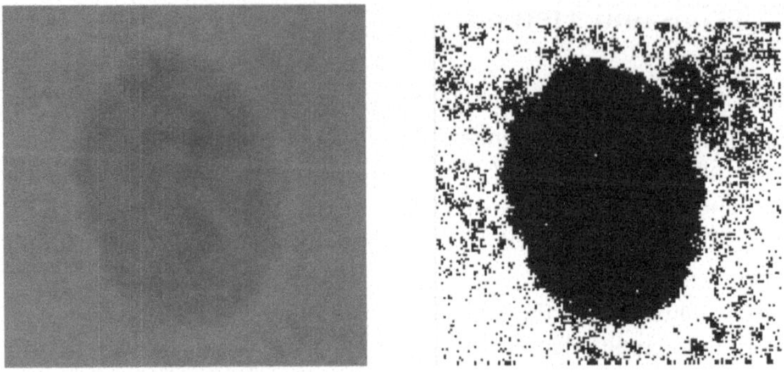

Fig. 4.1 Binarization of an image

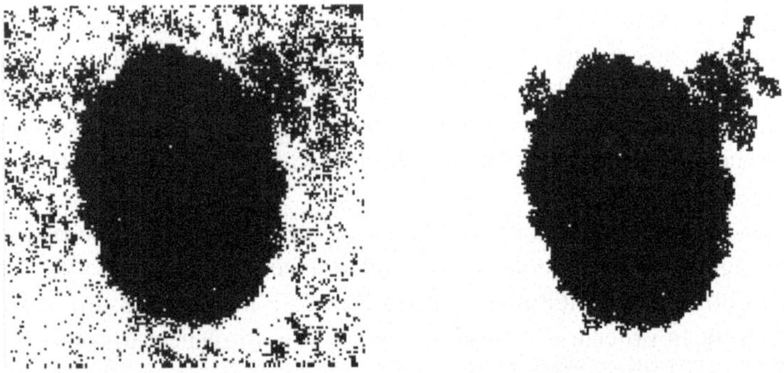

Fig. 4.2 Filtering of an image

Fig. 4.3 Cleaned image

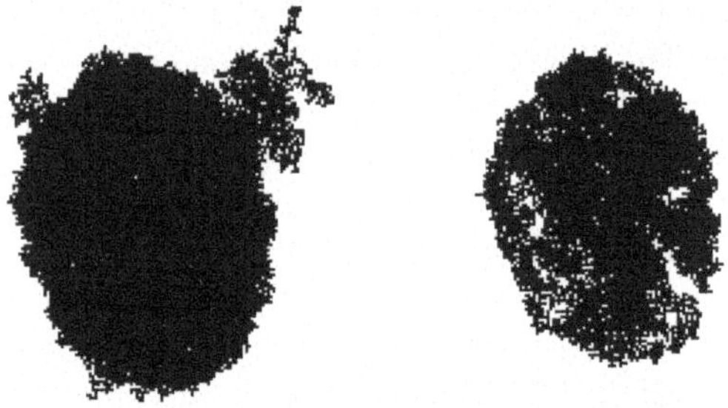

dimension D by the formula $H = 2 - D$. The Hurst exponent is calculated by the following algorithm [19].

1. Find the deviation of the values of the time series from the average value over a chosen segment of a sequence

$$\delta_{m,N} = \sum_{i=1}^{m} \left(x_i - \overline{x}_N \right), \tag{4.1}$$

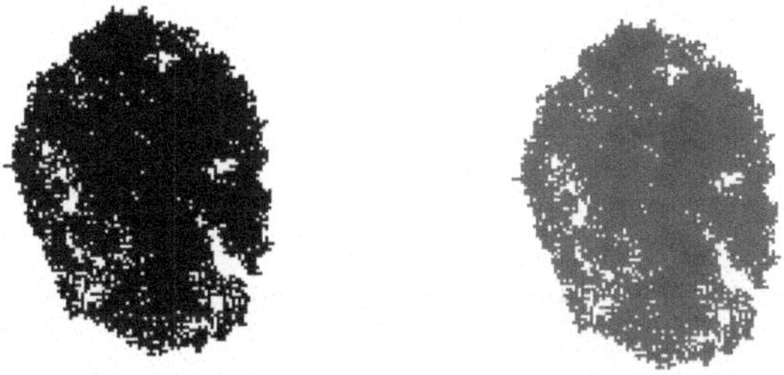

Fig. 4.4 Last stage of image cleaning

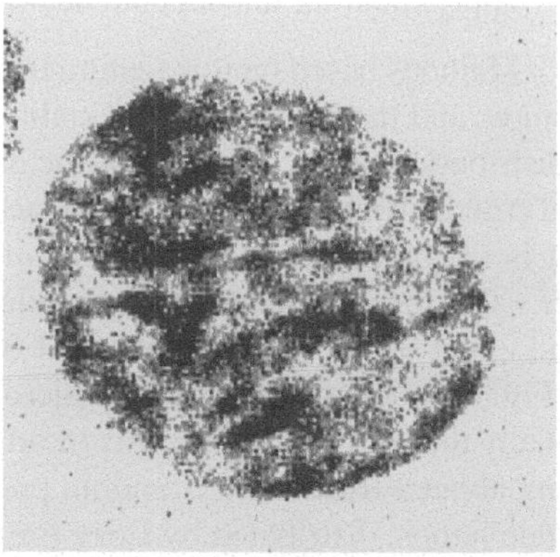

Fig. 4.5 Feulgen-stained nuclei of cell in buccal epithelium

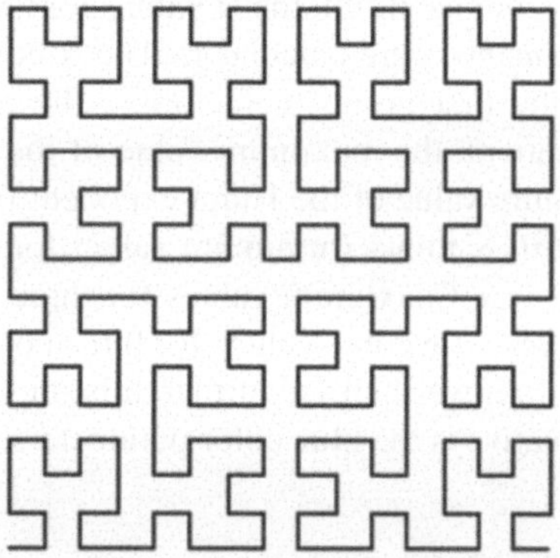

Fig. 4.6 Hilbert curve of fourth order

where N is the length of the segment varying from 2 up to the full length of the sequence, m is the upper limit of summing varying from 1 to $N - 1$, x_i is an element of the data sequence, $\overline{x}_N$ is the average value of the segment. Thus, we have $N - 1$ values $\delta_{2,N}, \ldots, \delta_{N-1,N}$.

2. Find the range of deviations

$$R = \max_{m=2,\ldots,N} \delta_{m,N} - \min_{m=2,\ldots,N} \delta_{m,N} \tag{4.2}$$

3. Normalize the range of deviation

$$Q = \frac{R}{s}, \tag{4.3}$$

   where s is the standard deviation of the data sequence.
4. Find lg$Q$ and lg$N$ and compute the linear approximation of the dependence of lg$Q$ on lg$N$.
5. Find the Hurst exponent, which is the tangent of the angle of the slope of the line approximating the dependence of lg$Q$ on lg$N$.

Methods based on this feature have minimal assumptions about the system under study, and they are extremely stable. The Hurst exponent characterizes the chaotic distribution of the elements of the data sequence. If $0 < H < 0.5$, then the sequence is ergodic (Fig. 4.7), i.e., if the system shows growth in the previous period of time, it is likely that the next moment of time will begin to decline, and vice versa. If $H = 0.5$, then the sequence is chaotic (Fig. 4.8), i.e., the values of the sequence have no effect on subsequent values. If $0.5 < H < 1.0$, then the sequence is trend-stable (Fig. 4.9), i.e., if the sequence increases or decreases in the previous segment, it is likely that it will continue this trend in the next segment. If $H > 1$, then we are talking about a fractal Levy random process (Fig. 4.10). There are independent amplitude jumps, distributed by Levy for in the segment determined by the magnitude of the jump, and increasing with it.

For each cell, the H values for the data sequence of the red, blue, and green components were calculated. The following features were calculated for every patient (the first group of features): the average value of the Hurst exponent for every patient, the maximum value of the Hurst exponent of every patient, and the minimum value of the Hurst exponent for every patient. Therefore, we calculate $\min_{BH}$, $\min_{GH}$, $\min_{RH}$ (minimum values for three colors for all patient cells), $\max_{BH}$, $\max_{GH}$, $\max_{RH}$ (maximum values for three colors for all patient cells), and aver_{BH}, aver_{GH}, aver_{RH} (average values for three colors for all the patient's cells).

As we shall see further, this stage of the screening discovered that the most informative is the blue color parameters. Thus, for each patient the following descriptive

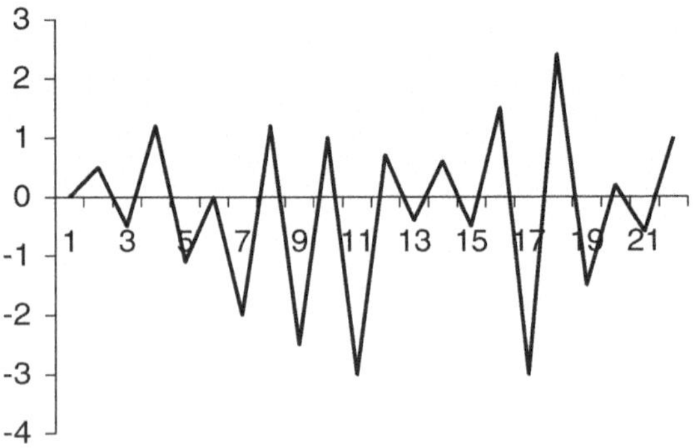

Fig. 4.7 Ergodic data sequence

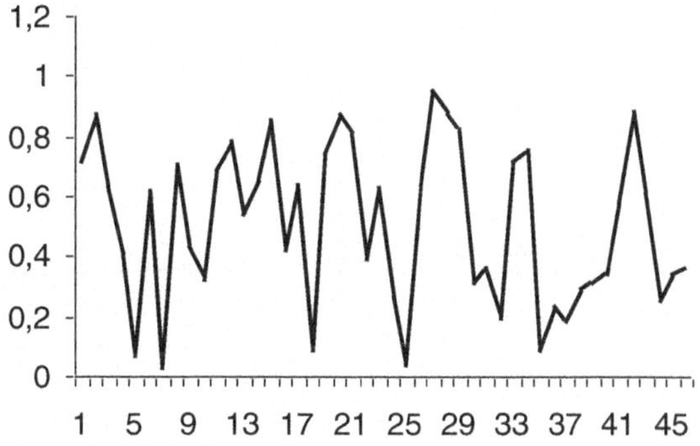

Fig. 4.8 Chaotic data sequence

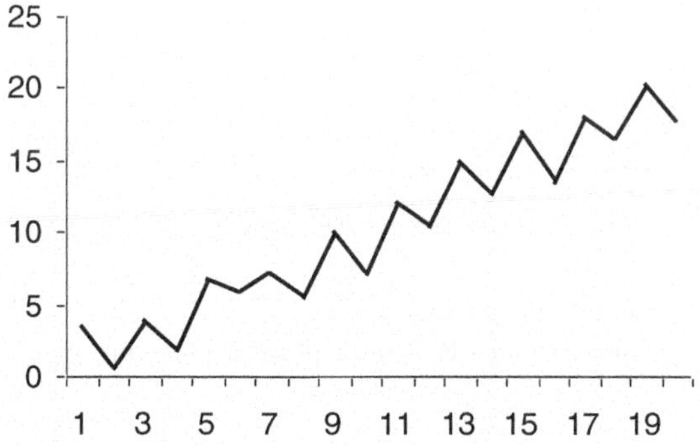

Fig. 4.9 Trend-stable data sequence

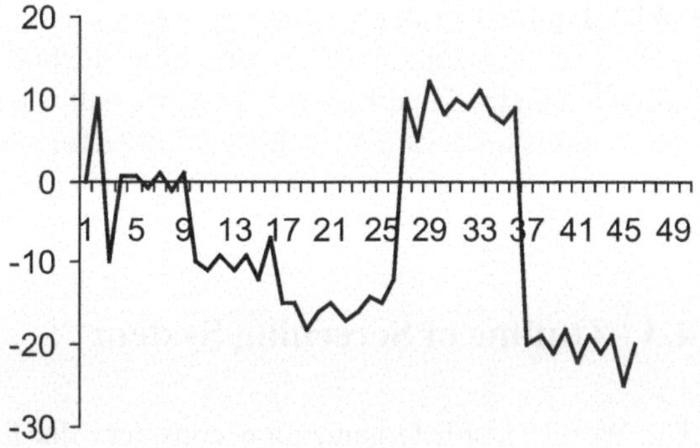

Fig. 4.10 Levy process

statistics of the Hurst exponent of the blue component for all the cells were calculated additionally (the second group of features).

1. Variance
2. Mean square
3. 75th empirical quartile
4. Median
5. Harmonic mean

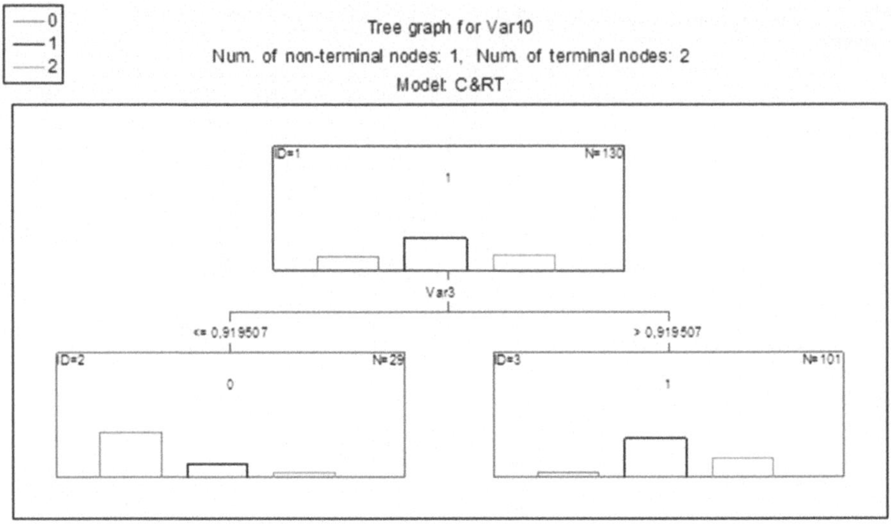

Fig. 4.11 Decision tree in CART model

6. Geometrical mean
7. Average cut-off value (including all but 5%)
8. Mean
9. Excess values

Classification of the data was made using the method of decision trees CART. Figure 4.11 demonstrates one of such tree.

To test the accuracy of the proposed method of screening we used the cross-validation method one-leave-out, i.e., we built a tree on all but one observation, then checked this observation on the resulting tree, and then repeated this procedure for every patient.

4.3 Outline of Screening System

The World Health Organization considers the fight against breast cancer, which includes prevention, early detection, diagnosis and treatment, rehabilitation, and palliative therapy, as one of its main tasks (see https://www.who.int/topics/cancer/breastcancer/ru/index3.html).

Prevention refers to the fight against the main risk factors for breast cancer, as well as the promotion of a healthy diet, physical activity, alcohol withdrawal, and the fight against obesity. Together, these activities help to reduce the incidence of breast cancer.

Often, preventive measures alone cannot significantly reduce the incidence of breast cancer due to the constraints associated with economic conditions in different countries. Therefore, the emphasis in the fight against breast cancer should be on its early detection, which can improve treatment efficacy and survival.

There are two types of early detection of breast cancer:

1. early diagnosis and treatment of cancer;
2. screening populations without visible symptoms to recognize people with suspected breast cancer.

One of the most important factors in the early spread of breast cancer is the early diagnosis of cancer. The more cancer is diagnosed, the more effective its treatment and patient survival.

Currently, the main components of screening are mammography and breast self-examination. Despite the fact that mammography is considered to be the only screening method that has proven its effectiveness, it is a complex and expensive method, which also involves the use of X-ray radiation. The effectiveness of breast self-examination has not yet been reliably evaluated, but its use increases the discipline and awareness of women and is therefore beneficial. So, mammography is considered the only screening method that has no alternatives as the main screening method. Nevertheless, its shortcomings are pushing researchers to look for other screening methods that are non-invasive, highly accurate, and easily implemented in practice using computer technology in particular, cloud platforms and IoT devices.

As shown above, the described screening method is associated with storing a large amount of graphic images and numerical data. Cloud platforms are increasingly being used to efficiently store and process such data such as AWS, Amazon, Google Cloud, Kaggle, etc.

An equally important part of screening is maintaining communication with the patient after the diagnosis. Since the processing of smears, their staining, drying, and photographing can take 2–3 h, the patient can leave the screening site and recover from their business and then get a report on the IoT device, in particular on a smart watch or fitness bracelet. It is also possible that to clarify the diagnosis, the patient will have to repeat the procedure, so maintaining contact with him is a very important component.

Modern IoT systems are created on the basis of data transfer protocols (CoAP, DTLS, Eddystone, HTTP, iBeacon, MQTT, PJON, STOMP, WebSocket, XMPP, etc.) for connecting end devices with cloud platforms (Azure IoT Suite, Amazon Web Services IoT, Kubernetics, OpenStack, etc.). We can develop the following scheme (Fig. 4.12).

A possible scenario of the screening may be follows:

1. Potential patient receives an invitation to visit a clinic and to pass a screening procedure through an IoT-gadget.
2. Patient visits a clinic and passes the analysis.
3. Patient goes away from a clinic and waits for results.

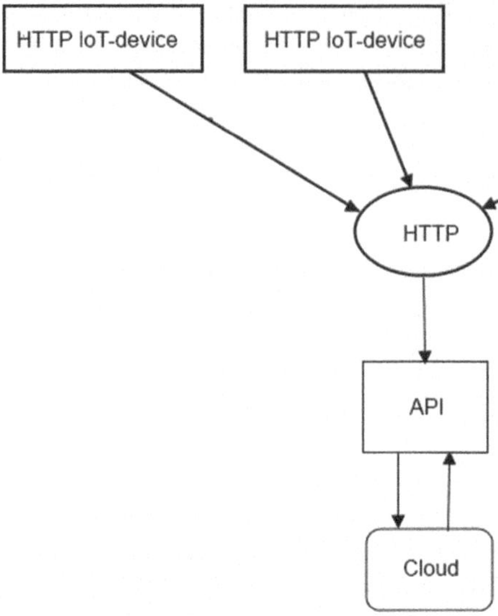

Fig. 4.12 Possible scheme of a screening system

4. Patient receives the results. Depending on the results she can obtain advice to visit invitation to mammologist, invitation to visit a clinic once more to refine the analysis or congratulations with favorable results and advises on healthy lifestyle.
5. Patient may program her IoT-gadget for systematic screening of mammary gland (one per 2–3 year) and use it for control of the health.

4.4 Results and Discussion

Classification based on the Hurst exponent depends on the properties of a data sequence. From the other hand, three channels of the model RGB can produce data sequences of different type. Thus, at the initial stage we must analyze type of data sequence and select a component which is potentially most useful for screening and produce a trend-stable data sequence (Tables 4.1, 4.2, and 4.3).

These results indicate the existence of a certain shift in the red and blue components: trend-stable data sequences are characteristic of all healthy and most patients with fibroadenomatosis and cancer, but some patients in the latter two groups fall into the extreme category of random processes with fractal time. However, it should be noted that for the two-sample Z-criterion and χ^2-criterion with significance levels of 0.05, this difference is not statistically significant. According to the green component, such a division does not exist at all. Therefore, these diseases are not subject to simple classification by type of data sequence although the hypothesis of the presence of a shift gives grounds for the application of more complex methods of

Table 4.1 Distribution of data sequence types in the groups of patients for red component

Type/diagnosis	Healthy	Breast cancer	Fibroadenomatosis
Ergodic	0	0	0
Chaotic	0	0	0
Trend-stable	29	54	27
Fractal	0	14	6

Table 4.2 Distribution of data sequence types in the groups of patients for green component

Type/diagnosis	Healthy	Breast cancer	Fibroadenomatosis
Ergodic	0	0	0
Chaotic	0	0	0
Trend-stable	2	6	6
Fractal	27	62	27

Table 4.3 Distribution of data sequence types in the groups of patients for blue component

Type/diagnosis	Healthy	Breast cancer	Fibroadenomatosis
Ergodic	0	0	0
Chaotic	0	0	0
Trend-stable	29	43	24
Fractal	0	25	9

discriminant analysis. Thus, the method of classification and regression trees (CART) and the blue component were chosen for classification.

We used two-stage classification. At the first stage, we constructed a decision tree and obtained a decision rule. Second, we classified patients using leave-one-out cross-validation, the Hilbert curve, and the first group of the features. Comparing the control group with breast cancer and fibroadenomatosis we randomly selected 51 patients with these diagnoses to prevent misbalancing (Figs. 4.13, 4.14, and 4.15; Tables 4.4, 4.5, 4.6, 4.7, 4.8, 4.9, and 4.10).

Further, assessing the quality of the model for its accuracy, we will use the traditional scale: excellent (0.9–1.0), very good (0.8–0.9), good (0.7–0.8), average (0.6–0.7), and unsatisfactory (0.5–0.6).

Summarizing these results, we can state that our method using the first group of the features differentiates control group and breast cancer with high sensitivity but modest specificity, almost does not distinguishes control group and fibroadenomatosis and has average accuracy comparing control group and joint group consisting of patients with breast cancer and fibroadenomatosis. The clear difference between control groups and breast cancer groups reflects the fact that the latter patients have significant malignancy-associated changes. The malignancy-associated changes in the patients with fibroadenomatosis are not so significant, and, as a result, the control group and fibroadenomatosis and the control groups and the joint group are distinguished not so good.

Consider the results obtained for the second groups of features consisting of descriptive statistics: variance, mean square, 75th empirical quartile, median,

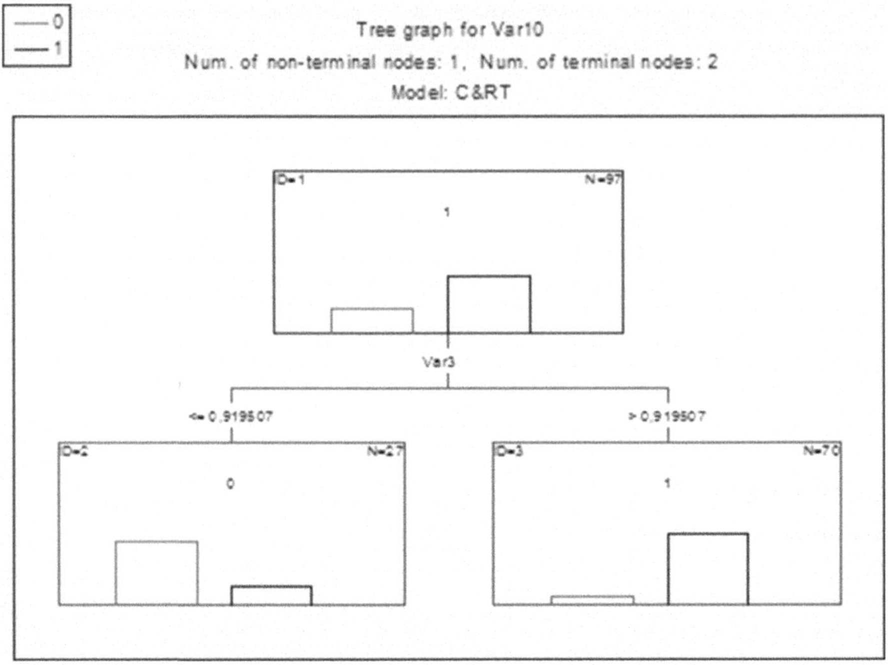

Fig. 4.13 Decision tree for control and breast cancer

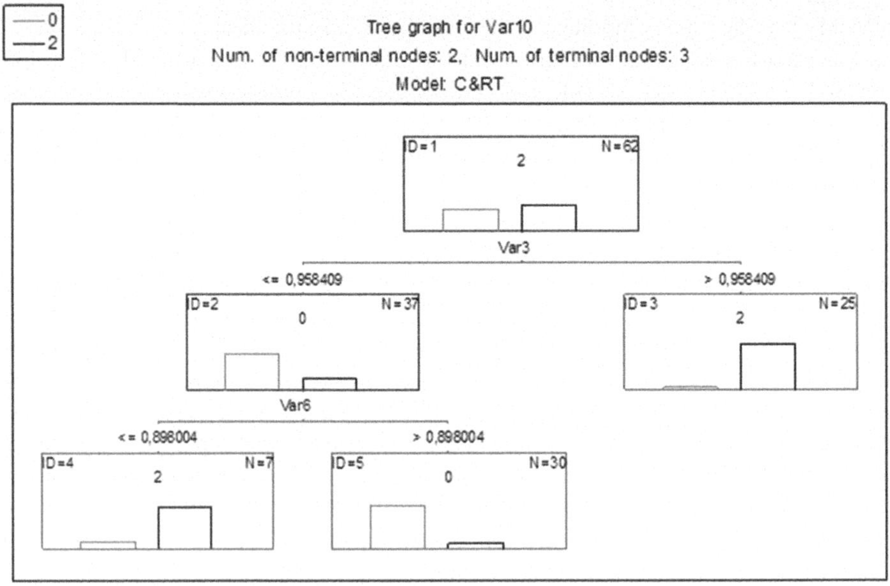

Fig. 4.14 Decision tree for control and fibroadenomatosis

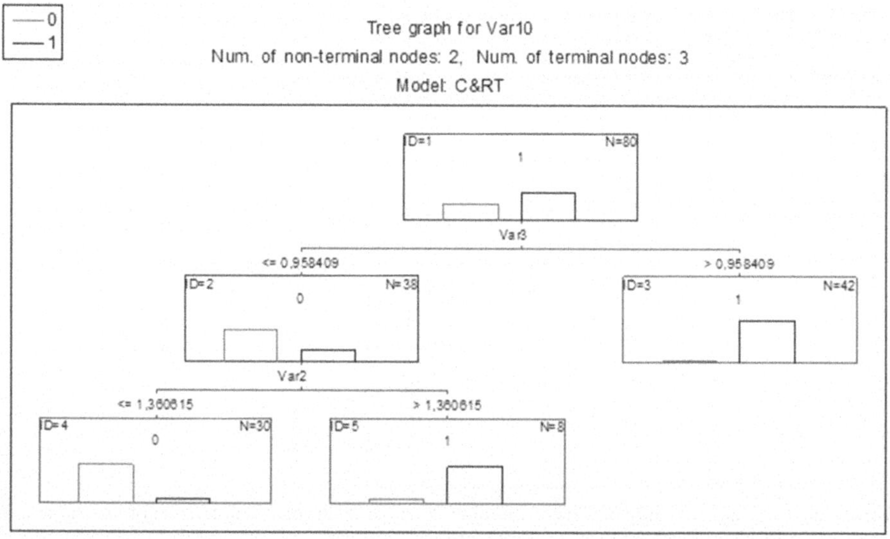

Fig. 4.15 Decision tree for control and joint group of breast cancer and fibroadenomatosis

Table 4.4 Contingency table of decision tree for differential diagnosis between control and breast cancer for the first group of features

Diagnosis	Control	Breast cancer	Total
Control	21	8	29
Breast cancer	6	62	68
Total	27	70	97

Table 4.5 Contingency table of cross-validation between control and breast cancer for the first group of features

Diagnosis	Control	Breast cancer	Total
Control	20	9	29
Breast cancer	5	63	68
Total	25	72	97

Table 4.6 Contingency table of decision tree for differential diagnosis between control and fibroadenomatosis for the first group of features

Diagnosis	Control	Fibroadenomatosis	Total
Control	27	2	29
Fibroadenomatosis	9	24	33
Total	36	26	62

Table 4.7 Contingency table of cross-validation between control and fibroadenomatosis for the first group of features

Diagnosis	Healthy	Fibroadenomatosis	Total
Healthy	18	11	29
Fibroadenomatosis	12	21	33
Total	30	32	62

Table 4.8 Contingency table of decision tree for differential diagnosis between control and joint group of breast cancer and fibroadenomatosis for the first group of features

Diagnosis	Control	BC&FAM	Total
Healthy	27	2	29
BC&FAM	3	48	51
Control	30	50	80

Table 4.9 Contingency table of cross-validation between control and joint group of breast cancer and fibroadenomatosis for the first group of features

Diagnosis	Healthy	BC&FAM	Total
Healthy	27	2	29
BC&FAM	14	37	51
Total	41	39	80

Table 4.10 Pairwise specificity, sensitivity, and accuracy of differential diagnosis for the first group of features

	Control vs breast cancer
Sensitivity, %	92.65
Specificity, %	68.97
Accuracy, %	85.57
	Control vs fibroadenomatosis
Sensitivity, %	66.67
Specificity, %	58.62
Accuracy, %	62.90
	Control vs BC&FAM
Sensitivity, %	72.00
Specificity, %	86.21
Accuracy, %	72.22

harmonic mean, geometrical mean, average cut-off value (including all but 5%), arithmetic mean, and excess values. We applied to these data the two-stage procedure described above: (1) construction of a decision tree; (2) classification using leave-one-out cross-validation, Hilbert curve, and the second group of the features. To avoid misbalancing, for comparison the control group with breast cancer and fibroadenomatosis we randomly selected 51 patients with BC and FAM into a joined group (Figs. 4.16, 4.17, and 4.18; Tables 4.11, 4.12, 4.13, 4.14, 4.15, 4.16, and 4.17).

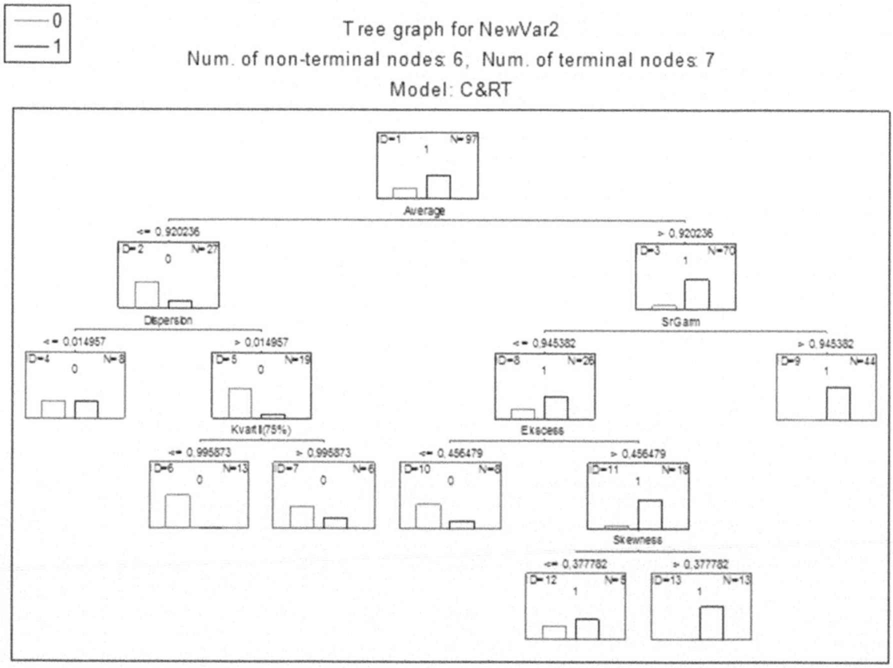

Fig. 4.16 Decision tree for control and breast cancer

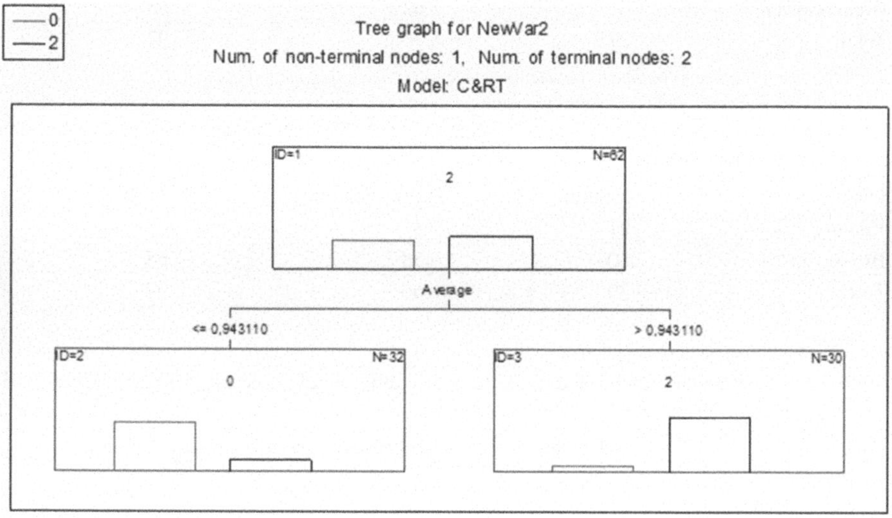

Fig. 4.17 Decision tree for control and fibroadenomatosis

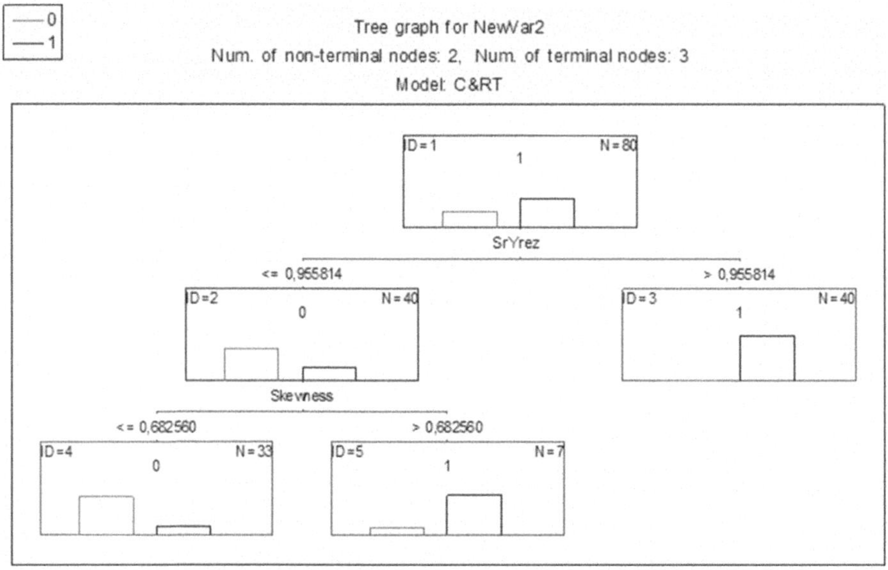

Fig. 4.18 Decision tree for control and joint group of breast cancer and fibroadenomatosis

Table 4.11 Contingency table of decision tree for differential diagnosis between control and breast cancer for the second group of features

Diagnosis	Healthy	Breast cancer	Total
Healthy	21	8	29
Breast cancer	6	62	68
Total	27	70	97

Table 4.12 Contingency table of cross-validation between control and breast cancer for the second group of features

Diagnosis	Healthy	Breast cancer	Total
Healthy	21	8	29
Breast cancer	10	58	68
Total	39	66	97

Table 4.13 Contingency table of decision tree for differential diagnosis between control and fibroadenomatosis for the second group of features

Diagnosis	Healthy	Fibroadenomatosis	Total
Healthy	26	3	29
Fibroadenomatosis	6	27	33
Total	53	9	62

Table 4.14 Contingency table of cross-validation between control and fibroadenomatosis for the second group of features

Diagnosis	Healthy	Fibroadenomatosis	Total
Healthy	25	4	29
Fibroadenomatosis	7	33	33
Total	32	37	62

Table 4.15 Contingency table of decision tree for differential diagnosis between control and joint group of breast cancer and fibroadenomatosis for the second group of features

Diagnosis	Control	BC&FAM	Total
Control	27	2	29
BC&FAM	6	45	51
Total	33	47	80

Table 4.16 Contingency table of cross-validation between control and joint group of breast cancer and fibroadenomatosis for the second group of features

Diagnosis	Control	BC&FAM	Total
Control	26	3	29
BC&FAM	10	41	51
Total	36	44	80

Table 4.17 Pairwise specificity, sensitivity, and accuracy of differential diagnosis for the second group of features

	Control vs breast cancer
Sensitivity, %	85.29
Specificity, %	72.41
Accuracy, %	81.44
	Control vs fibroadenomatosis
Sensitivity, %	81.82
Specificity, %	86.21
Accuracy, %	83.87
	Control vs BC&FAM
Sensitivity, %	78.43
Specificity, %	89.66
Accuracy, %	78.43

Summarizing these results, we can state that our method using the second group of the features differentiates control group and breast cancer with high sensitivity and good specificity, much better that the first group distinguishes the control group and fibroadenomatosis and has good accuracy comparing the control group and the joint group consisting of patients with breast cancer and fibroadenomatosis. Thus, the descriptive statistics of the distribution of the Hurst exponent is quite perspective features for differential diagnosis and screening breast cancer and fibroadenomatosis.

4.5 Conclusion

We were able to detect tumor-associated changes in the fractal structure of chromatin in people with fibroadenomatosis and breast cancer. This difference means that the information "encoded" in the cells has a certain coefficient of "chaos," and in healthy cells there is more "chaos" than in patients (Hurst exponent is closer to 0.5). The constructed classification models have very good, which allows to detect the presence of malignant or benign tumors in the human body during screening. At the same time, they cannot be used for the differential diagnosis of cancer and fibroadenomatosis, and this topic needs to be investigated by other methods.

References

1. Redon, C. E., et al. (2010). Tumors induce complex DNA damage in distant proliferative tissues in vivo. *Proceedings of the National Academy of Sciences, 107*(42), 17992–17997.
2. Lieberman-Aiden, E., et al. (2009). Comprehensive mapping of long-range interactions reveals folding principles of the human genome. *Science, 326*(5959), 289–193.
3. Bikou, O., et al. (2016). Fractal dimension as a diagnostic tool of complex endometrial hyperplasia and well-differentiated endometrioid carcinoma. *In Vivo, 30*, 681–690.
4. Bedin, V., et al. (2010). Fractal dimension of chromatin is an independent prognostic factor for survival in melanoma. *BMC Cancer, 10*, 260.
5. Adam, R., Silva, R., Pereira, F., et al. (2006). The fractal dimension of nuclear chromatin as a prognostic factor in acute precursor B lymphoblastic leukemia. *Cellular Oncology, 28*, 55–59.
6. Mashiah, A., Wolach, O., Sandbank, J., et al. (2008). Lymphoma and leukemia cells possess fractal dimensions that correlate with their interpretation in terms of fractal biological features. *Acta Haematologica, 119*, 142–150.
7. Losa, G. (2012). Fractals and their contribution to biology and medicine. *Medicographia, 34*, 365–374.
8. Metze, K. (2010). Fractal dimension of chromatin and cancer prognosis. *Epigenomics, 2*(5), 601–604.
9. Metze, K. (2013). Fractal dimension of chromatin: Potential molecular diagnostic applications for cancer prognosis. *Expert Review of Molecular Diagnostics, 13*(7), 719–735.
10. Nikolaou, N., & Papamarkos, N. (2002). Color image retrieval using a fractal signature extraction technique. *Engineering Applications of Artificial Intelligence, 15*(1), 81–96.
11. Ohri, S., Dey, P., & Nijhawan, R. (2004). Fractal dimension in aspiration cytology smears of breast and cervical lesions. *Analytical and Quantitative Cytology and Histology, 26*, 109–112.
12. Losa, G., & Castelli, C. (2005). Nuclear patterns of human breast cancer cells during apoptosis: Characterization by fractal dimension and (GLCM) co-occurrence matrix statistics. *Cell and Tissue Research, 322*, 257–267.
13. Muniandy, S., & Stanlas, J. (2008). Modelling of chromatin morphologies in breast cancer cells undergoing apoptosis using generalized Cauchy field. *Computerized Medical Imaging and Graphics, 32*, 631–637.
14. Susnik, B., Worth, A., LeRiche, J., & Palcic, B. (1995). Malignancy-associated changes in the breast: Changes in chromatin distribution in epithelial cells in normal-appearing tissue adjacent to carcinoma. *Analytical and Quantitative Cytology and Histology, 17*(1), 62–68.
15. Us-Krasovec, M., Erzen, J., Zganec, M., et al. (2005). Malignancy associated changes in epithelial cells of buccal mucosa: A potential cancer detection test. *Analytical and Quantitative Cytology and Histology, 27*(5), 254–262.

16. Andrushkiw, R. I., Boroday, N. V., Klyushin, D. A., & Petunin, Y. A. (2007). *Computer-aided cytogenetic method of cancer diagnosis*. Nova Publishers.
17. Boroday, N., Chekhun, V., Golubeva, E., & Klyushin, D. (2016). In vitro and in vivo densitometric analysis of DNA content and chromatin texture in nuclei of tumor cells under the influence of a nano composite and magnetic field. *Advances in Cancer Research & Treatment, 2016*, 1–12.
18. Sagan, H. (1994). *Space-filling curves*. Springer-Verlag.
19. Butakov, V., & Grakovskiy, A. (2005). Evaluation of arbitrary time series stochastic level by Hurst parameter. *Computer Modelling and New Technologies, 9*(2), 27–32.

Chapter 5
Smart IoT Treatment: Making Medical Care More Intelligent

Hena Iqbal and Udit Chawla

Abbreviations

AI	Artificial intelligence
ANOVA	Analysis of variance
BCI	Brain computer interface
CNN	Convolutional neural network
CT	Computed tomography
GPU	Graphics processing unit
IoMT	Internet of medical things
IoT	Internet of things
IT	Information technology
ML	Machine learning
PET	Positron emission tomography

5.1 Introduction

Modernization and Competition among the countries economically and technologically is taking the world toward a new revolution. Technological evolution is taking place at a high speed and continues progressing toward new heights with advancements. With these rising competitions, technologies have made much progress in the field of big data tools like Machine Learning (ML), AI, Internet of Things (IoT), etc. In order to evolve out of others, advance their position and to become a dominating force in success in the field of AI gave rise to a race among the countries worldwide. Apart from AI other tools like Internet of Things (IoT) is also gaining

H. Iqbal (✉)
Information Technology Department, Aldar University College, Dubai, UAE

U. Chawla
Future Institute of Engineering and Management, Kolkata, West Bengal, India

P. Siarry et al. (eds.), *The Fusion of Internet of Things, Artificial Intelligence, and Cloud Computing in Health Care*, Internet of Things,
https://doi.org/10.1007/978-3-030-75220-0_5

more and more attention widely, it has the capability to provide smart physical environments via cyberphysical services to the people [1]. In almost every field, big data tool like Machine Learning has been proved as an excellent tool for various complex researches requiring huge complex data by detecting its meaningful patterns [2]. Human activity recognition is also being adopted widely in recent years for healthcare monitoring, gait measurement, mental activities and functioning, and many more [3]. However, AI is not only limited to the field of machines and technology but is also spread across other fields as well. In the field of healthcare its application has given the world a way to better and healthy lifestyle.

According to various researches, there is lack of proper healthcare system in half of the world and near about 100 million people are penniless [4, 5]. In the data given by the WHO, it predicted that in the coming future, there will be shortage of proper medical facilities and experts by near about 129 million [6]. So, WHO started focusing on the improvement of the technologies in the field of healthcare by concentrating on the application of AI to improve the conditions of healthcare system. World Health Organization [7, 8]). Even the countries worldwide are contributing in AI to bring evolution in the field healthcare by spending investing considerable amount of money in it. There was an investment of around $20 billion by the United States, China, and United Kingdom in 2016 [9, 10].

Thus, AI is being implemented in order to remove the loopholes in the healthcare system in order to remove the disparities prevailing in healthcare globally [11]. AI is not just a machine-oriented term applicable on machines or in technological field but is widely distributed and is leading to growth of various other fields, functions, and technology. It can be generalized as well as narrow in its concept based on the quantity and richness of the data it uses, due to which there is no clear definition of the AI [9, 12]. In simplified terms, AI can be defined as the emulation of the human perception and intelligence, self-improvement, interconnection [13–15].

Incorporation of AI into the field of healthcare aims to reduce costs, improving healthcare services, medical decision-making, control the spreading diseases, and they provide required fallibilities for widespread health ailments, supporting, and improving the lifespan of the people specially aged ones, etc. [16, 17]. AI has progressed a lot by providing digital medical records along with digitalized curing techniques, health experts, etc. It also includes strategies in order to develop the infrastructure, research methods, opportunities, literacy, economic and legal policies [18–24].

AI is increasingly being used widely in healthcare, which stated few years back, and is having strong base in medical system [14, 15, 25–27]. According to an article, Journal Natural, published in 2017, a skin cancer was detected with the help of AI as effectively as a dermatologist [28], and in 2018, it was claimed by another article that the skin cancer was diagnosed much better than a dermatologist [29]. Similarly, there are various successful applications of it in other countries as well, like in France has been said that there can be replacement of medical experts, being radiologist and pathologist, to the AI system in healthcare and they are working enough to bring this change and to adapt it ([13] (SFR-IA Group, CERF, French Radiology Community, 2018; Dreyer & Geis, 2017).

Besides progressing, AI is facing some challenges as well in the field of healthcare with the makeable impact on the health system, services, organization, society, and the people [16, 17]. Though AI has been adopted widely in various fields of medicine, it has marked its visible positive outcomes in medicinal field with modifications and achievements by reducing cost of healthcare services to some extent and delivering quality and advanced healthcare facilities [14, 15, 30–32]. But there is lack of required information and its impact on healthcare services to some extent with limited idea about its outcomes of medicinal practice. Since application of AI in healthcare involves huge amount of quality, data are not possible to be carried out with limited investment which give rise to limited information, and variations in its applications as developing and underdeveloped countries may lack minimum required investment and infrastructure [4, 11]; (The Lancet Public Health, 2019).

In spite of being fewer practical implications of AI in medical field, it has positive outcomes, till now, of its applications. It can be further used and improved in order to bring out its wide applications, by minimizing the existing loopholes and unwanted variations of AI in medical field [33]. AI can be improved further with the implication of more investments in AI in healthcare, admitting more health experts and healthcare staffs, carrying out required researches in order to explore more of its practical implications, etc. For example, applications of AI in identification of various diseases and widespread complex health ailments with deeper researches on it.

5.2 Review of Literature

Data-based AI along with machine learning is one of the emerging tools currently, in various fields, in order to sort out various issues being faced in such fields [34–39]; (Le & Kong, 2011) and will be helpful in getting and maintaining relatively big data in this data-driven era. There have been many AI tools giving a transformation to the way a healthcare services are carried out, and it includes robotics, speech and scene recognition, language processing, sensory systems, etc., having a wide influence in different fields [40, 41]. AI has been applied not only in curing or treating in healthcare but also for providing various related services. It has helped in understanding languages and speeches, solved various issues, possible treatments, modeling, etc. Talking about some of the applications of AI, AI is helpful in recognition of various languages being used worldwide, to carry out researches based on previous data and information, and the robots being used nowadays are also the application of AI only, which is used to serve in every field worldwide [42].

Since we all are in the phase of vast revolution in industries and technology with the inclusion and combination of various types of technology, AI is prevailing in the field of medicines [43, 44]. Potential of AI is being welcomed by most of the parts of the society but along with it there are list of cautions as well to be taken care of. Once in news headlined "A.I. can be a boon to Medicine That Could Easily Go Rogue," it was said that AI being a gift for the society can become a curse as well [45]. Then also it is being widely accepted and used in medical field. In order to make use of AI efficiently, one should make predictions of its pros and cons with past applications and future requirements, etc., in medical stream [46]. There are probable chances of some mistakes, possibility of data manipulations, biasness in the data interpretation, data loss, cyber-crimes, unsuccessful implications of the data or the information, and many more.

In medical stream, AI is performing well enough thus boosting the medical science and pushing it toward growth, and it has helped a lot in investigating more about complex diseases that include ophthalmology, cancer detection, etc., which a human cannot do to certain extent [47–50]. AI is being used to detect various diseases in order get the idea about the disease, its symptoms, possible cures, etc., and to have a better understanding of its treatments and applicable medicines [14, 15, 51–56]. Due to its increasing use, it is predictable that there can be replacement of the clinical experts to this AI, so there is need of medical planning in order to maintain the ratio [14, 15, 54]. It is so because human mind cannot store and process such big data, neither humans can manipulate data to make out various outcomes not it can have the storage of medicinal records and information to large extent [57].

AI is being used in order to create data related to health or personal health of the people or the patients in the hospital. These data are created in various forms and are kept and used by the laboratories to carry out certain investigations, by the doctors to understand the patient's health conditions, etc. These data are not only used in the hospitals or the research laboratories but also by certain institutions or IT companies to carry out several research on healthcare or on application AI in various field with more wide scope [58]. Data available for various sets in healthcare are being used according to their models to be examined which determines the use of the data, purpose of the data to be used, information required, data to be used by whom, etc. An information is basically a set of data that are being used and kept by the organizations but nowadays these data are being used by the organizations or the institutions for the further analysis of the possible applications of the AI in healthcare (Data Governance Institute, n.d.) [59–61].

There are many cases where AI acted as a savior in order to carry out crucial or complex tasks in medical science when all other calculative or statistical tools were unable to perform the required tasks [62–64]. In medical field, AI has proved itself through various successful outcomes. With proper decisions and applications, AI has been used in cancer detection, recognizing persistent or incurable health issues, identifying possible curing methods for breast cancer, curing and predicting the reasons behind human mental illness, psychological disorders, fatigue, and many more [65–70].

AI is being used to carry out physical health detection but is not being applied to that extent in mental health detection [54, 71]. Mental health diagnosis requires large amount of complex data, not only quantitative but also qualitative, due to which AI has not been able to make more of mental health diagnosis. But there is large scope of AI in mental health diagnosis [72–77]. We are not so familiar with the complete interaction of the biological, social, and psychological system of the society and its people. Application of AI techniques and its other associated technological tools will help a lot to determine and understand these interactions more deeply which can take mental health diagnosis and its treatment to a level apart. For this, there is need to bring AI into mental health wellness as much as possible in order to make use of complex and big data through AI [77–79]. In order to detect and monitor the mental health of a person, Internet of Medical Things (IoMT) and Brain Computer Interface (BCI) are novel approach but are unexplored area for the research in the field of healthcare [80]. Brain tumors are the most serious ailment being faced nowadays as there is only 34.9% of survival rate is being determined in brain tumors. Thus, the early detection of the brain tumors is necessary for its diagnosis [81].

There was a time when image predictions and the interpretations of the complex data were carried out manually via human eyes and most of the information used to get missed. But the application of AI in medical imaging or the echocardiography has been very beneficial for the medical development. It is used to understand that in what way a ventral stream is organized with the use of Convolutional neural network (CNN). Such methods help to interpret large and complex data; apart from such complex methods, several other methods are also available like support vector machines, random forests, etc.; along with this, it has a drawback that it causes the problem of overfitting, load of computation, and required huge amount of memory and data [82–87]. In order to automatically process the data to learn and understand the sets of various medical data, blood tests and its images, clinical notes, etc., are made by using these methods. Not only solving the complex data and information, AI has been very advanced in medical imaging, thus giving it a new direction. In spite of all these, understanding medical imaging with the application of AI requires lots of training and experience to solve the complex issues or the abnormalities [83, 88]. Continuous development of medical imaging via computed tomography (CT), ultrasound, positron emission tomography (PET), etc., has led to rise in the amount of data being generated for interpretation. Since it requires proper experience and knowledge to interpret, the complex information is the only drawback of this method [89]. Institutions and various academic organizations are looking toward to solve the following loopholes by combining AI to various other technological tools in order to carry out analyzing, interpreting, categorization, notes on medical imaging by controlling computing costs, expanding GPU power, wide dataset for training purpose, financing for the institutions, etc., [90].

AI with the help of deep learning method (subpart of AI) can be helpful toward detecting and collecting information about the drugs or the medicines being used in healthcare. This could open the way for healthcare industry to much more developed healthcare system. Research is being carried out on developing, improving, creating the drugs though trials on the recruited patients, thus removing the possible uncertainties and the biasness in the process of detection [91–94]. There are various uses of AI in drug development like drug targeted association, protein characteristics, drug, combination, pharmacological properties, etc. [95–97]. Also, curing targets, developed medicines, creating links between drugs and the illness will lead Ai further in the field of drugs [17, 98]. Looking at the past performances of the technology in drug detection and development, due to AI and deep learning there is vast development in this field by investments, minimizing inaccuracies, proper researches, etc., which provided the ease of detection of probable issues and predicting the features and risks associated with the drugs [99–103].

Data kept by the organizations consist to complex data as well as the data related to the personal details or the personal heath of the people which are being used to be carried out through AI, and with this application of data for development and improvements AI in the field of healthcare, there is need of privacy of the data to be kept as well [104, 105]. There are several regulations being laid down by the government as well as by the researchers to maintain the standards of the data and other related infrastructures in order to facilitate the data interface [104–106]. Such data are based on several assumptions being made by the researchers which when applied may or may not give the positive outcomes; thus, there is chances of getting exploited or biased outcomes than required. So, there is need to be more precise and need of more relevant or accurate information of AI and the related technological tools being used in order to develop and improve the AI application in healthcare to bring out the changes in the methods and perspective of AI or technological applications [105, 107].

5.3 Objective

To identify a conceptual model for understanding the factors determining patient satisfaction for the use of artificial intelligence in healthcare.

5.4 Research Methodology

In the present study, USA, Canada, Australia, UAE, and China were chosen as a place of survey as these are the advanced countries and the use of AI is highest in these countries as compared to other countries. People in these countries prefer AI based treatments over other methods of treatment. Thus, 249 samples were collected from different locations in USA, Canada, Australia, UAE, and China with the help of structured questionnaire, which were sent to the respondents through email. Initially, around 40 quality parameters were identified for determining customers' awareness and preferences about AI in healthcare. Five-point Likert scale ranging from 1: strongly disagree to 5: strongly agree as used by Cronin and Taylor (1992) was introduced for the measurement of each parameter. Along with these parameters, demographic and psychographic variables were also recorded for the respondents. Data after proper cleaning and validation were used for several multivariate analyses to attain the objectives of the study.

5.5 Findings and Analysis

The value of Kaiser-Meyer-Olkin statistic is 0.898 (Table 5.1) and is also larger and greater than 0.5. The approximate Chi-square statistic is 3969.739 with 378 degree of freedom which is significant at 0.05 level.

Factor 1(Personal Touch) accounts for a variance of 9.504 which is 33.94% of the total variance (Table 5.2), likewise Factor 2 (Comprehensive Gap) accounts for a variance of 3.422 which is 12.22% of the total variance, Factor 3 (Answerability) accounts for a variance of 1.772 which is 6.329% of the total variance, Factor 4 (Nerve Racking) accounts for a variance of 1.560 which is 5.57% of the total variance, Factor 5 (Wrong Reporting) accounts for a variance of 1.231 which is 4.396% of the total variance, and Factor 6 (Enlightened) accounts for a variance of 1.145 which is 4.092% of the total variance, and thus, the first six factors combined account for 66.553. From the (Fig. 5.1), we can take factor whose eigenvalues are greater than one. An eigenvalues represent the amount of variance associated with the factor.

In the rotated factor matrix (Table 5.3), Factor 1 has high coefficient for the variables, V26—As a patient, I want to be treated as a person, not as a number, V28—It's important to ask questions while getting the result, V23—It is important to read how doctors work before getting a scan/reports, V24—Humans are essential, when discussing the results of a scan, V25—Personal contact is involved in getting the results, V27—Explanation would be missed, when a computer gives the result, V30—Humans and artificial intelligence can accompaniment each other, V16—It is important to have a good understanding of the results of a scan/reports. Therefore, this factor may be labeled as "Personal Touch." Factor 2 has high coefficient for the variables, V21—It is important to ask questions on the accuracy of the results, V22—It is important to be well informed about the process of scan being made, V19—It is important that a scan provides as much information about the body as possible, V18—It is important to talk with someone about the results of a scan/reports, V20—It is important to get the results of a scan as quickly as possible, V17—It is important to be able to ask questions personally about the results of a scan/reports. Therefore, this factor may be labeled as "Comprehensive Gap." Factor 2 has high coefficient for the variables, V12—It is unclear that how a computers will be used in evaluating scans/reports, V13—Although computers are better in evaluating scans, I will still prefer a doctor, V14—When artificial intelligence is used, personal data may go into the wrong hands, V11—It's quite worrisome that a computer does not take feelings into account. Therefore, this factor may be labeled as "Answerability." Factor 4 has high coefficient for the variables, V5—It's a matter of

Table 5.1 KMO and Bartlett's test

Kaiser-Meyer-Olkin measure of sampling adequacy		0.898
Bartlett's test of Sphericity	Approx. Chi-Square	3969.739
	Df	378
	Sig.	0.000

Table 5.2 Total variance explained

	Initial eigenvalues			Extraction sums of squared loadings			Rotation sums of squared loadings		
Component	Total	% of variance	Cumulative %	Total	% of variance	Cumulative %	Total	% of variance	Cumulative %
1	9.504	33.943	33.943	9.504	33.943	33.943	4.864	17.373	17.373
2	3.422	12.221	46.164	3.422	12.221	46.164	4.116	14.698	32.072
3	1.772	6.329	52.493	1.772	6.329	52.493	2.905	10.376	42.448
4	1.560	5.572	58.065	1.560	5.572	58.065	2.554	9.121	51.569
5	1.231	4.396	62.461	1.231	4.396	62.461	2.502	8.934	60.503
6	1.146	4.092	66.553	1.146	4.092	66.553	1.694	6.051	66.553
7	0.945	3.374	69.927						
8	0.787	2.809	72.737						
9	0.743	2.654	75.390						
10	0.645	2.303	77.693						
11	0.605	2.162	79.855						
12	0.598	2.135	81.990						
13	0.540	1.928	83.918						
14	0.460	1.641	85.560						
15	0.449	1.603	87.163						
16	0.420	1.501	88.665						
17	0.371	1.324	89.989						
18	0.368	1.316	91.305						
19	0.327	1.167	92.472						
20	0.322	1.150	93.622						
21	0.311	1.110	94.732						
22	0.270	0.964	95.696						
23	0.243	0.867	96.563						
24	0.232	0.829	97.393						
25	0.206	0.735	98.128						
26	0.196	0.699	98.827						
27	0.174	0.622	99.448						
28	0.154	0.552	100.000						

Extraction Method: Principal Component Analysis

awe that how a computer can give the results of a scan/reports, V6—Doctors get lazy due to Artificial intelligence, V3—Humans can get a better overview than the computers on what happens in my body, V4—It's a matter of worry when a computers analyze scans/reports without humans intrusion. Therefore, this factor may be labeled as "Nerve Racking." Factor 5 has high coefficient for the variables, V15—Artificial intelligence may prevent errors, V9—A computer should never be trusted blindly, V7—Reports/Scans are not ready for evaluating by implementing artificial intelligence. Therefore, this factor may be labeled as "Wrong Reporting." Factor 6 has high coefficient for the variables, V36—If cost is not the matter, then a computer should be used to make a full body scan instead of looking at specific body

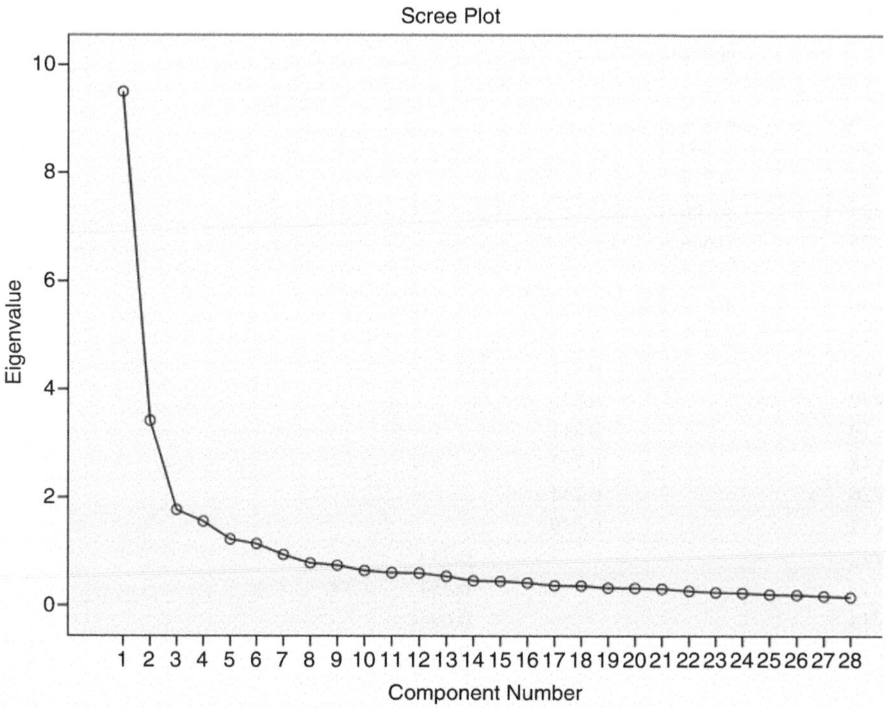

Fig. 5.1 Scree plot

parts, V33—Due to the use of artificial intelligence, few number of doctors are required, V39—If a computer can predict about the disease that we can get in the future, I want to know that no matter what. Therefore, this factor may be labeled as "Enlightened." Table 5.4 helps to identify which factors have been extracted.

$$H_0 : B_1 = 0$$

The null hypothesis implies that there is no linear relationship between Patient Satisfaction and the factors "Personal Touch," "Comprehensive Gap," "Answerability," "Nerve Racking," "Wrong Reporting," and "Enlightened."

$$H_1 : B_1 != 0$$

The alternative hypothesis implies that there is relationship, positive or negative, between Patient Satisfaction and the factors "Personal Touch," "Comprehensive Gap," "Answerability," "Nerve Racking," "Wrong Reporting," and "Enlightened."

In the above Table *R*-square (Table 5.5) value is 0.395 which indicates 39.5% of the total variation in the dependent variable, overall satisfaction can be explained by the independent variables, "Personal Touch," "Comprehensive Gap," "Answerability," "Nerve Racking," "Wrong Reporting," and "Enlightened."

Table 5.3 Rotated component matrix

	Component					
	1	2	3	4	5	6
V26	0.813					
V28	0.809					
V23	0.748					
V24	0.706					
V25	0.666					
V27	0.661					
V30	0.612					
V16	0.438					
V21		0.871				
V22		0.832				
V19		0.811				
V18		0.792				
V20		0.734				
V17		0.689				
V12			0.754			
V13			0.754			
V14			0.695			
V11			0.607			
V5				0.765		
V6				0.718		
V3				0.592		
V4				0.575		
V15					0.781	
V9					0.752	
V7					0.633	
V36						0.839
V33						0.767
V39						0.484

Extraction Method: Principal Component Analysis
Rotation Method: Varimax with Kaiser Normalization
[a]Rotation converged in 7 iterations

From the above ANOVA table (Table 5.6), we can see that the regression model predicts the dependent variable significantly well and it is statistically significant as *p*-value is less than 0.05. Thus H_1 is rejected, whereas H_0 is accepted.

The coefficient table (Table 5.7) helps to predict overall satisfaction from "Personal Touch," "Answerability," "Nerve Racking," "Wrong Reporting," and "Enlightened," and from the table, these factors are statistically significant to the regression model. The factor "Comprehensive Gap" is statistically not significant in the coefficients table.

Table 5.4 Factors Extracted determining patient satisfaction for the use of artificial intelligence in healthcare

Personal touch	As a patient, I want to be treated as a person, not as a number
	It's important to ask questions while getting the result
	It is important to read how doctors work before getting a scan/reports
	Humans are essential, when discussing the results of a scan
	Personal contact is involved in getting the results
	Explanation would be missed, when a computer gives the result
	Humans and artificial intelligence can accompaniment each other
	It is important to have a good understanding of the results of a scan/reports
Comprehensive gap	It is important to ask questions on the accuracy of the results
	It is important to be well informed about the process of scan being made
	It is important that a scan provides as much information about the body as possible
	It is important to talk with someone about the results of a scan/reports
	It is important to get the results of a scan as quickly as possible
	It is important to be able to ask questions personally about the results of a scan/reports
Answerability	It is unclear that how a computers will be used in evaluating scans/reports
	Although computers are better in evaluating scans, I will still prefer a doctor
	When artificial intelligence is used, personal data may go into the wrong hands
	It's quite worrisome that a computer does not take feelings into account
Nerve racking	It's a matter of awe that how a computer can give the results of a scan/reports
	Doctors gets lazy due to artificial intelligence
	Humans can get a better overview than the computers on what happens in my body
	It's a matter of worry when a computers analyze scans/reports without humans intrusion
Wrong reporting	Artificial intelligence may prevent errors
	A computer should never be trusted blindly
	Reports/scans are not ready for evaluating by implementing artificial intelligence
Enlightened	If cost is not the matter, then a computer should be used to make a full body scan instead of looking at specific body parts
	Due to the use of artificial intelligence, few number of doctors are required
	If a computer can predict about the disease that we can get in the future, I want to know that no matter what

Table 5.5 Regression model summary

Model	*R*	*R* square	Adjusted *R* square	Std. error of the estimate
1	0.628[a]	0.395	0.380	0.7137

Table 5.6 ANOVA

Model	Sum of squares	Df	Mean square	F	Sig.
Regression	80.346	6	13.391	26.293	0.000[b]
Residual	123.252	242	0.509		
Total	203.598	248			

[a]Predictors: (Constant), Enlightened, Wrong_Reporting, Nerve_Racking, Answerability, Comprehensive_Gap, Personal_Touch
[b]Dependent Variable: SAT

Table 5.7 Coefficient

	Unstandardized coefficients		Standardized coefficients		
Model	B	Std. error	Beta	T	Sig.
(constant)	3.707	0.045		81.962	0.000
Personal_Touch	0.225	0.045	0.248	4.968	0.000
Comprehensive_Gap	−0.038	0.045	−0.042	−0.832	0.406
Answerability	−0.157	0.045	−0.174	−3.470	0.001
Nerve_Racking	−0.112	0.045	−0.124	−2.470	0.014
Wrong_Reporting	0.207	0.045	0.228	4.557	0.000
Enlightened	0.438	0.045	0.484	9.668	0.000

[a]Dependent Variable: SAT

$$\text{Patient Satisfaction} = 3.707 + 0.248 * (\text{Personal Touch}) - 0.174 * (\text{Answerability})$$
$$-0.124 * (\text{Nerve Racking}) + 0.228 * (\text{Wrong Reporting}) + 0.484 * (\text{Enlightened})$$

5.6 Managerial Implications

Artificial Intelligence has grown leaps and bounds, it has advanced steadily fast over the last few years, and thus, healthcare sector will be transformed significantly. Many people do the speculation about the changes and the impact it will have on the lives of the doctors and the patients. It is to see how patients would react about such a big transformation. It's very important from patient point of view to ask questions while getting the result through artificial intelligence. It's very significant to read and understand how doctors work before getting a scans and reports. Humans' interactions are too very essential, when discussing the results of a scan or reports. Personal contact of personnel should be involved in getting and discussing the results. It has also come into the light that due to the use of artificial intelligence, few number of doctors and personnel are required for the treatment and less human errors. Computers can predict about the disease that we can get in the future and it helps us to realize its pitfalls. Overall, we have to take cautious approach by balancing high end technology and human touch.

References

1. Fortino, G., & Trunfio, P. (Eds.). (2014). *Internet of things based on smart objects: Technology, middleware and applications*. Springer Science & Business Media.
2. Savaglio, C., Ganzha, M., Paprzycki, M., Bădică, C., Ivanović, M., & Fortino, G. (2020). Agent-based internet of things: State-of-the-art and research challenges. *Future Generation Computer Systems, 102*, 1038–1053. https://doi.org/10.1016/j.future.2019.09.016
3. Wang, Z., Wu, D., Gravina, R., Fortino, G., Jiang, Y., & Tang, K. (2017). Kernel fusion based extreme learning machine for cross-location activity recognition. *Information Fusion, 37*, 1–9. https://doi.org/10.1016/j.inffus.2017.01.004
4. Sallstrom, L., Morris, O., & Mehta, H. (2019). Ethical considerations: Artificial intelligence in Africa's healthcare.
5. World Bank and World Health Organization. (2017). Half the world lacks access to essential health services, 100 million still pushed into extreme poverty because of health expenses.
6. Global Health Workforce Alliance and World Health Organization. (2013). Auniversal truth: No health without a workforce.
7. World Health Organization. (2017). Big data and artificial intelligence for achieving universal health coverage: An international consultation on ethics: Meeting report.
8. World Health Organization. (n.d.). Draft global strategy on digital health 2020–2024.
9. House of Lords. (2018). *AI in the UK: Ready, willing and able?* House of Lords.
10. National Science and Technology Council. (2016). *Preparing for the future of artificial intelligence*. Executive Office of the President.
11. Wahl, B., Cossy-Gantner, A., Germann, S., & Schwalbe, N. R. (2018). Artificial intelligence (AI) and global health: How can AI contribute to health in resource-poor settings? *BMJ Global Health, 3*(4), e000798.
12. Russell, S., & Norvig, P. (2016). *Artificial Intelligence: A modern approach* (3rd ed.). Pearson.
13. Jha, S., & Topol, E. J. (2016). Adapting to artificial intelligence: Radiologists and pathologists as information specialists. *JAMA, 316*(22), 2353–2354.
14. Topol, E. J. (2019a). High-performance medicine: The convergence of human and artificial intelligence. *Nature Medicine, 25*(1), 44–56.
15. Topol, E. J. (2019b). *Deep medicine: How artificial intelligence can make healthcare human again* (1st ed.). Basic Books.
16. Bughin, J., Hazan, E., Ramaswamy, S., et al. (2017). *Artificial intelligence: The next digital frontier*. McKinsey Global Institute.
17. Hamet, P., & Tremblay, J. (2017). Artificial intelligence in medicine. *Metabolism, 69*(S36), S40.
18. Canadian Institute for Advanced Research. (2018). CIFAR Pan-Canadian artificial intelligence strategy.
19. China Institute for science and technology policy at Tsinghua University. (2018). *China development report*. Tsinghua University.
20. European Commission. (2018). *Artificial intelligence for Europe*. European Commission.
21. Martinho-Truswell, E., Miller, H., NtiAsare, I., et al. (2018). *Towards an AI strategy: Harnessing the AI revolution*. Mexico City.
22. National Institution for Transforming India Aayog. (2018). *National strategy for artificial intelligence*. National Institution for Transforming India.
23. Strategic Council for AI Technology. (2017). *Artificial intelligence technology strategy*. Strategic Council for AI Technology.
24. Villiani, C., Bonnet, Y., Rondepierre, et al. (2018). *For a meaningful artificial intelligence: Towards a French and European strategy*. Conseil National Du Numérique.
25. Bibault, J.-E., Giraud, P., Housset, M., Durdux, C., Taieb, J., Berger, A., et al. (2018). Deep learning and radiomics predict complete response after neoadjuvant chemoradiation for locally advanced rectal cancer. *Scientific Reports, 8*(1), 12611.

26. Erlich, Y., Shor, T., Pe'er, I., & Carmi, S. (2018). Identity inference of genomic data using long-range familial searches. *Science, 362*(6415), 690–694.
27. Miller, D. D., & Brown, E. W. (2018). Artificial intelligence in medical practice: The question to the answer? *The American Journal of Medicine, 131*(2), 129–133.
28. Esteva, A., Kuprel, B., Novoa, R. A., Ko, J., Swetter, S. M., Blau, H. M., et al. (2017). Dermatologist-level classification of skin cancer with deep neural networks. *Nature, 542*(7639), 115–118.
29. Haenssle, H. A., Fink, C., Schneiderbauer, R., Toberer, F., Buhl, T., Blum, A., et al. (2018). Man against machine: Diagnostic performance of a deep learning convolutional neural network for dermoscopic melanoma recognition in comparison to 58 dermatologists. *Annals of Oncology, 29*(8), 1836–1842.
30. Berwick, D. M., Nolan, T. W., & Whittington, J. (2008). The triple aim: Care, health, and cost. *Health Affairs, 27*, 759–769.
31. Bodenheimer, T., & Sinsky, C. (2014). From triple to quadruple aim: Care of the patient requires care of the provider. *Annals of Family Medicine, 12*, 573–576.
32. Esteva, A., Robicquet, A., Ramsundar, B., Kuleshov, V., DePristo, M., Chou, K., et al. (2019). A guide to deep learning in healthcare. *Nature Medicine, 25*, 24–29.
33. McGlynn, E. A., McDonald, K. M., & Cassel, C. K. (2015). Measurement is essential for improving diagnosis and reducing diagnostic error: A report from the institute of medicine. *Journal of the American Medical Association, 314*, 2501–2502.
34. Tan, L.T., & Kong, H.Y. (2012). A novel and efficient mixed-signal compressed sensing for wide-band cognitive radio. In Proceedings of IFOST.
35. Tan, L.T., & Le, L.B. (2015). Compressed sensing based data processing and MAC protocol design for smartgrids. In Proceedings of IEEE WCNC.
36. Tan, L. T., & Le, L. B. (2016). Joint data compression and MAC protocol design for smart grids with renewable energy. *Wireless Communications and Mobile Computing, 16*(16), 2590–2604.
37. Tan, L. T., & Hu, R. Q. (2018). Mobility-aware edge caching and computing framework in vehicle networks: A deep reinforcement learning. *IEEE Transactions on Vehicular Technology, 67*(11), 10190–10203.
38. Tan, L. T., Hu, R. Q., & Hanzo, L. (2019). Twin-timescale artificial intelligence aided mobility-aware edge caching and computing in vehicular networks. *IEEE Transactions on Vehicular Technology, 68*, 3086–3099.
39. Thanh, T. L., Yun, K. H., & Quoc, B. V. N. (2010). Projected Barzilai-Borwein methods applied to distributed compressive spectrum sensing. In Proceedings of IEEE DySPAN.
40. Kakkad, V., Patel, M., & Shah, M. (2019). Biometric authentication and image encryption for image security in cloud framework. *Multiscale and Multidisciplinary Modeling, Experiments and Design, 2*, 233–248.
41. Pannu, A. (2015). Artificial intelligence and its application in different areas. *International Journal of Engineering Innovative Technology, 4*(10), 79–84.
42. Parekh, V., Shah, D., & Shah, M. (2020). Fatigue detection using artificial intelligence framework. *Augmented Human Research, 5*, 5.
43. Pang, Z., Yuan, H., Zhang, Y.-T., & Packirisamy, M. (2018). Guest editorial health engineering driven by the industry 4.0 for aging society. *IEEE Journal of Biomedical and Health Informatics, 22*(6), 1709–1710.
44. Schwab, K. (2017). *The fourth industrial revolution. First* (p. 192). Currency.
45. Metz, C., & Smith, C. S. (2019). A.I. can be a boon to medicine that could easily go rogue. The New York times. B5.
46. Kim, J. W., Jones, K. L., & Angelo, E. D. (2019). How to prepare prospective psychiatrists in the era of artificial intelligence. *Academic Psychiatry, 43*, 1–3.
47. Brinker, T. J., Hekler, A., Hauschild, A., Berking, C., Schilling, B., Enk, A. H., et al. (2019). Comparing artificial intelligence algorithms to 157 German dermatologists: The melanoma classification benchmark. *European Journal of Cancer, 111*, 30–37.

48. Hosny, A., Parmar, C., Quackenbush, J., Schwartz, L. H., & Aerts, H. J. W. L. (2018). Artificial intelligence in radiology. *Nature Reviews. Cancer, 18*(8), 500–510.
49. Sengupta, P. P., & Adjeroh, D. A. (2018). Will artificial intelligence replace the human echocardiographer? *Circulation, 138*(16), 1639–1642.
50. Vidal-Alaball, J., RoyoFibla, D., Zapata, M. A., Marin-Gomez, F. X., & Solans, F. O. (2019). Artificial intelligence for the detection of diabetic retinopathy in primary care: Protocol for algorithm development. *JMIR Research Protocols, 8*(2), e12539.
51. Beam, A. L., & Kohane, I. S. (2016). Translating artificial intelligence into clinical care. *Journal of the American Medical Association, 316*(22), 2368–2369.
52. Bishnoi, L., & Singh, N. S. (2018). Artificial intelligence techniques used in medical sciences: A review (pp. 106–113).
53. Fogel, A. L., & Kvedar, J. C. (2018). Artificial intelligence powers digital medicine. *NPJ Digital Medicine, 1*(1), 3–6.
54. Jiang, F., Jiang, Y., Zhi, H., Dong, Y., Li, H., Ma, S., et al. (2017). Artificial intelligence in healthcare: Past, present and future. *Stroke and Vascular Neurology, 2*(4), 230–243.
55. Miotto, R., Wang, F., Wang, S., Jiang, X., & Dudley, J. T. (2017). Deep learning for healthcare: Review, opportunities and challenges. *Briefings in Bioinformatics, 19*(6), 1236–1246.
56. Reddy, S., Fox, J., & Purohit, M. P. (2019). Artificial intelligence-enabled healthcare delivery. *Journal of the Royal Society of Medicine, 112*(1), 22–28.
57. Graham, S., Depp, C., Ellen, E. L., Nebeker, C., Tu, X., Kim, H. C., & Jeste, D. V. (2019). Artificial intelligence for mental health and mental illnesses: An overview. *Current Psychiatry Reports, 21*, 116.
58. Winter, J. S., & Davidson, E. (2019). Governance of artificial intelligence and personal health information. *Digital Policy, Regulation and Governance, 21*(3), 280–290.
59. Khatri, V., & Brown, C. V. (2010). Designing data governance. *Communications of the ACM, 53*(1), 148–152.
60. Perkmann, M., & Schildt, H. (2015). Open data partnerships between firms and universities: The role of boundary organizations. *Research Policy, 44*(5), 1133–1143.
61. Susha, I., Janssen, M., & Verhulst, S. (2017). Data collaboratives as 'bazaars'? A review of coordination problems and mechanisms to match demand for data with supply. *Transforming Government: People Process and Policy, 11*(1), 157–172.
62. Campbell, C. (2014). Machine learning methodology in bioinformatics. In N. Kasabov (Ed.), *Springer handbook of bio−/neuroinformatics* (pp. 185–206). Springer.
63. Gross, E. (2011). Artificial neural networks and predictive medicine: A revolutionary paradigm shift. In K. Suzuki (Ed.), *Artificial neural networks—Methodological advances and biomedical applications* (pp. 139–150). InTech.
64. Inza, I., Calvo, B., Armañanzas, R., Bengoetxea, E., Larrañaga, P., & Lozano, J. A. (2010). Machine learning: An indispensable tool in bioinformatics. *Methods in Molecular Biology, 593*, 25–48.
65. Bennett, C. C., & Hauser, K. (2013). Artificial intelligence framework for simulating clinical decision-making: A Markov decision process approach. *Artificial Intelligence in Medicine, 57*, 9–19.
66. Daoud, M., & Mayo, M. (2019). A survey of neural network-based cancer prediction models from microarray data. *Artificial Intelligence in Medicine, 97*, 204–214.
67. Delen, D., Walker, G., & Kadam, A. (2004). Predicting breast cancer survivability: A comparison of three data mining methods. *Artificial Intelligence in Medicine, 34*, 113–127.
68. Lamy, J., Sekarb, B., Guezennec, G., Bouaud, J., & Séroussia, B. (2019). Explainable artificial intelligence for breast cancer: A visual case based reasoning approach. *Artificial Intelligence in Medicine, 94*, 42–53.
69. Pereira, C. R., Pereira, D. R., Weber, S. A. T., Hook, C., de Albuquerquee, V. H. C., & Papa, J. P. (2019). A survey on computer-assisted Parkinson's disease diagnosis. *Artificial Intelligence in Medicine, 95*, 48–63.

70. Shaikhina, S., Lowe, D., Daga, S., Briggs, D., Higgins, R., & Khovanova, N. (2015). Machine learning for predictive modelling based on small data in biomedical engineering. IFAC Paper Online. 48–20. pp. 469–474.
71. Miller, D. D., Facp, C. M., & Brown, E. W. (2018). Artificial intelligence in medical practice: The question to the answer ? *The American Journal of Medicine, 131*(2), 129–133.
72. Gabbard, G. O., & Crisp-Han, H. (2017). The early career psychiatrist and the psychotherapeutic identity. *Academic Psychiatry, 41*(1), 30–34.
73. Iniesta, R., Stahl, D., & Mcguf, P. (2016). Machine learning, statistical learning and the future of biological research in psychiatry. *Psychological Medicine, 46*(May), 2455–2465.
74. Janssen, R. J., Mourão-Miranda, J., & Schnack, H. G. (2018). Making individual prognoses in psychiatry using neuroimaging and machine learning. *Biological Psychiatry: Cognitive Neuroscience and Neuroimaging, 3*(9), 798–808.
75. Luxton, D. D. (2014). Artificial intelligence in psychological practice: Current and future applications and implications. *Professional Psychology: Research and Practice, 45*(5), 332–339.
76. Mohr, D., Zhang, M., & Schueller, S. M. (2017). Personal sensing: Understanding mental health using ubiquitous sensors and machine learning. *Annual Review of Clinical Psychology, 13*, 23–47.
77. Shatte, A. B. R., Hutchinson, D. M., & Teague, S. J. (2019). Machine learning in mental health: A scoping review of methods and applications. *Psychological Medicine, 49*, 1–23.
78. Bzdok, D., & Meyer-Lindenberg, A. (2018). Machine learning for precision psychiatry: Opportunities and challenges. *Biological Psychiatry: Cognitive Neuroscience and Neuroimaging, 3*(3), 223–230.
79. Jeste, D. V., Glorioso, D., Lee, E. E., Daly, R., Graham, S., Liu, J., et al. (2019). Study of independent living residents of a continuing care senior housing community: Sociodemographic and clinical associations of cognitive, physical, and mental health. *The American Journal of Geriatric Psychiatry, 27*(9), 895–907.
80. Chatterjee, R., Maitra, T., Islam, S. H., Hassan, M. M., Alamri, A., & Fortino, G. (2019). A novel machine learning based feature selection for motor imagery EEG signal classification in internet of medical things environment. *Future Generation Computer Systems, 98*, 419–434. https://doi.org/10.1016/j.future.2019.01.048
81. Khan, S. R., Sikandar, M., Almogren, A., Din, I. U., Guerrieri, A., & Fortino, G. (2020). IoMT-based computational approach for detecting brain tumor. *Future Generation Computer Systems, 109*, 360–367. https://doi.org/10.1016/j.future.2020.03.054
82. Ismail, W. N., Hassan, M. M., Alsalamah, H. A., & Fortino, G. (2020). CNN-based health model for regular health factors analysis in internet-of-medical things environment. *IEEE Access, 8*, 52541–52549. https://doi.org/10.1109/ACCESS.2020.2980938
83. Lee, J. G., Jun, S., Cho, Y. W., et al. (2017). Deep learning in medical imaging: General overview. *Korean Journal of Radiology, 18*(4), 570–584.
84. Mahmoud, A., Bansal, M., & Sengupta, P. P. (2017). New cardiac imaging algorithms to diagnose constrictive pericarditis versus restrictive cardiomyopathy. *Current Cardiology Reports, 19*(5), 43.
85. Mayr, A., Binder, H., Gefeller, O., et al. (2014). The evolution of boosting algorithms. From machine learning to statistical modelling. *Methods of Information in Medicine, 53*(6), 419–427.
86. Meherwar Fatima, M. P. (2017). Survey of machine learning algorithms for disease diagnostic. *Journal of Intelligent Learning Systems and Applications, 9*(1), 1–16.
87. Narula, S., Shameer, K., Salem Omar, A. M., et al. (2016). Machine-learning algorithms to Automate morphological and functional assessments in 2D echocardiography. *Journal of the American College of Cardiology, 68*(21), 2287–2295.
88. Darcy, A. M., Louie, A. K., & Roberts, L. W. (2016). Machine learning and the profession of medicine. *Journal of the American Medical Association, 315*(6), 551–552.

89. Pelka, O., Nensa, F., & Friedrich, C. M. (2018). Annotation of enhanced radiographs for medical image retrieval with deep convolutional neural networks. *PLoS One, 13*(11), e0206229.
90. Gilbert, F. J., Smye, S. W., & Schonlieb, C. B. (2019). Artificial intelligence in clinical imaging: A health system approach. *Clinical Radiology, 75*(1), 3–6.
91. Huang, Z., Juarez, M. J., & Li, X. (2017). Data mining for biomedicine and healthcare. Journal of Healthcare Engineering. Article ID 7107629. 2 p.
92. Mamoshina, P., Vieira, A., Putin, E., & Zhavoronkov, A. (2016). Applications of deep learning in biomedicine. *Molecular Pharmaceutics, 13*(5), 1445–1454.
93. Seddon, G., Lounnas, V., McGuire, R., van den Bergh, T., Bywater, R. P., Oliveira, L., & Vriend, G. (2012). Drug design for ever, from hype to hope. *Journal of Computer-Aided Molecular Design, 26*(1), 137–150.
94. Zhang, Y., Zhang, G., & Shang, Q. (2017). Computer-aided clinical trial recruitment based on domain-specific language translation: a case study of retinopathy of prematurity. *Journal of Healthcare Engineering, 2017*. 9 pages.
95. Klopman, G., Chakravarti, S. K., Zhu, H., Ivanov, J. M., & Saiakhov, R. D. (2004). ESP: A method to predict toxicity and pharmacological properties of chemicals using multiple MCASE databases. *Journal of Chemical Information and Computer Sciences, 44*(2), 704–715.
96. Menden, M. P., Iorio, F., Garnett, M., McDermott, U., Benes, C. H., Ballester, P. J., & Saez-Rodriguez, J. (2013). Machine learning prediction of cancer cell sensitivity to drugs based on genomic and chemical properties. *PLoS One, 8*(4), e61318.
97. Nascimento, A. C., Prudêncio, R. B., & Costa, I. G. (2016). A multiple kernel learning algorithm for drug-target interaction prediction. *BMC Bioinformatics, 17*(1), 46.
98. Matthews, H., Hanison, J., & Nirmalan, N. (2016). "Omics"-informed drug and biomarker discovery: Opportunities, challenges and future perspectives. *Proteomes, 4*(3), 28.
99. Duch, W., Swaminathan, K., & Meller, J. (2007). Artificial intelligence approaches for rational drug design and discovery. *Current Pharmaceutical Design, 13*(14), 1497–1508.
100. Emig, D., Ivliev, A., Pustovalova, O., Lancashire, L., Bureeva, S., Nikolsky, Y., & Bessarabova, M. (2013). Drug target prediction and repositioning using an integrated network-based approach. *PLoS One, 8*(4), e60618.
101. Hughes, J. P., Rees, S., Kalindjian, S. B., & Philpott, K. L. (2011). Principles of early drug discovery. *British Journal of Pharmacology, 162*(6), 1239–1249.
102. Katsila, T., Spyroulias, G. A., Patrinos, G. P., & Matsoukas, M. T. (2016). Computational approaches in target identification and drug discovery. *Computational and Structural Biotechnology Journal, 14*, 177–184.
103. Mohs, R. C., & Greig, N. H. (2017). Drug discovery and development: Role of basic biological research. *Alzheimer's & Dementia: Translational Research & Clinical Interventions, 3*(4), 651–657.
104. Hripcsak, G., Bloomrosen, M., Flately Brennan, P., Chute, C. G., Cimino, J., Detmer, D. E., Edmunds, M., Embi, P. J., Goldstein, M. M., Hammond, W. E., Keenan, G. M., Labkoff, S., Murphy, S., Safran, C., Speedie, S., Strasberg, H., Temple, F., & Wilcox, A. B. (2014). Health data use, stewardship, and governance: Ongoing gaps and challenges: A report from AMIA's 2012 health policy meeting. *Journal of the American Medical Informatics Association: JAMIA, 21*(2), 204–211.
105. Rosenbaum, S. (2010). Data governance and stewardship: Designing data stewardship entities and advancing data access. *Health Services Research, 45*(5 pt 2), 1442–1455.
106. Blumenthal, D. (2010). Launching HITECH. *New England Journal of Medicine, 62*, 382–385.
107. Harper, E. M. (2013). The economic value of health care data. *Nursing Administration Quarterly, 37*(2), 105–108.

Chapter 6
Privacy and Security Concerns in IoT-Based Healthcare Systems

Joseph Bamidele Awotunde, Rasheed Gbenga Jimoh, Sakinat Oluwabukonla Folorunso, Emmanuel Abidemi Adeniyi, Kazeem Moses Abiodun, and Oluwatobi Oluwaseyi Banjo

6.1 Introduction

In recent years, the healthcare system and technology have been deeply entangled. As the outcome of fast-paced growth in the areas of the Internet of Things (IoT), new opportunities are now arising. Furthermore, with the adoption of wearable biosensors by the people across the globe, there are newly emerged applications for individualized telemedicine and mobile health. This new emergence of these technologies is a result of their high availability, simplicity to personalize, and easy accessibility, thus enabling the providers to deliver personalized content cost-effectively on large scale easily. Also, big data analytics and IoT are progressively gaining more attraction for the next generation of mHealth and eHealth facilities. Despite the new fields evolving rapidly, they also have their shortcomings, particularly when the goal is healthcare systems with a complicated problem, difficult in energy-efficient, safe, flexible, suitable, and consistent solutions. More especially when it comes to the issue of security and privacy of IoT generally. It has been projected that IoT will rise to a market scope of $300B by 2022 in healthcare covering the medical devices, systems, applications, and services sectors [1].

J. B. Awotunde (✉) · R. G. Jimoh
Department of Computer Science, University of Ilorin, Ilorin, Nigeria
e-mail: awotunde.jb@unilorin.edu.ng; jimoh_rasheed@unilorin.edu.ng

S. O. Folorunso · O. O. Banjo
Department of Mathematical Science, Olabisi Onabanjo University, Ago-Iwoye, Nigeria
e-mail: sakinat.folorunso@oouagoiwoye.edu.ng; banjo.tobi@oouagoiwoye.edu.ng

E. A. Adeniyi · K. M. Abiodun
Department of Computer Science, Landmark University, Omu Aran, Nigeria
e-mail: adeniyi.emmanuel@lmu.edu.ng; moses.abiodun@lmu.edu.ng

P. Siarry et al. (eds.), *The Fusion of Internet of Things, Artificial Intelligence, and Cloud Computing in Health Care*, Internet of Things,
https://doi.org/10.1007/978-3-030-75220-0_6

IoT allows a broad range of intelligent applications and resources to solve the problems facing individuals or the healthcare sector [2]. For instance, P to D (Patient-to-Doctor), P to M (Patient to Machine), S to M (Sensor to Mobile), M to H (Mobile to Human), D to M (Device to Machine), O to O (Object to Object), D to M (Doctor to Machine), and T to R (Tag to Reader) have dynamic IoT link capabilities. This brings people, computers, smart devices, and complex systems together intelligently to ensure a productive healthcare system [3, 4]. The healthcare system that depends on IoT assists the individuals and aid their vital everyday life activities. Remote patient monitoring is one such technology, common for the diagnosis, treatment, and care of patients.

These IoT devices connect to cloud infrastructures such as Google Cloud Computing, Microsoft Azure Cloud, Amazon Web Services, or any other custom web services capturing storage and analytics information. Furthermore, IoT services include remote medical observation of persons with chronic or long-term situations. These systems can monitor elderly patient treatment instructions and track the position of patients who are placed on wearable healthcare tools in hospitals and clinics. The collected health information can then be delivered to their care provider. Medical devices that can be integrated or deployed as IoT technology are infusion pumps that attach to analytical dashboards and hospital beds with sensors that measure the vital signs of patients. The IoT receives its maximum capabilities through the use of objects, i.e., "Smart" objects, which use multiple sensors and actuators fully prepared to learn in their context, and through the use of embedded communication infrastructure to communicate with any possible alternatives; it is not enough to collect a huge of data alone, and it must be turned to use materials that can help organizations to revolutionize their business processes.

While IoT has produced extraordinary prospects that aid in increasing income, decrease costs, and improve efficiencies, it is very important to put all the huge amounts of data into use. Enterprises need to build a network where a large amount of sensor data can be processed, handled, and analyzed robustly and cost-effectively way to generate benefits from IoT [5]. In this context, it is important to use a big data tool that can help ingest and read different data sources as well as facilitate the process of data integration. Integration and review of data allow businesses to revolutionize their business processes. In particular, these companies may transform a huge sum of money of sensor-collected data on valuable observation using data analytics software.

The IoT systems not only monitoring patients health status in real-time but can also be used to mining information collected from patients through IoT devices. The sensor-fitted devices are most data collection tools in the IoT setting that require data distribution service and message queue telemetry transport called custom protocols. The IoT sensors are expected to produce an immense volume of data because these devices are almost found in all fields. The data created from IoT objects can be used to investigate the impact of any events or decisions, treatment, diagnosis, prediction of any illness, and finding potential research trends. The generated data are processed using different data analytic tools [6].

In the field of healthcare, IoT devices such as satellites could have diverse applications, such as heart beat monitoring, blood sugar level monitoring, and capsule endoscopy [7]. The combination of sensors and actuators, as well as other mobile technology equipment, will transform the medical industry's functioning especially during any infectious disease outbreak [8]. Such systems, known as the Internet of Medical Things (IoMT), are a coupled structure of healthcare smart devices that receive information subsequently offered by web communications systems to healthcare IT systems [9, 10]. Currently, 3.7 million therapeutic equipment is already in practice then linked to and monitored by different portions of the body to notify medical resolutions [11].

Cloud computing enables businesses to easily handle enormous data and extract valuable data from the collected data, which are the fundamental obstacles facing big data technologies. To ensure the consistency of the software, the cloud offers enormous space for data storage and processing. However, cloud storage is impacted by the number of leaks and outflows. The structure should be built to protect data secrecy. To avoid data theft by unauthorized users, encryption methods might be more useful [12]. To make the system more autonomous and effective, the decentralized techniques should include different data and research division. This improves the precision of analysis that ensures a stable data-cloud platform. In the cloud-based world, protection is the main challenge and new technology can develop to guarantee data security and privacy in the cloud environment [13].

These IoT devices connect to cloud infrastructures such as Google Public Computing, Microsoft Azure Cloud, Amazon Web Services, or any other custom web services capturing storage and analytics information. Furthermore, IoT services include remote medical observation of persons with chronic or long-term situations. These systems can monitor elderly patient treatment instructions and track the position of patients who are placed on wearable healthcare tools in hospitals and clinics.

The use of IoT in monitoring patient healthcare using sensors and devices comes with tremendous security concerns. The recent sophisticated attacks like data integrity, data breaching, and data collusion are major safety and confidentiality concerns of IoT in IoT-based healthcare monitoring systems. During data communication of patients' health monitoring data, there are conventional solutions presented. But they are unable to deal with complex attacks at the period of data transfer and fail to fight the recent attacks on IoT-based healthcare system. The safety of data collected from IoT sensors and devices such as blood glucose, body temperature, fetal monitors, and ECG are crucial to patient's lives. Hence, it has become paramount for the IoT community, computer experts, and healthcare providers to secure each sensor/device in the IoT environment with the integrity of its data that will guarantee the device's security and privacy.

The safety and security of IoT devices are greatly affected by cyber-attacks and threats, yet the protection and comfort of the daily health of patients depend on this data gathering. Also, the privacy of patients' sensitive data can be affected. Popular forms of attacks in healthcare are ransomware, DDoS attacks, insider, email breach, and deceit scams [14]. Besides, there are other types of communication attacks such as data credibility, data breach, eavesdropping, impersonation, and conspiracy, among others. Specifically, these security and privacy of the new threats/attacks pose problems, such that the data may be breached during data communication [15], thus making patient personal data to be exposed. Similar conditions preclude the awareness of patents in the future of IoT healthcare because these issues are not treated in a timely and proper manner.

Although there are numerous security protocols, like encryption and other security implementations, MAC techniques, public-key cryptography, k-anonymity, and many more [16–20], to secure data from threats/attacks. When relating them to IoT-based health systems, they also have distinctive boundaries in terms of processor enactment, energy cost, device cost, etc. While many current works provide data privacy protection over contact to patients, when a cloud service has been agreed upon, they do not protect the data, particularly when a cloud service is under threat by an insider or service vendor. The IoT model also needs appropriate clarifications to safeguard patient information from Internet threats/strikes from sensing devices to healthcare providers. This study consequently discusses the issues of privacy and security in IoT healthcare systems and provides an overview of IoT, including its architectural design. This chapter also suggested a framework to secure healthcare information in the IoT environment.

The rest of this chapter is prearranged as follows: Section 6.2 discusses the overview of the Internet of Things. Section 6.3 presents the Internet of Things solution for the healthcare system. Section 6.4 presents the security and privacy of the Internet of Things in healthcare applications. Section 6.5 presents the architecture for the secure transmission of healthcare information in an IoT-based environment. Lastly, Section 6.6 concludes the chapter and discusses future works for the realization of efficient uses of the framework in healthcare systems.

6.2 Overview of Internet of Things

The rapid merging and technological expansions of micro-electro-mechanical digital electronics and wireless communication technologies resulted in the advent of IoT Internet of Things. The IoT has given birth to the recent growth in the number of sensors and devices connected, and an increase in the data collected from these devices is called big data. The consumption reflects how the evolution of big data naturally overlays with IoT-based devices. These give upsurge to non-trivial worries about processing data, data analysis, security, and the managing of big data in an uninterruptedly escalating system [21]. The scientists have studied the issues connected with the effective utilization of IoT to address these concerns. The convergence of these has created several opportunities despite different studies on big data, analytics, and IoT for the flourishing of big data and analytics in IoT systems [21].

The report from Cisco has it that the quantity of items coupled through the Internet has passed the number of human beings globally [22, 23]. Internet-connected gadgets that make up IoT networks include laptops, PCs, tablets,

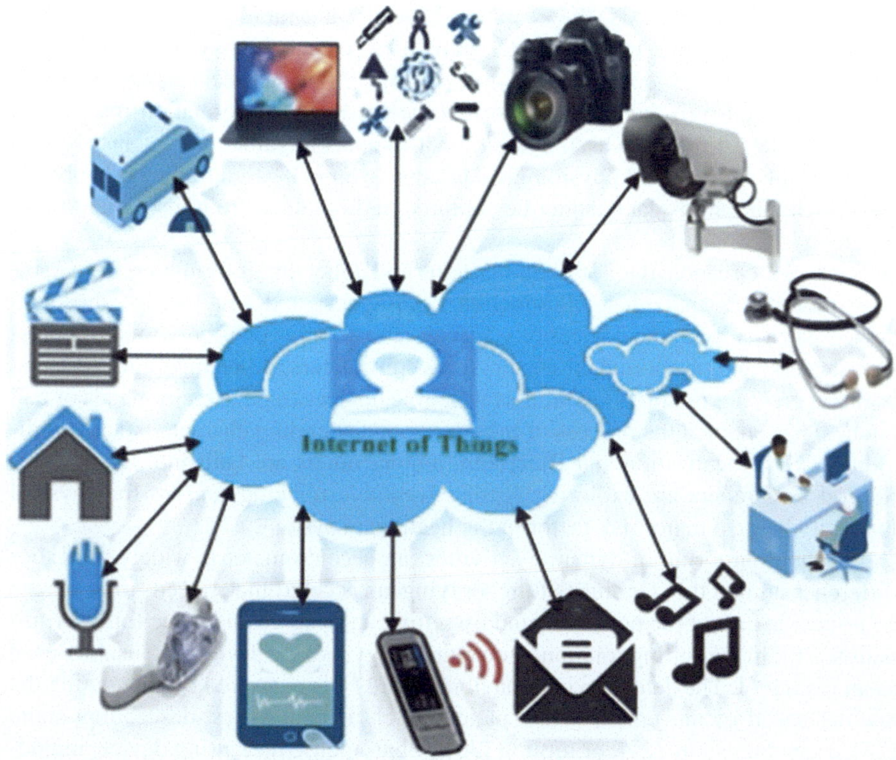

Fig. 6.1 Internet of Things with different devices

WiFi-enabled detectors, wearable devices, medical instruments, and home appliances, among others, as seen in Fig. 6.1. According to estimates, the volume of Internet-connected users is projected to increase from 22.9 billion in 2016 to 50 billion by 2020 [24].

6.2.1 The Physical Objects IoT-Based Components

The concepts of IoT include a collection of technologies that allow a broad variety of devices and objects to use networking technologies to link, communicate, and interact. The initial solution for the implementation of the IoT-based systems is the radio-frequency identification (RFID) technology. The IoT-based wearable devices have proved to be cost-effective and have been promoted in recent years in sensing technologies. The idea of customized IoT-based healthcare systems has been introduced and is becoming increasingly popular. The use of a series of interconnected devices has been used by patients to create an IoT network dedicated to healthcare evaluation in healthcare networks system. Physical artifacts (also known as physical devices): In these contexts, they capture, classify, and monitor information. This involves machines that track the vital signs of a patient (body temperature, heart rate, blood glucose, blood pressure, everyday life). Physical devices are linked to the Internet and turn the physical world's patient-related information into digital data. Physical artifacts are used in their environments to gather, track, classify, and provide data about patient physiological effects. In an IoT-based framework, objects are very important as data cannot be captured and obtained from the patient without them.

Sensors are responsible for defining items and collecting information from cameras, identifiers, and others. Production of low-cost and small-scale embedded devices such as wearable devices (e.g., accelerators, gyroscopes or barometric pressure sensors) and physiological sensors (e.g., spirometers, skin temperature sensors, or blood pressure monitors) as well as wearable devices (e.g., exercise bands or cell phones) has enabled the process of measuring and sounding characteristics of individuals. GPS localization and Bluetooth, among others are built into the devices. Several researchers are exploring regular wearable tracking sensors for physical inactivity being a major risk factor in the healthcare system.

For the monitoring of dynamic activities, an accelerometer is widely used. For difference among the standing, sitting, or lying, an accelerometer needs to be placed on a specific part of the body [25] and by setting a threshold and value for discrimination [26]. In measuring rotational movements, gyroscope devices are usually used as an extra tool. The detection of behaviors like [27], is measured by calculating the angular speed of movement of the patient, such as bent knees, descending stairs [28], ascending stairs [29], or turning [30]. A barometric measuring device, including an accelerometer, is also useful for monitoring the activity of the stairs [31] and fall detection [32]. Wearable devices are also goods for wristbands that monitor the number of steps, distance, and calories burned. Such wearable devices communicate through Bluetooth with a mobile phone using relevant mobile applications. Smartwatches and cell phones are now substitutes for traditional sensors that are portable.

6.3 Internet of Things Solutions for Healthcare Systems

Although the IoT-enabled healthcare system technologies are still at an early stage, potential industry applications are rapidly emerging and increasing. Many healthcare-enabled research projects and industrial cases relevant to IoT have been developed and deployed.

IoT-based frameworks will simplify healthcare procedures and increase the efficiency of patient care by allowing various organizations to cooperate [33]. In specific, Ambient-assisted living aims to ease the daily lives of people with disabilities and serious health conditions. Many ground-breaking services can be provided by the use of IoT in this field, such as the gathering of critical health information through a sensor network, the transfer of data to a cloud medical facility for storing and analysis, and the effective regulation of sensor data [8, 33].

A significant advantage of the IoT Healthcare system's incorporation is that it delivers low-cost and ubiquitous health services of high quality. A large quantity of sensor network information that needs to be handled for additional data processing is created by pervasive healthcare systems [34, 35]. This represents a solution for the efficient management of patient medical data collected through the sensor network and enables the abstraction of technical information, removing the need for technological infrastructure expertise [22, 24]. Besides, it results in the simple computerization of the data collection and distribution process at a cheap cost. It would also allow mobile devices suitable for entry, distribution, retrieval, and communication of health information [36].

By improving the protection of therapeutic data and the accessibility and redundancy of resources, Cloud enables this application scenario to face common challenges such as safety, secrecy, and consistency. It is essential to provide live-assisted facilities in real time due to the efficient operation of sensor data [37]. The IoT-based cloud also allows the safe execution of cloud-based multimedia-based health services, which can solve the problem of running large multimedia on some devices with limited computing and low battery capabilities. It also offers a versatile storage and management technology for streaming data generated in healthcare body sensor networks, both online and offline. The wearable monitoring systems can be implemented in a group of people due to the use of the IoT Health model and can produce vast quantities of contextual data that are collected, processed, and analyzed in a scalable manner [38, 39]. The use of IoT technology in healthcare systems has several advantages, and the resulting services can be separated into categories for monitoring individuals (e.g., patients and staff) and artifacts, patient recognition, and authentication, sensing, and automated collection of data in sensor networks.

6.3.1 Categories of IoT Applications in Healthcare Systems

Self-management services in telemonitoring and AAL settings have become a heated facial study and implementation point in recent years, designed to meet the particular demand of the patients to increase the effectiveness and performance of a treatment (e.g., adjusting the dosage of the patient). The processes offer an alternative approach to improving patients' quality of life (QoL) through contact between patients, doctors, and caregivers. These systems can deal with a range of patient situations using sensor technology, objective and subjective methods of diagnosis, care plans, and recommendations, providing patients with personalized information and guidance based on their input. When gathering and storing appropriate health data, the "Closed Loop Principle" is the practice of the service and then transmitting feedback to the patient [40].

Healthcare Monitoring System

In current wearable fitness applications, heart rate monitors, ECG monitors, glucose monitoring, pulse oximeters, and blood pressure monitors are used. Micro- and nanochemical sensors are planned to be complemented shortly to include a continuous medical diagnosis. Additional chemical signals, e.g., in air and sweat, which can be translated into medical surveillance (e.g., people with asthma, other cardiovascular conditions, skin infections, and pharmacokinetics of drugs) can be identified by these miniaturized smart sensors.

Monitoring is the environment where IoT devices and applications have been used to track patient health status and overall well-being. Examples include assisted living in the environment, active aging, therapy and entertainment, contact and social events, health status tracking, diet, and body weight. Community control, enhancing the quality of life, and encouraging living comfortably and independently are the key goals of this group of applications. Monitoring is the most common application field for many individuals and encourages healthy and independent living. It is the most common example of methods of tracking aged care [41]. It has been noticed that the elderly tended to sit at home and to accept technologies if it helps them to live independently [42]. One prominent use in this section is Ambient-Assisted Living (AAL), which is a term used to track and enable aged people to live peacefully and conveniently. AAL systems track the everyday activities of the patient to recognize abnormal circumstances and emergencies and facilitate the daily life of the patient. AAL can enhance both the patient and the caregiver's quality of life by doing so.

IoT applications for tracking and helping patients with severe disorders such as diabetes mellitus and cardiovascular diseases are included in this field. In the implementation of home-based clinical screening services for aged people with chronic conditions, these applications can be extended to disabilities who want to preserve their independent lifestyle [43]. For elderly villages or homes, this could be a perfect solution as it could support the simultaneous monitoring of many individuals [44]. It is suggested that the use of remote monitoring can not only minimize the rate of mortality and hospital referral and admittance, but also be efficient in the treatment of infectious diseases. An example of this is a smartphone program named MAHI, which can collect Bluetooth glucometer blood glucose data and post data on the web for recommendations to the caregiver [45]. Besides, once elderly mental health conditions became persistent, such as stress and anxiety, long-term data could be detected by evaluating small behavioral improvements [46].

Node Physical Characteristics

Different characteristics may be needed for the sensor and devices involved: type factor, height, weight, and energy usage; flexibility and ergonomic criteria; a degree of IP & IK protection, battery capacity; Internet access; processing and location prerequisites; multimodality and range of interaction; performance and latency limitations; self-healing and EMC criteria; and implementation cost.

Recognition of Human Activity

Human Behavior Identification (HAR) and Tracking of the everyday life of the elderly is another essential feature. The device can detect abnormal circumstances by constantly tracking the behaviors of elderly people and can decrease the effects of unexpected events such as sudden falls [47]. To avoid straying, HAR may also identify the position of the aged and the availability of communication aid. The positioning of artifacts will support the aged people to quickly locate their personal and household objects [48].

Clinical Applications

Inpatient healthcare, IoT clinical applications include disease detection and diagnostics, prediction of disease, and treatment. A more accurate diagnosis and efficient treatment of several diseases [49] can be provided by technology. The device can detect seizures and alert the patient, for example, and send warnings to caregivers [45]. Telehealth and its sub-categories, like teleconsultation and telediagnosis, give specialist consultation by communication devices to patients who are unable to come to medical centers [50].

Preventive Measures

The IoT will track and avoid the occurrence of such harmful conditions. In older patients with chronic disease, for example, the risk of contracting pressure ulcers is high, which can lead to lifelong illness, and the patients may die from ulcers [51]. The use of pressure sensors to recognize the pressure points of older patients based on different positions and to prevent the development of pressure ulcers will solve this kind of issue. Also, pressure distribution data for elderly people with chronic diseases can be used in the design of mattresses and wheelchairs [52].

Mental Health

IoT technology is used to track, anticipate, and take care of elderly patients' mental disorders [46]. It has been mentioned that by analyzing changes in everyday activities in long term surveillance, several forms of mental health disorders could be observed or even predicted. A common field in this application category is dementia. Technology is used in these systems to support people with dementia or other mental illnesses. For instance, by mitigating anxiety, promoting a positive disposition, and minimizing isolation, an intelligent robot is quite beneficial as a companion to older people with dementia [53, 54]. This lets them have a social life that is more involved.

Rehabilitation

The use of wearable devices can promote many facets of recovery facilities, such as providing input to patients and health workers, or measuring the efficacy of the rehabilitation process [55], or supporting incapacitated patients. Sharma et al. [54, 56] noted that elderly adults and stroke patients would benefit from autonomous exoskeletons of the hip joint, which can support individuals during recovery.

Accessibility to Healthcare Facilities

Mobile health innovations can be used to offer patients living in hard-to-reach areas with quicker healthcare facilities [57]. Besides, older persons can acquire a lot about health knowledge and advancement programs [58], allowing certain disease problems to be self-managed. In patients with osteoarthritis of the knee, the use of pedometer driven exercise guidance from a study in self-management was shown to be more successful than health education alone [59].

Accessibility for Caregivers

Together with smartphones, wearable technology enables healthcare professionals to provide real-time monitoring and treatment for patients remotely [45, 54]. Physicians can access the patient's health data and provide input through a web browser. To recognize emergencies such as falls, elevated heart rate, and send warnings to the caregiver as well as the emergency center, the mobile may also be programmed [45].

6.4 IoT Healthcare Protection and Privacy Technologies

The major problems facing today's healthcare systems include population aging, the prevalence of chronic illnesses, the shortage of healthcare professionals, and the unpredictable growth in healthcare costs, among other factors. Public and private sector actors should work to solve these challenges and find more innovative and accessible solutions that can be applied in out-of-hospital settings. Recent technological developments have greatly changed the understanding of an individual's conventional way of conducting day-to-day operations. In the real world, including the healthcare background, the Internet of Things has to be a rising trend in different segments. This rapid IoT revolution, however, has also generated some uncertainties and concerns about the protection of data that is stored in different connected items. If the number of items such as sensors and computers increases, it becomes more difficult to maintain robust protection and the privacy of sensitive data.

These protection and privacy problems are the product of worsening the efficacy of healthcare systems dependent on the Internet of Things (IoT) and adversely affecting the confidential health information of individuals. Since healthcare data is important and sensitive, the IoT healthcare paradigm's protection of security and privacy makes matters even more problematic. While evolving IoT paradigms in the medical system contributes significantly to the advancement of current healthcare systems, end-users need to address many privacy and security concerns. When they grant authorization for potentially insecure or leaky third-party applications, end-users may be susceptible to malicious threats. Since the data are transmitted to the cloud, it moves through unsafe communication networks, many of which have security issues. Besides, when the data project into the cloud storage facility of the owner, there are alternate data breach issues.

To enhance the comfort of patients concerning the protection and secrecy dangers they pose to the lives of patients and other effects, such as privacy breaches and financial threats, safe and protected IoT healthcare applications are needed. Through reviewing the components of the technology platform in-depth, this chapter focuses on privacy and security challenges in IoT healthcare systems.

Remote patient management processes and warning systems are assisted by health care providers and applications. Data are the most valuable asset of these applications as knowledge obtained through these processes is known to be vulnerable [60, 61].

Besides, it is important to ensure the confidentiality and availability of such data. Sensitive data should be protected, as should protect against unlawful entry, other challenges, and risks. Conversely, due to the amount of data provided by the wearable sensors and the constant interaction between the devices in the system [60], these are difficult areas in the IoT ecosystem. Healthcare practitioners and software developers have worked together in recent years to create stable IoT healthcare applications to solve these problems [61].

Also, the inherent difficulties impede the services offered by IoT technology. The problems often prevent patients from implementing smart healthcare systems, taking into account the problems posed by privacy and security issues [62]. In a device concerned with confidential data, trust is also a crucial factor. Therefore, it would increase the performance of the programs and loyalty between clients by creating a layout that addresses the entire threat landscape. As a result, IoT healthcare will encourage more individuals to benefit from it [60].

6.4.1 Security Concern in IoT Healthcare Applications

In a wide variation of healthcare applications, the IoT plays an important role, from chronic disease treatment at one end of the continuum to disease prevention at the other end. This involves gathering physiological data using sensors, analyzing and archiving the information using gateway devices and the cloud, and then wirelessly sending the scrutinized data to healthcare authorities for additional study and evaluation [63]. Not only can these applications enhance access to treatment while increasing the quality of care, but they will also decrease the cost of care. Publishing new technology without considering protection in healthcare applications leaves patient privacy vulnerable; a person's physiological data are highly sensitive.

Modern healthcare would need ubiquitous health tracking with the least real contact between doctors and patients, which can be accomplished by the IoT definition. Wearable, implantable, or wearable wireless medical sensors can be combined with different forms of wireless communication motes (such as Mica2, MicaZ, Telos, etc.) [64]. Such wireless medical sensors have gathered/generated large quantities of information that must be protected from security attacks. When transmitting to remote locations, we can escape several malicious data attacks by implementing protection algorithms/techniques [65]. Security is also a primary prerequisite for healthcare applications. For ethical and legal purposes, the effectiveness of healthcare applications depends primarily on patient protection and privacy [63, 65].

However, in terms of information safety and confidentiality, the sum of related gadgets and the huge sum of impressionable datasets gathered by those gadgets have brought novel challenges. Cyber-attacks have also changed along with the rapid development of IoT and had created a recent avenue of invasion and risk to the whole medical industry. Many studies explored IoT's numerous privacy and protection issues and device weaknesses in cloud and fog computing settings relevant to IoT-based medical management gadgets [66, 67] and [66] analyzed the IoMT protection and confidentiality taxonomy in detail.

The safety and confidentiality of records relating to patients are twofold essential notions. When we refer to record safety, this signifies that records are securely stowed and transmitted to ensure their absoluteness, genuineness, and legitimacy. Record confidentiality signifies that records can solitary be obtained by individuals who are authorized to sight and utilized it [68, 69]. More rational security measures may be established with different objectives and specifications in mind. The extensive utilization of IoT gadgets offers an improved assurance of an individual's health [70], but it also places a great deal of demand on record safety and concealment.

Consequently, efficacious IoT advancement needs to accept safety and confidentiality as an essential concentration. Although most healthcare establishments don't devote sufficient funds to shield safety and confidentiality [68], there isn't any hesitation that safety and confidentiality perform a significant function in IoT. IoT gadgets create a growing amount of ever more complex real-time records, which is extremely delicate. On one side, the failure of health organization or system security may have catastrophic consequences. On the other hand, privacy information for the patient is accessible at all levels of record processing, record transfer, cloud storage, and record republication.

Since IoT gadgets don't possess enough reminiscence, computation, and information transmission abilities, they need an efficient, accessible high-performance computation and a large storage system for real-time computation and record stowage. Several IoT organizations currently deposit the health records collected and extend their application servers into the cloud. The apps will get their medical activities uploaded into the cloud appropriately. Cloud facilities enable a hopeful clarification for the effectual administration of ubiquitous medical records through their resistance and capacity to obtain public resources and mutual infrastructure in a pervasive and universal manner.

The diversity of IoT components makes the security concerns of IoT applications more complex for users. Thus, it is the main concern for the production of these IoT applications to recognize and deal with these security problems. Confidentiality, integrity, and availability (CIA) can be summarized as the minimum security criteria for the applications.

Security Issues for Communication Technologies

Security risks and connectivity technologies problems in IoT-based healthcare networks come in several forms. For instance, the activation of DoS/DDoS attacks, comprising of flood attacks, black hole attacks, and home attacks, is a safety problem for these technologies [4]. These systems are also susceptible to secure coupling, interface, usability, power usage, and exploration mode switching on/off, leveraging main ex-change function, baritone loss, identity fraud, monitoring, surveillance, suspicious activities, and linkage interference [71]. Intrusion 27 to track suspicious activations, identity-based authentication, anti-jamming, and packet filtering to block unauthorized users from accessing are the security strategies that should be implemented in this community. The encryption of all wireless traffic often guarantees that the data transmitted through wireless networks are confidential. Also, to prevent the alteration of communications, strong authentication is necessary.

Trusted Third-Party Auditing

The information from sensors may somehow be skewed at sources though appear right during transmission, or intentionally changed by malware by an unauthorized user in the IoT system through the Internet. These distorted data could then be used to make decisions on life and death. Hence, trusting the data provided to us may be questionable, and the issue is yet to be handle properly. Compassionate therapy is linked to another form of trust. Caring is about the relationship between the patient, their families and community, nurses, and other health providers, one that is being forged. Compassionate care for the sick is a duty for all healthcare providers, but kindness depends on trust.

Nursing, for instance, has been ranked as the most truthful, ethical career for the 14th straight year [72]. This high rating was based on a relationship with patients and the public that starts with confidence and a personal connection. Besides, technology has helped to transform health care by enabling better diagnosis, surveillance, and treatment. Nurses must incorporate technologies at many levels with the implementation of IoT in healthcare and decide about the right use for their practice and how to use technology to achieve better patient outcomes. The same would have to be done by other healthcare practitioners.

Cloud servers aren't completely reliable. Where data manipulation, as well as erasure, occurs lacking consumer authorization, the quality and accuracy of healthcare records deposited in the cloud may be in jeopardy. The data standards are usually particularized by the consumer for security reasons so that the server supplier isn't in an undeviating connection with the record basis. Furthermore, the reputable trusted third party (TTP), which delivers the impartial audit outcomes, could be properly presented to allow cloud service providers to be accountable and to shield the authentic advantages of cloud operators [68]. Trusted third party inspects to enhance security in cloud storage. The TTP's work a wireless transmission issues consist of complex audits, batch auditing, and performance measurement auditing.

Data Anonymization

Clinician-delicate information can be divided into three categories: specific identifiers, quasi-identifiers, and privacy attributes. An explicit identification, such as an ID number, name, and mobile phone number, may be used to identify a patient distinctly. An amalgamation of quasi-identifiers may also provide a specific indication of a patient, such as age, birth information, and address. Privacy information ascribes to a patient's delicate characteristics, which includes sickness and profits. While considering the allocation features of the earliest data in the procedure of data publication, it's crucial to guarantee that the personal characteristics of the novel dataset are accurately treated to assure the confidentiality of the patient.

Currently, haphazardperturbation expertise and anonymous data technology are typically utilized to resolve such issues as k-anonymity, l-diversity, and confidence bounding. The conventional k-anonymity is particularly extensively utilized. The disadvantage, however, is that it doesn't restrict delicate records, and invaders may utilize steadiness invasion and contextual information invasion to recognize delicate information and individual communication, resulting in privacy loss [68].

Security and privacy for IoT devices remain huge issues that bring a whole new degree of user privacy concerns online. This is because such apps can only collect personal information, such as the names of users and telephone numbers, but cannot also track user behaviors (e.g., when users are in their homes and what they had at lunchtime). It is therefore very important to build an IoT based on security and privacy to ensure trust and privacy for users during the use of IoT.

Security Issues for Application

Several organizations have widely accepted IoT and big data analytics. These pieces of machinery are, however, yet in their first phases. It has not yet tackled several current work challenges. Big data analysis is a crucial dispute for several utilizations owing to the nature of data and the scalability of fundamental procedures that support these methods [73, 74]. This segment thus poses some difficulties in the big data analytics focused on IoT.

Data security concerns occur where a network is corrupted by the utilization of big data analytics techniques to infer or reestablish individual information, while data are created by anonymous users. The confidentiality matter has to turn out to be a central concern in the data mining province with the advent of big data analytics tools employed in IoT. Consequently, most consumers are hesitant to rely on such networks, which do not have firm terms of service-level agreement (SLA) concerning abuse or misuse of personal information by customers. Users' sensitive information must be undisclosed and safeguarded from outside intrusion.

Although provisional identity, concealment, and encryption offer numerous means to implement data protection, ethical considerations, for instance, what to employ, how to utilize, and why employ engendered big data in IoT, must be determined [75]. Alternative safety jeopardy connected with IoT data is the variety of system kinds employed and the complexity of data produced, for instance, fresh computers, data formats, and procedures for communication. These systems are intended to interact with supportive utilization and can have various extents and forms external to the system. Therefore, to authenticate these devices, each unit should be issued by an IoT system with a non-repudiable identification scheme. Besides, organizations will sustain a meta-archive of these related tools for analyzing consideration. This composite architecture of IoT is innovative to safekeeping experts, resulting in elevated security risks. Any intrusion in this case thus violates network stability and disconnects interconnected equipment.

Security and privacy are crucial problems in the collection and storing of vast volumes of data in the setting of IoT-based Big Data Analytics. Similarly, these schemes depend seriously on third party facilities and infrastructure to conduct critical processes and host secluded data. Therefore, unprecedented growth in data volume causes difficulties in obtaining every single part of vital data. There are no long-standing security mechanisms that provide full security in IoT-based Big Data scenarios [76–78]. Current algorithms are not meant for complex data interpretation and are thus not implemented effectually. Legacy data protection approaches are primarily designed for static datasets, while the actual data specifications dynamically alter [76, 79, 80]. Therefore, it is difficult to deploy these safety resolutions for energetically cumulative data.

Data Search

Sensitivedata must be scrambled before contracting out to preserve data confidentiality, which obsolescence the current use of data built on readable keyword searches. Allowing an encoded record pursuit service in the cloud is thus of utmost significance. The main approaches for searchable encryption comprise searchable symmetric encryption (SSE) and keyword search public-key encryption (PEKS). It should also be remembered that the further sophisticated the encryption methods, the easier it is to scan the data, and the easier it is to verify the accuracy of the search results. If the results of the search cannot be enforced appropriately, then all protection and privacy safeguards have less value [68].

Access Control

Access control is the way an information scheme determines an individual's uniqueness and predefined rules that prohibit unauthorized individuals from retrieving resources [68]. Access control involves various encryption methods, such as private key encryption (PKE), public-key encryption (PKE), and attribute-based encryption (ABE) [68].

Security Issues for Physical Objects

Physical entity vulnerability concerns include

Physical attacks: The majority of IoT computers, such as constrained utility nodes, are small and wirelessly connected. Thus, it is essential to protect confidential data held in IoT devices and provide IoT-related safe storage resources. There seems to be an elevated risk of threats since more data are believed to be in flow than in traditional architectures and unintended access to data transmitted [81, 82]. On the other hand, the edge technology layer can be defined as an intermediate layer that each has its safety specifications [83].

IntegratingRFIDinto IoT: In IoT applications for users, RFID technology has been used for identifying, tracking, and tracing disabled users. However, because of resource limitations, RFID systems are vulnerable to being targeted. The RFID system, virtualization system, and the Internet are the three basic components of the IoT-based RFID systems [84]. Numerous securities refer to modules such as eavesdropping, middle attack, denial of service, spoofing, copying, monitoring, tag misuse, and wireless connectivity threats. [85]. That's why we ought to secure and restrict access to RFID tag information. To avoid peer-to-peer eavesdropping [86]. As RFID technology does not involve a line of sight, if it is not encoded, unauthorized RFID readers can obtain the data. In addition, by using elliptic curve cryptography [87], authentication in IoT applications based on RFID is enhanced.

IntegratingWSNsinto IoT: There are minimal computing and energy resources in those technologies. They are operated by batteries, and via lossy connections, they are linked. They are still fragile enough to be targeted by any rival. An intruder can install malicious nodes that can operate together to inflict harm to the system. Another problem is how a sensor node and an Internet host can protect the channel [88]. WSNs have been used for healthcare in many delicate IoT systems, so if WSNs protection is attacked, it can result in human harm and loss of resources [89]. Therefore, such security requirements for WSNs must be taken into accounts, such as the encryption and measurement for data confidentiality and integrity of the Message Authentication Code (MAC), security protocols for a safe location, and accessibility.

Denial of Service (DoS) attacks: DoS attacks on IoT systems are the most common and simplest attacks to introduce. They can be seen in many ways and are defined as an attack that can compromise the ability of the network or systems to perform anticipated functions. The IoT has been widely criticized since its conception for the lack of attention given to safety concerns in the design and implementation of its hardware, software, and infrastructure components. This negligent approach has led to numerous vulnerabilities that have already been successfully exploited by hackers and cybercriminals to compromise IoT elements so that they can be misused for different purposes, including the staging of Denial of Service and DoS threats [90]. DoS attacks and DoS (DDoS) sharing allow network facilities/data inaccessible for users. When DoS attacks have been compromised by various nodes, it is known as a DDoS attack. Despite their often sophisticated and commercially appealing exterior design, many IoT devices are built from cheap generic hardware components. These chips and firmware usually contain security vulnerabilities that are essentially built-in and thus difficult for owners and operators to track. Also, the infrastructure and coordination of firmware and software updates for the wireless problem are still at a primitive level. So, it is also hard to update or repair these unsecured IoT computers.

6.4.2 Privacy Issues in IoT Healthcare Applications

The most critical problem is data privacy in the IoT. The patient's body carries the sensors used in the IoT. These sensors are sensed by all significant information about the patient. So, sensitive information of the patient should not be leaked to the external world. The sensor nodes in IoT-based healthcare applications collect the patient's sensitive data and forward it to a coordinator node. If the sensitive information is overheard by an attacker and the data are used for any illicit reason, then the patient may be seriously harmed. It is not enough to only protect secrecy [91]. Data should also be safe from outside modifications. In this case, if a patient's sensitive and essential data have been corrupted, this changed data will be transmitted to the coordinator. For life-critical patients, this lack of honesty results in serious harm. Data loss can also occur in poor communication environments. In terms of performance and security, the implementation of emerging technology poses many challenges, and thus, applications for the IoT must be secured. It can have deadly consequences to reveal any part of an IoT healthcare system to a hacker, whether a terrorist, disgruntled individual, blackmailer, or any other malicious actor. Many researchers are fully working on the issue of protecting IoT systems, but since no system can be 100 percent safe, it is important to identify and measure appropriate risk by ethicists and medical, legal, security, and financial professionals.

Risk of Patients Privacy Exposure

Health information (HI) is a broad term that includes both safe health information (PHI), which includes unique identifiers that can be uniquely connected to the patient, and not easily identifiable de-identified health information (DHI) [92]. It is necessary to clarify here that DHI is not necessarily anonymous data; in fact, data can vary from completely anonymous to fully identifiable, varying according to the degree to which identity is retained, masked, or eliminated, depending on the effort, capacity, time, and cost needed for full identification [93].

In the data, a minimum degree of identification is also required so that health researchers can aggregate datasets or perform efficiency or policy analysis for greater social benefits. HIPAA's Privacy Rule offers detailed guidance for alternative methods of de-identification [94] to establish this safety level of identifiability, thus minimizing privacy risks for patients and allowing secure data sharing practices. Therefore, data processed for de-identification using the above methods, i.e., DHI, are considered safer to share than PHI. Vendors and product manufacturers who have collaborated with healthcare service providers are also subject to HIPAA regulations as protected organizations (CEs) or business associates (BAs), as mentioned earlier. Non-partnered persons are not subject to HIPAA legislation and are deemed to be non-covered organizations (NCEs).

Data Encryption

Universal dataencryption could be executed at three communication phases: connection encoding, node encoding, and end-to-end encoding. The communication acquired from the earlier connection will be decoded into a readable form for any transitional node in associated encryption, and the readable text will thereafter be encoded into scrambled text by utilizing the undisclosed key of the following connection [68, 91]. Unlike liaison encryption, node encryption doesn't require plaintext communications in the system node. So, node encryption can deliver huge network data protection. When utilizing end-to-end encryption, the message is not decrypted until it is forwarded to the destination. Since communications are continually existing as scrambled text all through to protect eHealth public services, vital organization procedures execute a significant function in the protection method. Nevertheless, the communication frequency could be greatly altered by intricate encryption systems or transmission protocols, and also fail to perform data transmission. They must use important medical services that are not accessible. Scientific and cautious steps are needed to solve the hard equilibrium between safety, protection, and system application consumption [68, 91]. Protection matters have been key impediments to eHealth systems that deliver unremarkable assistance to the aging and weak individuals owing to the inadequate funds obtainable and confidentiality apprehensions.

Data Eavesdropping and Data Confidentiality

It is a form of threat that brings security threats to the protection of the medical records of patients. This involves the sniffing of vital medical information conveyed by the IoT sensor/device resulting in privacy risks in communication. Assume that unsecured medical data were distributed by an IoT sensor/device to adjacent or upstream nodes. By using a sniffing software tool, an intruder will eavesdrop on the health information by sniffing it. To collect the health data of the patients, any unauthorized person can use a powerful transmitted signal like a sniffer. In general, the patient's medical records are maintained in compliance with legal confidentiality obligations and are given access only to licensed caregivers. It is necessary to prevent intercepted storage or spying data as it flows through wireless connections [90].

Identity Threats and Privacy of Stored Data

The following guidelines should be considered to protect the privacy of information storage. Only the least possible amount of information that is required should be retained. In the event of compulsory retention, only personal information is preserved, and the based on "need-to-know" knowledge is taken out. Pseudonymization and anonymization may be used to hide the real identity connected to the stored data. A database could allow access only to statistical data (sum, average, count, etc.) without revealing any particular record. The appropriate technique could be to ensure that the output (typically aggregate queries) is independent of the absence or presence of a specific record, adding noise called differential privacy [95].

Threats of Cyber-Attacks on Privacy

Attacks are actions taken using different techniques and methods to damage a device or interrupt regular operations by leveraging vulnerabilities. Attackers initiate assaults, for either personal satisfaction or compensation, to achieve goals. Cyber-attacks will inject false information into a system, which causes IoT applications to suffer critical harm. In smart healthcare applications, it is important to provide the patient with the required degree of defense from cyber threats. The resource constrained existence of many IoT devices present in a smart home environment does not, however, allow standard security solutions to be implemented. Due to rising threats and government regulations, cyber protection systems that protect networks and computers from cyber-attacks are becoming widespread. At the same time, the vast volume of information collected by cyber security systems poses a significant threat to the privacy of those who are secured by them.

Location Privacy

Location privacy is concerned with threats to the privacy of locations and eavesdropping on the location of a device. By routing to a randomly chosen intermediate node (RRIN), location privacy in WSNs, precisely hiding the location of the message sender, can be accomplished [96]. The Location Privacy Routing (LPR) protocol, which uniformly distributes the directions of incoming and outgoing traffic at sensor nodes, will prevent packet dropping and tracing [97]. Phantom single-path routing ensures that packets follow different paths to the Base Station (BS) in such a way that each packet generated by a source follows a different random path to the BS [98].

6.5 Framework for Secure Transmission of Healthcare Information on IoT-Based Platform

The IoT provides computing tools as extremely flexible as web services. With the rapid growth of IoT and cloud computing technology, a growing number of individuals, organizations, and businesses prefer IoT and cloud platforms for storing and manipulating their data. Cloud computing has major benefits including cloud storage, connectivity, data sharing, and hardware and software cost savings. Many security challenges attributed to the IoT environment, however, have not yet been addressed, especially in traditional computer environments [66, 67]. Moreover, protection and privacy concerns have been observed to seriously limit the practical implementations of IoT technologies [66]. To tackle these major problems, it is important to propose and develop new algorithms and methods to secure the IoT platform and infrastructure.

The safety and confidentiality of records relating to patients are twofold essential notions. When we refer to record safety, this signifies that records are securely stowed and transmitted to ensure their absoluteness, genuineness, and legitimacy. Record confidentiality signifies that records can solitary be obtained by individuals who are authorized to sight and utilized it [68, 69]. More rational security measures may be established with different objectives and specifications in mind. The extensive utilization of IoT gadgets offers an improved assurance of an individual's health [70], but it also places a great deal of demand on record safety and concealment.

Consequently, efficacious IoT advancement needs to accept safety and confidentiality as an essential concentration. Although most healthcare establishments don't devote sufficient funds to shield safety and confidentiality [68, 99], there isn't any hesitation that safety and confidentiality perform a significant function in IoT. IoT gadgets create a growing amount of ever more complex real-time records, which is extremely delicate. On one side, the failure of health organization or system security may have catastrophic consequences. On the other hand, privacy information for the patient is accessible at all levels of record processing, record transfer, cloud storage, and record republication.

In this section, this chapter suggested an enhanced novel method built on an amalgamation of security procedures in each layer to hide the undisclosed message into a cover object to deliver satisfactory fortification for the concealed message transmission utilizing a standard IoT transmission channel. This approach will positively achieve the targeted standard of certain critical characteristics such as information confidentiality, efficiency and sturdiness, proof of the outstanding performance, and efficient application of this method. The primary goal of protection can be reached in the field of data transmission through the IoT-based system.

The secure transmission of medical information on the IoT environment was displayed in Fig. 6.2. The framework comprises certification manager, information manager, personal medical information encryption, security access control, and medical data confidentiality for the smart healthcare system. The framework consists of a service provider who updates healthcare data locally and transmits it through certification manager smart healthcare (medical institution). The authentication institution is called a healthcare certification manager, and they are in charge of key creation, management, and distribution including the role of intermediate for information and endorsement. The information manager in smart healthcare responsible for verification establishment that encrypts provides personal and medical information for storing data in the cloud database. The main function of the layer is for the independence of data provided by medical institutions to separate the function of smart healthcare information manager block. The layer also performing the encryption and authentication of the data, which in turn provides information decryption.

6.6 The Results and Discussion

The functions of the layers in the proposed framework are discussed in this section: the framework will be able to secure the medical information on the IoT-based platform.

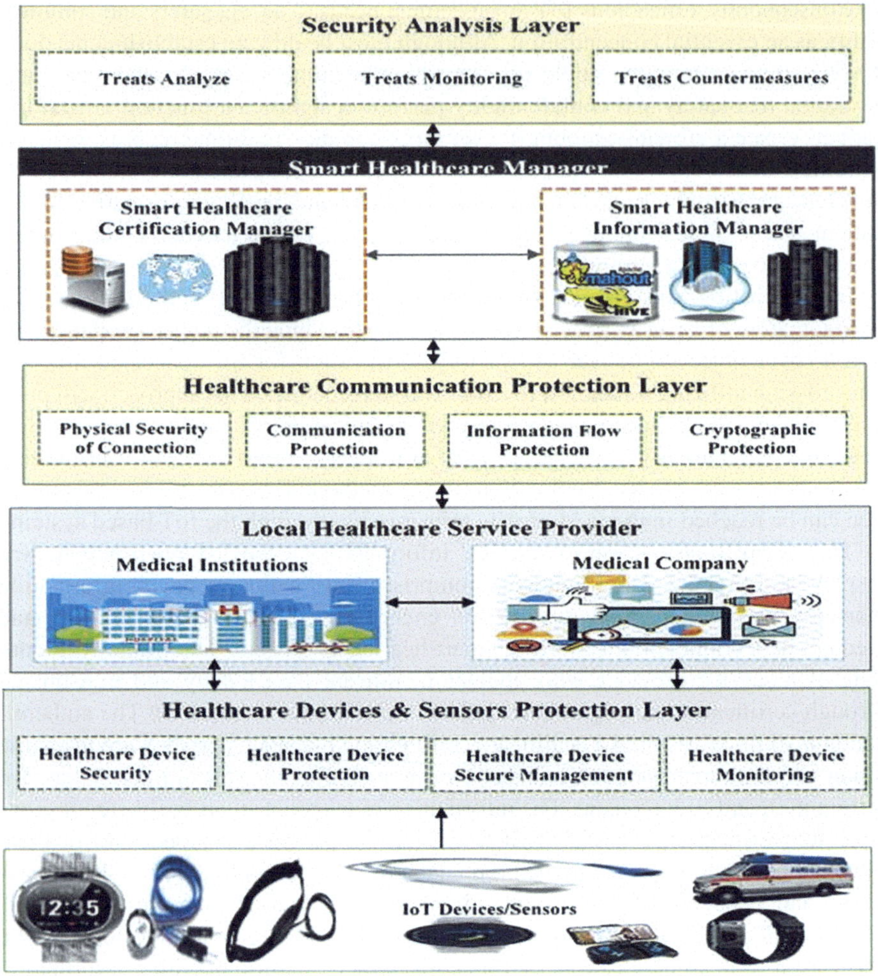

Fig. 6.2 The framework of a secure medical information on IoT-based environment

6.6.1 *Healthcare Device Protection Layer*

The protection layer employed anti-theft and intrusion mechanisms to prevent alteration and removal of the terminal. The confidentiality, integrity, and availability are maintained in this layer, by seeing to the functionality of the smart devices. This security was able to prevent the uncontrollable alteration of an attached device from the IoT platform by providing physical protection function using the provided techniques. The device monitoring scrutinized the process and the status of the terminal, error detection using equivalent data, and established countermeasures. Integrity review, malicious usage pattern identification, service denial operations are tracked and scrutinized to trace its security routine directory. The terminal integrity was protected by the device protection by ensuring that the terminal is working under the settings required to perform within specified utilities. For the integrity of the terminal functions, the boot phase of the terminal and the execution of the terminal operation is tested.

6.6.2 *Healthcare Communication Protection Layer*

Information exchange between terminals of the IoT-based system was supported by the communication protection layer. This was made possible with the communication feature that provides interoperability between different devices. As threats to such information sharing, the degree of security needed for the communication role of IoT services needs to be prepared. Link physical protection covers the layers of physical links (e.g., cables) in the network. Security functions like encryption are given by the communication security block between terminals. Most IoT apps analyze features, including authentication and encryption, and use standardization protocols that have been reviewed. To secure the reliability of the communication, encryption technology with the integrity and confidentiality of communication records is used on the communication organizations. The destination device and network are transferred by the information flow protection block on the message types and content permitted using network integration and borderline fortification tools. All components of the network are being managed by the network management block monitor updates and maintain entirely communication protection policies, including network breakdown, password protected communication settings, and configuration of the firewall.

6.6.3 *Security Analysis Layer*

The layer analyzed data collected from the overall status data from terminals in addition to the network traffic to identify responses to security breaks or coercions to the system. This was done to identify in real-time some attack circumstances to device trends and set up countermeasures against such situations. This can be done using the intrusion activity pattern with an access control strategy from the gathered protection status data from the IoT-based environment. The analysis feature looks for events or patterns that may cause a particular device to have security vulnerabilities or threats. Malicious conduct analysis and rule-based analysis are performed at this level. The malicious behavior analysis discovers abnormal activities by scrutinizing usage trends in the system after studying normal activities. The events that do not occur in a normal system were analyzed using rule-based and, according to the established rules, define security threats. In the case of a security incident, it analyzes intrusion actions and suggests countermeasures. Before a security attack happens, this feature prepares for security incidents by security policies. The identification and recovery of threats work to detect an existing safety incident and to restore the damage to normal status. In the event of an attack or security incident, the security forensics feature examines basic vulnerabilities and abuse cases.

The communication layer with numerous radar gadgets and items which can be linked over a radio receiver link supports information exchange between terminals. This radio receiver link could be separate from WiFi, ultra-wideband, RFID, ZigBee, and Bluetooth. The IoT gateway tolerates cyberspace and numerous networks to connect. The upper level is about big data analytics, where vast volumes of data obtained from radars are processed in the cloud and accessible by big data analytics apps. These frameworks provide API monitoring and a dashboard to aid in managing engine communication.

6.7 Conclusion

The integration of computer and biomedical technologies in medical systems has supported healthcare events, for instance, real-time disease analysis, remote monitoring of patients, and real-time drug prescriptions, among others. The methods have significantly helped to store both patients' personal information and their symptoms on the cloud, which can help during contagious diseases. This aids the quality of services provided by the physicians, thereby improving patients' satisfaction. But there are still security and privacy challenges face by IoT-based healthcare system, and many users are not ready to use the IoT-based platform. Therefore, this chapter presents a summary of the IoT-based architecture by discussing the privacy and security issues in IoT healthcare applications. This chapter also proposed a framework to secure healthcare information on the IoT-based platform. This chapter also demonstrates the architecture of the extensive healthcare system based on IoT, the technological problems, and some standard implementations relevant to comprehensive healthcare. Data safety, privacy, and confidentiality were looked into IoT-based security and privacy in healthcare systems. The proposed architecture has four layers; this was proposed in other to fully secure the IoT environments at all levels of the healthcare system. To provide verification, entry control, network, and device protection, integrity, and confidentiality, the framework model uses the features of the IoT environment. To eliminate all security threats in advance may be very difficult due to the use of diverse devices and technological rudiments of sensors used in healthcare systems, the security specifications suggested in this study are intended to contribute to the creation of secure IoT environments. This chapter concluded that the current framework will go a long way to help in protecting the sensors and devices use in the IoT-based environment at a different level of the system. The full implementation of the proposed scheme will be tested in future work.

References

1. Firouzi, F., Rahmani, A. M., Mankodiya, K., Badaroglu, M., Merrett, G. V., Wong, P., & Farahani, B. (2018). Internet-of-things and big data for smarter healthcare: From device to architecture, applications, and analytics.
2. Medaglia, C. M., & Serbanati, A. (2010). An overview of privacy and security issues on the internet of things. In *The internet of things* (pp. 389–395). Springer.
3. Yang, P., Wu, W., Moniri, M., & Chibelushi, C. C. (2012). Efficient object localization using sparsely distributed passive RFID tags. *IEEE Transactions on Industrial Electronics, 60*(12), 5914–5924.
4. Adeniyi, E. A., Ogundokun, R. O., & Awotunde, J. B. (2021). IoMT-based wearable body sensors network healthcare monitoring system. In *IoT in healthcare and ambient assisted living* (pp. 103–121). Springer.
5. Riggins, F. J., & Wamba, S. F. (2015, January). Research directions on the adoption, usage, and impact of the internet of things through the use of big data analytics. In 2015 48th Hawaii international conference on system sciences (pp. 1531–1540). IEEE.
6. Yaqoob, I., Hashem, I. A. T., Gani, A., Mokhtar, S., Ahmed, E., Anuar, N. B., & Vasilakos, A. V. (2016). Big data: From beginning to the future. *International Journal of Information Management, 36*(6), 1231–1247.
7. Pramanik, P. K. D., Upadhyaya, B. K., Pal, S., & Pal, T. (2019). Internet of things, smart sensors, and pervasive systems: Enabling connected and pervasive healthcare. In *Healthcare data analytics and management* (pp. 1–58). Academic.
8. Darwish, A., Ismail Sayed, G., & Ella Hassanien, A. (2019). The impact of implantable sensors in biomedical technology on the future of healthcare systems. Intelligent pervasive computing systems for smarter healthcare (pp. 67–89).
9. Joyia, G. J., Liaqat, R. M., Farooq, A., & Rehman, S. (2017). Internet of medical things (IOMT): Applications, benefits, and future challenges in the healthcare domain. *The Journal of Communication, 12*(4), 240–247.
10. Manogaran, G., Chilamkurti, N., & Hsu, C. H. (2018). Emerging trends, issues, and challenges on the internet of medical things and wireless networks. *Personal and Ubiquitous Computing, 22*(5–6), 879–882.
11. Qadri, Y. A., Nauman, A., Zikria, Y. B., Vasilakos, A. V., & Kim, S. W. (2020). The future of healthcare internet of things: A survey of emerging technologies. *IEEE Communications Surveys and Tutorials, 22*(2), 1121–1167.
12. Akhtar, P., Khan, Z., Rao-Nicholson, R., & Zhang, M. (2019). Building relationship innovation in global collaborative partnerships: Big data analytics and traditional organizational powers. *R&D Management, 49*(1), 7–20.
13. Chan, M. M., Plata, R. B., Medina, J. A., Alario-Hoyos, C., Rizzardini, R. H., & de la Roca, M. (2018). Analysis of behavioral intention to use cloudbased tools in a MOOC: A technology acceptance model approach. *Journal of Universal Computer Science, 24*(8), 1072–1089.
14. Zhang, P., Zhou, M., & Fortino, G. (2018). Security and trust issues in fog computing: A survey. *Future Generation Computer Systems, 88*, 16–27.
15. Karati, A., Islam, S. H., Biswas, G. P., Bhuiyan, M. Z. A., Vijayakumar, P., & Karuppiah, M. (2017). Provably secure identity-based signcryption scheme for the crowdsourced industrial internet of things environments. *IEEE Internet of Things Journal, 5*(4), 2904–2914.
16. Solomon, M., & Elias, E. P. (2018). Privacy protection for wireless medical sensor data. *International Journal of Scientific Research in Science and Technology, 4*, 1439–1440.
17. Frustaci, M., Pace, P., Aloi, G., & Fortino, G. (2017). Evaluating critical security issues of the IoT world: Present and future challenges. *IEEE Internet of Things Journal, 5*(4), 2483–2495.
18. Shen, J., Gui, Z., Ji, S., Shen, J., Tan, H., & Tang, Y. (2018). Cloud-aided lightweight certificates authentication protocol with anonymity for wireless body area networks. *Journal of Network and Computer Applications, 106*, 117–123.

19. Roy, S., Chatterjee, S., Das, A. K., Chattopadhyay, S., Kumari, S., & Jo, M. (2017). Chaotic map-based anonymous user authentication scheme with user biometrics and fuzzy extractor for crowdsourcing internet of things. *IEEE Internet of Things Journal, 5*(4), 2884–2895.
20. Luo, E., Liu, Q., & Wang, G. (2016). Hierarchical multi-authority and attribute-based encryption friend discovery scheme in mobile social networks. *IEEE Communications Letters, 20*(9), 1772–1775.
21. ur Rehman, M. H., Yaqoob, I., Salah, K., Imran, M., Jayaraman, P. P., & Perera, C. (2019). The role of big data analytics in industrial internet of things. *Future Generation Computer Systems, 99*, 247–259.
22. Pace, P., Aloi, G., Gravina, R., Caliciuri, G., Fortino, G., & Liotta, A. (2018). An edge-based architecture to support efficient applications for healthcare industry 4.0. *IEEE Transactions on Industrial Informatics, 15*(1), 481–489.
23. Ahmed, E., Yaqoob, I., Gani, A., Imran, M., & Guizani, M. (2016). Internet-of-things-based smart environments: State of the art, taxonomy, and open research challenges. *IEEE Wireless Communications, 23*(5), 10–16.
24. Pace, P., Aloi, G., Caliciuri, G., Gravina, R., Savaglio, C., Fortino, G., … & Mortara, M. (2019, April). Inter-health: An interoperable IoT solution for active and assisted living healthcare services. In 2019 IEEE 5th world forum on internet of things (WF-IoT) (pp. 81–86). IEEE.
25. Veltink, P. H., Bussmann, H. J., De Vries, W., Martens, W. J., & Van Lummel, R. C. (1996). Detection of static and dynamic activities using uniaxial accelerometers. *IEEE Transactions on Rehabilitation Engineering, 4*(4), 375–385.
26. Lyons, G. M., Culhane, K. M., Hilton, D., Grace, P. A., & Lyons, D. (2005). A description of an accelerometer-based mobility monitoring technique. *Medical Engineering & Physics, 27*(6), 497–504.
27. Luštrek, M., & Kaluža, B. (2009). Fall detection and activity recognition with machine learning. *Informatica, 33*(2).
28. Pappas, I. P., Popovic, M. R., Keller, T., Dietz, V., & Morari, M. (2001). A reliable gait phase-detection system. *IEEE Transactions on Neural Systems and Rehabilitation Engineering, 9*(2), 113–125.
29. Paganelli, F., & Giuli, D. (2007, May). An ontology-based context model for home health monitoring and alerting in chronic patient care networks. In 21st international conference on advanced information networking and applications workshops (AINAW'07) (Vol. 2, pp. 838–845). IEEE.
30. Salarian, A., Russmann, H., Wider, C., Burkhard, P. R., Vingerhoets, F. J., & Aminian, K. (2007). Quantification of tremor and bradykinesia in Parkinson's disease using a novel ambulatory monitoring system. *IEEE Transactions on Biomedical Engineering, 54*(2), 313–322.
31. Moncada-Torres, A., Leuenberger, K., Gonzenbach, R., Luft, A., & Gassert, R. (2014). Activity classification is based on inertial and barometric pressure sensors at different anatomical locations. *Physiological Measurement, 35*(7), 1245.
32. Bianchi, F., Redmond, S. J., Narayanan, M. R., Cerutti, S., & Lovell, N. H. (2010). Barometric pressure and triaxial accelerometry-based fall event detection. *IEEE Transactions on Neural Systems and Rehabilitation Engineering, 18*(6), 619–627.
33. Darwish, A., Hassanien, A. E., Elhoseny, M., Sangaiah, A. K., & Muhammad, K. (2019). The impact of the hybrid platform of the internet of things and cloud computing on healthcare systems: Opportunities, challenges, and open problems. *Journal of Ambient Intelligence and Humanized Computing, 10*(10), 4151–4166.
34. Mukherjee, P., & Mukherjee, A. (2019). Advanced processing techniques and secure architecture for sensor networks in ubiquitous healthcare systems. In *Sensors for health monitoring* (pp. 3–29). Academic.
35. Ismail, W. N., Hassan, M. M., Alsalamah, H. A., & Fortino, G. (2020). CNN-based health model for regular health factors analysis in internet-of-medical things environment. *IEEE Access, 8*, 52541–52549.

36. Wang, N., Deng, Z., Wen, L. M., Ding, Y., & He, G. (2019). Understanding the use of smartphone apps for health information among pregnant Chinese women: Mixed methods study. *JMIR mHealth and uHealth, 7*(6), e12631.
37. Le Kernec, J., Fioranelli, F., Ding, C., Zhao, H., Sun, L., Hong, H., ... Romain, O. (2019). Radar signal processing for sensing in assisted living: The challenges associated with the real-time implementation of emerging algorithms. *IEEE Signal Processing Magazine, 36*(4), 29–41.
38. Farahani, B., Firouzi, F., & Chakrabarty, K. (2020). Healthcare IoT. In *Intelligent internet of things* (pp. 515–545). Springer.
39. Padmavathi, S. (2020). A fog-based approach for real-time analytics of IoT-enabled healthcare. In *The internet of things use cases for the healthcare industry* (pp. 43–66). Springer.
40. Dohr, A., Modre-Opsrian, R., Drobics, M., Hayn, D., & Schreier, G. (2010, April). The internet of things for ambient assisted living. In 2010 seventh international conference on information technology: new generations (pp. 804–809). IEEE.
41. Brownsell, S., & Hawley, M. (2004). Fall detectors: Do they work or reduce the fear of falling? *Housing, Care, and Support, 7*(1), 18.
42. Wagner, F., Basran, J., & Dal Bello-Haas, V. (2012). A review of monitoring technology for use with older adults. *Journal of Geriatric Physical Therapy, 35*(1), 28–34.
43. Nguyen, H. H., Mirza, F., Naeem, M. A., & Nguyen, M. (2017, April). A review of IoT healthcare monitoring applications and a vision for transforming sensor data into real-time clinical feedback. In 2017 IEEE 21st international conference on computer supported cooperative work in design (CSCWD) (pp. 257–262). IEEE.
44. Kalid, N., Zaidan, A. A., Zaidan, B. B., Salman, O. H., Hashim, M., & Muzammil, H. (2018). Based on real-time remote health monitoring systems: A review on patients' prioritization and related "big data" using body sensors information and communication technology. *Journal of Medical Systems, 42*(2), 30.
45. Ayo, F. E., Ogundokun, R. O., Awotunde, J. B., Adebiyi, M. O., & Adeniyi, A. E. (2020, July). Severe acne skin disease: A fuzzy-based method for diagnosis. Lecture notes in computer science (including subseries Lecture Notes in Artificial Intelligence and Lecture Notes in Bioinformatics), 2020, 12254 LNCS (pp. 320–334).
46. Azimi, I., Rahmani, A. M., Liljeberg, P., & Tenhunen, H. (2017). Internet of things for remote elderly monitoring: A study from a user-centered perspective. *Journal of Ambient Intelligence and Humanized Computing, 8*(2), 273–289.
47. Fortino, G., Gravina, R., & Galzarano, S. (2018). *Wearable computing: From modeling to implementation of wearable systems based on body sensor networks*. John Wiley & Sons.
48. Zheng, M., Liu, P. X., Gravina, R., & Fortino, G. (2018). An emerging wearable world: New gadgetry produces a rising tide of changes and challenges. *IEEE Systems, Man, and Cybernetics Magazine, 4*(4), 6–14.
49. Fortino, G., Giannantonio, R., Gravina, R., Kuryloski, P., & Jafari, R. (2012). Enabling effective programming and flexible management of efficient body sensor network applications. *IEEE Transactions on Human Machine Systems, 43*(1), 115–133.
50. Fortino, G., Guerrieri, A., Bellifemine, F., & Giannantonio, R. (2009, October). Platform-independent development of collaborative wireless body sensor network applications: SPINE2. In 2009 IEEE international conference on systems, man and cybernetics (pp. 3144–3150). IEEE.
51. Lee, S. Y., Chou, C. L., Hsu, S. P., Shih, C. C., Yeh, C. C., Hung, C. J., ... Liao, C. C. (2016). Outcomes after stroke in patients with previous pressure ulcer: A Nationwide matched retrospective cohort study. *Journal of Stroke and Cerebrovascular Diseases, 25*(1), 220–227.
52. Jaul, E., & Menzel, J. (2014). Pressure ulcers in the elderly, as a public health problem. *Journal of General Practice, 2*, 5.
53. Pal, D., Triyason, T., & Funikul, S. (2017, December). Smart homes and quality of life for the elderly: A systematic review. In 2017 IEEE international symposium on multimedia (ISM) (pp. 413–419). IEEE.
54. Tun, S. Y. Y., Madanian, S., & Mirza, F. (2020). Internet of things (IoT) applications for elderly care: A reflective review. *Aging Clinical and Experimental Research*, 1–13.

55. Shany, T., Redmond, S. J., Marschollek, M., & Lovell, N. H. (2012). Assessing fall risk using wearable sensors: A practical discussion. *Zeitschrift für Gerontologie und Geriatrie, 45*(8), 694–706.
56. Sharma, C. A., Kumar, A. K. S. V., Prasad, A., Begum, R., Sharvani, G. S., & Manjunath, A. E. (2018, January). Multifaceted bio-medical applications of exoskeleton: A review. In 2018 2nd international conference on inventive systems and control (ICISC) (pp. 11–15). IEEE.
57. Oladele, T. O., Ogundokun, R. O., Awotunde, J. B., Adebiyi, M. O., & Adeniyi, J. K. (2020, July). Diagmal: A malaria coactive neuro-fuzzy expert system. Lecture notes in computer science (including subseries lecture notes in artificial intelligence and lecture notes in bioinformatics), 2020, 12254 LNCS (pp. 428–441).
58. Yein, N., & Pal, S. (2017, January). Technological assistance for falls among the aging population: A review. In *International conference on research into design* (pp. 409–419). Springer.
59. De Bruin, E. D., Hartmann, A., Uebelhart, D., Murer, K., & Zijlstra, W. (2008). Wearable systems for monitoring mobility-related activities in older people: A systematic review. *Clinical Rehabilitation, 22*(10–11), 878–895.
60. Amaraweera, S. P., & Halgamuge, M. N. (2019). Internet of things in the healthcare sector: Overview of security and privacy issues. In *Security, privacy, and trust in the IoT environment* (pp. 153–179). Springer.
61. Tao, H., Bhuiyan, M. Z. A., Abdalla, A. N., Hassan, M. M., Zain, J. M., & Hayajneh, T. (2018). Secured data collection with hardware-based ciphers for IoT-based healthcare. *IEEE Internet of Things Journal, 6*(1), 410–420.
62. Uddin, M. A., Stranieri, A., Gondal, I., & Balasubramanian, V. (2018). Continuous patient monitoring with a patient-centric agent: A block architecture. *IEEE Access, 6*, 32700–32726.
63. Vermesan, O., & Friess, P. (Eds.). (2014). *Internet of things-from research and innovation to market deployment* (Vol. 29). River Publishers.
64. Malan, D. J., Fulford-Jones, T., Welsh, M., & Moulton, S. (2004). Codeblue: An ad hoc sensor network infrastructure for emergency medical care. In International workshop on wearable and implantable body sensor networks.
65. Kumar, P., & Lee, H. J. (2012). Security issues in healthcare applications using wireless medical sensor networks: A survey. *Sensors, 12*(1), 55–91.
66. Abdulraheem, M., Awotunde J. B., Jimoh, R. G., & Oladipo, I. D. (2021). An efficient lightweight crypotographic Algorithm for IoT security. *Communication in Computer and Information Science, 1350*, 444–456.
67. Mutlag, A. A., Ghani, M. K. A., Arunkumar, N. A., Mohammed, M. A., & Mohd, O. (2019). Enabling technologies for fog computing in healthcare IoT systems. *Future Generation Computer Systems, 90*, 62–78.
68. Sun, W., Cai, Z., Li, Y., Liu, F., Fang, S., & Wang, G. (2018). Security and privacy in the medical internet of things: A review. *Security and Communication Networks, 2018*.
69. Tang, J., Liu, A., Zhao, M., & Wang, T. (2018). An aggregate signature based trust routing for data gathering in sensor networks. *Security and Communication Networks, 2018*.
70. Sun, W., Cai, Z., Liu, F., Fang, S., & Wang, G. (2017, October). A survey of data mining technology on electronic medical records. In 2017 IEEE 19th international conference on e-health networking, applications and services (Healthcom) (pp. 1–6). IEEE.
71. Thomas, C. (2020). Introductory chapter: Computer security threats. In *Computer security threats*. IntechOpen.
72. Jones, J. C. (2016). Nurses rank as most honest, ethical profession for 14th straight year.
73. Burhan, M., Rehman, R. A., Khan, B., & Kim, B. S. (2018). IoT elements, layered architectures, and security issues: A comprehensive survey. *Sensors, 18*(9), 2796.
74. Alassaf, N., Gutub, A., Parah, S. A., & Al Ghamdi, M. (2019). Enhancing speed of SIMON: A light-weight-cryptographic algorithm for IoT applications. *Multimedia Tools and Applications, 78*(23), 32633–32657.
75. Tsai, C. W., Lai, C. F., Chao, H. C., & Vasilakos, A. V. (2015). Big data analytics: A survey. *Journal of Big Data, 2*(1), 1–32.

76. Marjani, M., Nasaruddin, F., Gani, A., Karim, A., Hashem, I. A. T., Siddiqa, A., & Yaqoob, I. (2017). Big IoT data analytics: Architecture, opportunities, and open research challenges. *IEEE Access, 5*, 5247–5261.
77. Fortino, G., Guerrieri, A., Bellifemine, F. L., & Giannantonio, R. (2009, July). SPINE2: Developing BSN applications on heterogeneous sensor nodes. In 2009 IEEE international symposium on industrial embedded systems (pp. 128–131). IEEE.
78. Iyengar, S., Bonda, F. T., Gravina, R., Guerrieri, A., Fortino, G., & Sangiovanni-Vincentelli, A. (2008, March). A framework for creating healthcare monitoring applications using wireless body sensor networks. In proceedings of the ICST 3rd international conference on body area networks (pp. 1–2).
79. Fortino, G., Galzarano, S., Gravina, R., & Li, W. (2015). A framework for collaborative computing and multi-sensor data fusion in body sensor networks. *Information Fusion, 22*, 50–70.
80. Aloi, G., Caliciuri, G., Fortino, G., Gravina, R., Pace, P., Russo, W., & Savaglio, C. (2016, April). A mobile multi-technology gateway to enable IoT interoperability. In 2016 IEEE first international conference on internet-of things design and implementation (IoTDI) (pp. 259–264). IEEE.
81. Dedeoglu, V., Jurdak, R., Dorri, A., Lunardi, R. C., Michelin, R. A., Zorzo, A. F., & Kanhere, S. S. (2020). Blockchain technologies for IoT. In *Advanced applications of blockchain technology* (pp. 55–89). Springer.
82. Suresh, A., Nandagopal, M., Raj, P., Neeba, E. A., & Lin, J. W. (2020). *Industrial IoT application architectures and use cases*. CRC Press.
83. Glaroudis, D., Iossifides, A., & Chatzimisios, P. (2020). The survey, comparison, and research challenges of IoT application protocols for smart farming. *Computer Networks, 168*, 107037.
84. Nie, X., & Zhong, X. (2013, March). Security in the internet of things based on RFID: Issues and current countermeasures. In *Proceedings of the 2nd international conference on computer science and electronics engineering*. Atlantis Press.
85. Fathy, M., Samouti, S. A., Samouti, A., & Senior, I. T. (2016). NFC threats and attacks: Applying a low cost algorithm for secure channel using Twofish. *Bulletin de la Société Royale des Sciences de Liège, 85*, 1475–1486.
86. Sfar, A. R., Natalizio, E., Challal, Y., & Chtourou, Z. (2018). A roadmap for security challenges in the internet of things. *Digital Communications and Networks, 4*(2), 118–137.
87. Bayat, M., Beheshti-Atashgah, M., Barari, M., & Aref, M. R. (2019). Cryptanalysis and improvement of a user authentication scheme for the internet of things using elliptic curve cryptography. *IJ Network Security, 21*(6), 897–911.
88. Puthal, D., Yang, L. T., Dustdar, S., Wen, Z., Jun, S., Moorsel, A. V., & Ranjan, R. (2020). A user-centric security solution for the internet of things and edge convergence. *ACM Transactions on Cyber-Physical Systems, 4*(3), 1–19.
89. Anand, S., & Sharma, A. (2020). Assessment of security threats on IoT based applications. *Materials Today: Proceedings*.
90. Ayo, F. E., Folorunso, S. O., Abayomi-Alli, A. A., Adekunle, A. O., & Awotunde, J. B. (2020). Network intrusion detection is based on deep learning model optimized with rule-based hybrid feature selection. *Information Security Journal: A Global Perspective, 29*, 1–17.
91. Abikoye, O. C., Ojo, U. A., Awotunde, J. B., & Ogundokun, R. O. (2020). A safe and secured iris template using steganography and cryptography. *Multimedia Tools and Applications, 79*(31–32), 23483–23506.
92. Banerjee, S., Hemphill, T., & Longstreet, P. (2018). Wearable devices and healthcare: Data sharing and privacy. *The Information Society, 34*(1), 49–57.
93. Nelson, G. S. (2015). Practical implications of sharing data: A primer on data privacy, anonymization, and de-identification. In SAS global forum proceedings (pp. 1–23).
94. Portability, I. (2012). Guidance regarding methods for de-identification of protected health information in accordance with the health insurance portability and accountability act (HIPAA) privacy rule.

95. Hall, R., Rinaldo, A., & Wasserman, L. (2013). Differential privacy for functions and functional data. *Journal of Machine Learning Research, 14*(Feb), 703–727.
96. Gupta, S., Kumar, P., Singh, J. P., & Singh, M. P. (2016). Privacy preservation of source location using phantom nodes. In *Information technology: New generations* (pp. 247–256). Springer.
97. Yao, L., Kang, L., Shang, P., & Wu, G. (2013). Protecting the sink location privacy in wireless sensor networks. *Personal and Ubiquitous Computing, 17*(5), 883–893.
98. Manjula, R., & Datta, R. (2018). A novel source location privacy preservation technique to achieve enhanced privacy and network lifetime in WSNs. *Pervasive and Mobile Computing, 44*, 58–73.
99. Huang, M., Liu, A., Wang, T., & Huang, C. (2018). Green data gathering under delay differentiated services constraint for the internet of things. *Wireless Communications and Mobile Computing, 2018*.

Chapter 7
IoT Healthcare Applications

Sunitha Lingam

Abbreviations

CGM	Continuous glucose monitoring
CYCORE	Cyber infrastructure for comparative effectiveness research
ADAMM	Automated device for *asthma monitoring*
GPS	Global positioning system
IoT	Internet of Things
PPG	Photoplethysmography
QR	Quick response

7.1 What Is the IoT Healthcare System?

IoT stands for Internet of Things. Simply put, it can connect numerous devices to send data to each other through the internet. These devices are usually embedded with various technologies, sensors or related software. The significant advantage is that the devices work without human intervention. The tools can learn through the data collected under data analytics.

IoT has found its application [1] in multiple fields in recent times; healthcare is just one of them. In the upcoming times, IoT will continue to be implemented within healthcare and is guaranteed to increase productivity and data analysis drastically. These technological advancements will enhance medical devices [2] and produce better outcomes and improved analytics, which is likely to be accomplished promptly.

Quite often, cloud technology is coupled closely with IoT technology because both require internet access. Examples of this are our smartphones and smartwatches. Our smartphones can connect to our home security systems, cars and

S. Lingam (✉)
Department of CSE, Koneru Lakshmaiah Education Foundation, Deemed to be University, Hyderabad, India

P. Siarry et al. (eds.), *The Fusion of Internet of Things, Artificial Intelligence, and Cloud Computing in Health Care*, Internet of Things,
https://doi.org/10.1007/978-3-030-75220-0_7

kitchen appliances. Through the concept of IoT, imagine preparing a meal from your phone while driving home from work.

The healthcare-specific IoT produces a massive amount of data generated by these connected devices which hold the potential to transform healthcare. Hospital staff are overwhelmed with patient monitoring devices: pulse oximeters, CPAPs, ventilators, infusion pumps, ECG machines and the list goes on. Combining patient data from the various machines can provide a much more rich and accurate story about the patient's condition. IoT connectivity can centralize this data; it can be analysed and communicated to all healthcare [3] providers through smart technology.

There are many medicines for various health problems and conditions common man is hardly aware of in the market. Many pharmaceutical industries are working to produce genuine drugs. IoT can be beneficial in this regard. QR code or IoT infrastructures can help individuals to assess how good their medicines are. One can know about the manufacturer and become knowledgeable on how legitimate their purchases are.

IoT is a four-step process.

- IoT System Construction is an interconnected device consisting of sensors, actuators, detectors, monitors and camera devices to collect the data next.
- Data collected from sensors [4] and other technologies within these devices are in analogue form. These signals are integrated and converted to the digital format for pre-processing.
- Once the data are pre-processed, it is aggregated and standardized. These data are then transferred to the data centre or cloud.
- Finally, data are managed and analysed at the required level. Advanced analytics is applied to these data for effective decision-making.

These stages are interconnected since the yield of processing one step is the input for the following steps.

IoT also helps track the real-time location of various hospital equipment such as oxygen cylinders, wheelchairs and nebulizers. These devices are tracked with sensors embedded within, which help in tracking their location. Medical staff working from various geographical regions can be tracked in real time (Fig. 7.1).

Many healthcare specialized companies are moving towards investing in IoT intensively. Currently, be it X-ray machines or biosensors there in connectivity in most tech devices with Bluetooth or WiFi. When medical devices enabled with IoT, assist the jobs performed by health practitioners by providing them with critical data. This inclusion of IoT im-proves outcomes of healthcare facilities and reduces the burden of health practitioners. It becomes easier to monitor patients and make observations on the progress of a treatment or even housing vaccines with devices with IoT specialized in medicine [5].

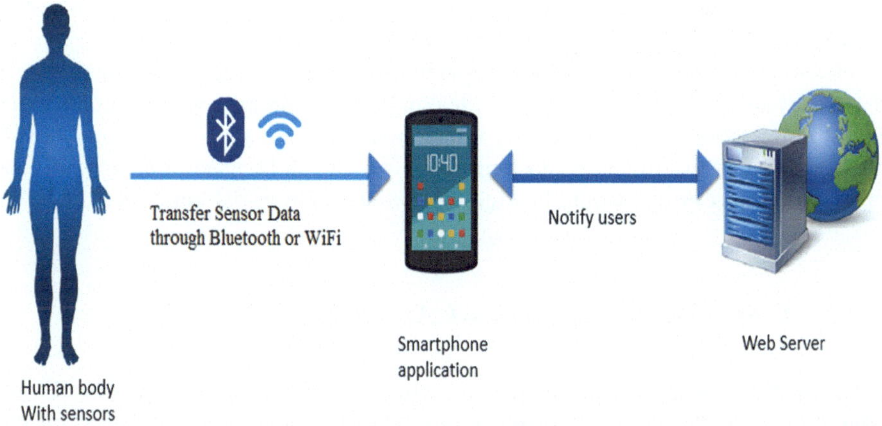

Fig. 7.1 IoT architecture

7.2 Cloud-Based IoT Healthcare Applications

Cloud-based IoT guarantees distributed-location-based services. The platform can be used to periodically collect and broadcast data. IoT is widely applied in various fields, such as the medical healthcare system. On the other hand, cloud computing offers on-demand computing resources as a service from mobile devices to supercomputers. Cloud computing is a method for large data storage and analytics. The combination of IoT and cloud computing will enable monitoring services and processing of sensory datasets.

The cloud eventually serves as the brain to improved decision-making and optimized Internet-based interactions.

Cloud computing paradigm is one of the trending topics in the recent year information technology field. It has mobility, security, efficiency, reliability and scalability advantages. Users are provided with storage, applications, services, servers, hardware and networks, which are the most demanded resources. For IoT systems, cloud computing serves as a backbone, according to researchers. Sharing of information amongst patients, caretakers, and professionals is more organized and structured with cloud computing. Cloud secures the medical records and reduces risks of these getting lost. As a result, healthcare services and applications have benefited from developing IoT and cloud computing technologies.

Authorized users can access important information for treating patients and research purpose. This integration would make information exchange simpler and cheaper between practitioners or even hospitals.

Let us understand in brief with the example of a Smart Fridge which addresses vaccine management issues. Weka developed it to deal with vaccine storage which is done at an apt temperature. Errors can lead to spoilage of vaccine. With Smart Fridge, vaccines can be monitored and stored at the recommended temperature, from remote locations. Inventory management services are automated, which makes it easier for clinicians to stay updated regarding vaccine storage.

Health practitioners can log in and specify the vaccine needed. The Smart Fridge then gives access to the vial requested leaving the remaining inventory unaffected. Smart Fridge eliminates unnecessary interaction work that needs to be done. It also allows us to analyse the data and find trends which can be used to design vaccine programs. Smart Fridge would be highly beneficial in high-risk rural areas.

7.2.1 Cloud-Based IoT Network Architecture

IoT stronglyassociated with cloud computing, a cloud used as front end. Cloud computing provides several advantages to IoT. Cloud computing is based on the concept of allowing users to perform regular computing tasks using services delivered entirely on the internet.

Cloud-based IoT [6] has bestowed us with data collection and broadcasting services. Despite being geographically separated, the cloud has helped to access these facilities periodically. While combining IoT and Cloud, healthcare practitioners must understand how these facilities are exceptional and useful. Memory and space requirements can be minimized if an application [7] is hosted on the Internet (Fig. 7.2).

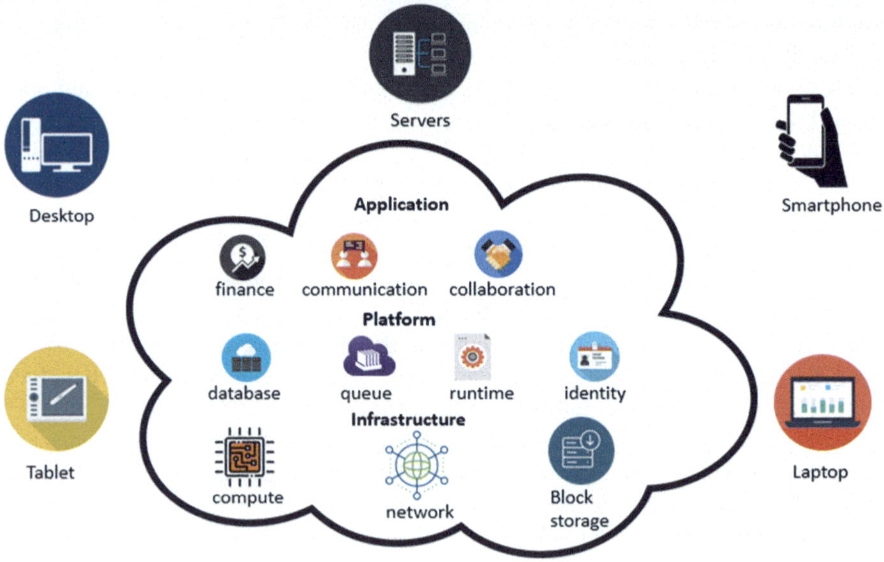

Fig. 7.2 Cloud computing

7.3 Opportunities in IoT Healthcare

Before introducing IoT into healthcare, doctors or health workers couldn't interact with patients and monitor their health conditions regularly. Treatment was discrete. With IoT, these communications are made easy and possible. The scenarios of huge hospital stay and getting admitted have reduced guaranteeing customer satisfaction.

Better outcomes are expected at much lower costs. It has always been observed that the introduction of technology with innovative strategies has benefitted business models. With improved customer engagement, asset management, cost reduction, reduction in theft possibility and customer engagement, IoT has proved beneficial for businesses and marketing in the current times.

IoT, machine learning, block-chain technologies and big data analytics, are expected to be the future trend. With IoT devices get smarter.

7.3.1 Functional Fields

Technical developers work with Arduino or raspberry pi modules, net-work connections and cable connections. Having accurate and precise sensors is very important to produce correct and reliable results. Specialists in sensor technology and integration would have to work on improving their working. Communication between various devices facilitates that data are transmitted from one location to others, storing or retrieving. It is essential to have fast communication networks [8] with a good number of participants.

The application used should be updated and maintained regularly considering the evolution of system hardware and system software. Software Development Engineers, therefore, are pivotal for handling the application. Cloud design and management are planning for efficient usage of resources. Cloud architecture [9] needs to be understood at various levels of comprehension.

Data collected from various devices and various individuals after being stored are analysed to find patterns. Data analysts have a very crucial role to play when it comes to handling big data and exploiting it in cost-efficient ways. Processing extensive data with a minimal amount of hardware is an economical idea. By making predictions using various algorithms, IoT devices can help determine conditions deviated from the normal situation. They can prove to be very valuable in life-threatening situations.

7.3.2 *Non-functional Attributes*

Apart from functional features, non-functional attributes are also of utmost importance. Non-functional attributes include security, reliability, privacy, scalability, adaptability and portability. These are even more crucial as failing to meet any one of them can prove dangerous and fatal.

It becomes necessary to maintain confidentiality of information such as patient details, diagnosis information, treatment procedure or any other confidential information. Not everyone can access all or part of the information. Authentication stages need to be defined. Cyber security experts need to work on the protection of information stored. Transfer of data needs to be secure. Block-chain can be an apt solution for the same considering that the current and previous systems are vulnerable.

7.4 IoT Solutions for the Disabled in Healthcare

Around 650 million people in this world are disabled. IoT can ease the lives of these people and make them more independent.

7.4.1 *Smart Homes*

Oneapproach can be to automate their homes. The idea of smart homes enhances the quality of living of the specially abled people. Features of their residence can be specialized for the individual's care. Various tasks can be performed by connecting devices such as speakers, oven, television, air conditioners and other electrical appliances. This would be of exceptional help to individuals with mobility impairments. Voice assistants such as Siri, Google and Alexa can also be used for controlling the house. Voice commands can be used to lock and open the doors, turn lights on and off and even adjust the thermostat. Smart lights can be used to alert deaf individuals when there are visitors at the door.

The various components of smart homes are given as follows:

- Sensors: Sensors are installed within the house to collect internal data to analyse conditions at home. They are attached to various devices, and finally, the data collected are transmitted to the IoT server with the help of a local network.
- Processors: IoT server after receiving the data processes it. There are various software designed appropriately to translate the data collected by sensors to perform necessary actions.
- Actuators: These are the components which would control the working mechanism and movement of a device or machine. The commands sent by the server are executed by performing needed action.

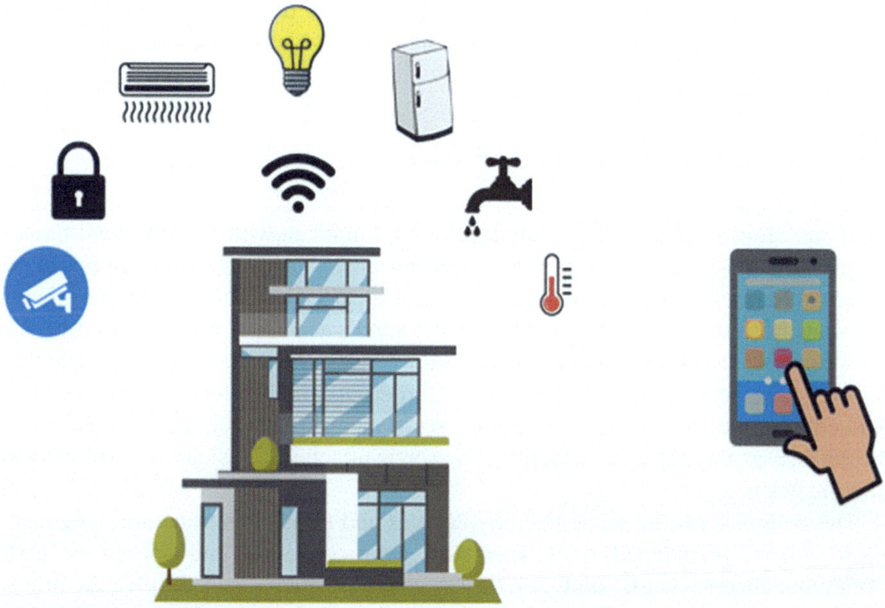

Fig. 7.3 Smart homes

- Smartphone App: The conditions can be handled with the help of an android app. Various devices or electronic devices can be controlled by a fixed schedule or by this app.
- Cloud: The data collected from sensors stored in a database over the cloud. The collected data could be analysed and made use of in future.

As we observe, the necessary steps, as in Sect. 7.1, are very similar to the four stages in smart homes (Fig. 7.3).

7.4.2 Travelling Made Easy

A few more ideas can ensure safety outside their homes.

There is a Crosswalk IoT system in Dutch. Sensors are embedded in traffic lights and streetlights. There is an android application that connects various individuals and tracks their geographical location. The app tracks down if any specially abled individuals or older adults are waiting at the pavement to cross the road. The traffic lights remain red and allow pedestrians movement for a more extended period to safely cross the street.

Cloud Vision API is made available to developers by Google to creating apps which can be used to design IoT devices for visually impaired people using image recognition algorithms. The device captures the surroundings with the camera and uses this to identify objects, landmarks or places. The device can work like smart glasses where the user is to told what is around through a hearing unit.

7.4.3 Communication Made Easier

Deaf and blind people use sign language to communicate with various hand movements. This language has its grammar. Special gloves enabled with sensors can be designed to track hand motion and record it as electrical signals. An accelerometer is one such sensor that can be used to find the hand's acceleration by considering the x,y,z coordinates and the change in the position due to motion or vibration. The flex sensor is another sensor that can be used to measure the bending or the amount of deflection of the gloves. The flex sensor's resistance varies when there is bending in the surface of the object to which the sensor is attached. This can be exploited to find the gesture.

These signals can be recognized by devices and translate into natural language. Each gesture is mapped to a word and then converted into speech or text. Communication at work, study, or to use voice assistants gets simpler. At times, devices or appliances can be handled by gestures. Gadgets can be controlled with hand movement without any human intervention.

A Bluetooth module can be used to transmit the signals data to a target device where the output in the form of text or speech can be given. If it's text, then text-to-speech conversion software can be used to translate the data into audio finally.

Since gloves are lightweight, they can be carried easily even while travelling. This would bridge the communication gap between specially abled people with the traditional world (Fig. 7.4).

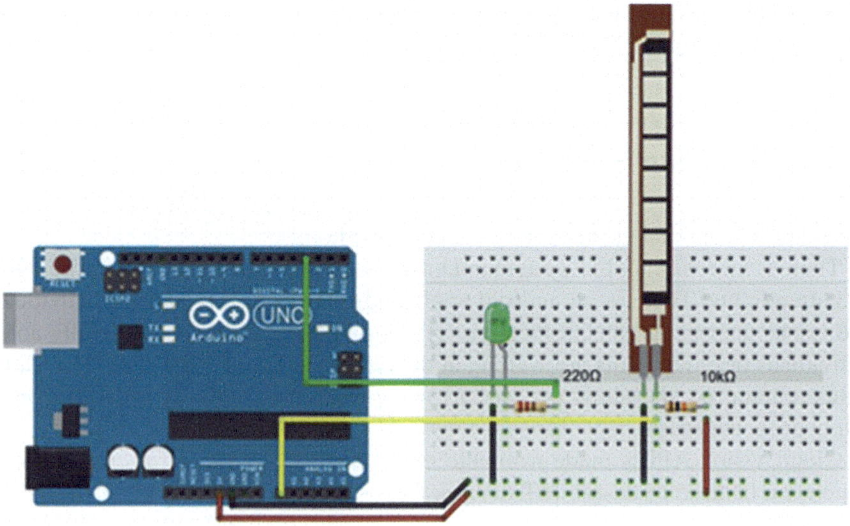

Fig. 7.4 Flex sensor

7.5 Research Challenges

IoT in healthcare is an emerging field of study and hence has challenges [10, 11], few of which we might be known now, and few we might discover in future.

7.5.1 *Patient Comfort*

IoT devices work with a lot of sensors and devices. Excessive usage of embedded systems make patients uncomfortable. Also, so much hardware makes the system costly but effective. It becomes essential to design comfortable sensors at lesser costs.

7.5.2 *Noise Removal*

The data collected from sensors are then transmitted to a connected device through WiFi or Bluetooth and then to a monitoring centre if needed. This can affect the quality of the data. Noise removal thus becomes essential. New, better architectures are required to enhance data transmission quality and reduce noise. Researchers need to find out improves techniques for the same.

7.5.3 *Data Storage and Analysis*

There are massive amounts of data that are to be stored and analysed. Storage of such vast quantities of information and retrieving them is a challenge. We need suitable storage devices that are reliable and large enough to store extensive details. There are millions of people who use the application simultaneously. Every second huge record needs to be updated into the database. For data analytics, the stored documents need to be retrieved. We need faster mediums to access information. The transfer of data requires to be quicker and correct.

7.5.4 *Power Consumption*

Since the number of sensors and devices connected through a network increases, the amount of power leakage also increases, leading to higher energy consumption. Hardware improvement becomes more crucial. It is relatively more essential to design better optimization algorithms and software that manage hardware efficiently instead of reducing energy usage.

7.5.5 Security

There are a lot of people accessing the data of the devices. Different authentication techniques, therefore, become necessary. For instance, doctors can assess the patient's medical records along with the sensor readings, vaccine or medication information, or any other confidential documents. Since the networks [12] used to connect can be public, they are unstable, and it is possible that there can be a man who can interrupt the connection and get unwanted access. Privacy is paramount, and these devices are very vulnerable to attack.

Hence, there is a need for more good encryption techniques and authentication steps before giving users, be it patients or practitioners access to the data and devices.

When IoT uses the cloud, new issues arise which needs new network architectures that integrate them. The critical concerns during integration are quality of service and quality of experience and data security, privacy and reliability.

7.6 IoT Healthcare Applications: Case Studies

7.6.1 IoT in Diabetes Treatment

A person with high blood sugar levels is said to have diabetes. It is due to improper secretion of insulin by the pancreas. Around 422 million people worldwide, irrespective of their age group, have diabetes, and nearly 1.6 million deaths annually are attributed directly to diabetes. IoT has found its way to help patients suffering from diabetes problem.

Smart Continuous Glucose Monitoring (CGM)

Diabetes patients need to be administered and monitored regularly for treatment. CGM device has been designed to monitor glucose levels in the blood continuously. Readings are taken after regular time intervals. CGM then sends these data to an application [5] over the smartphone or smartwatches where it can be checked easily. This information can be then analysed to detect trends. Health practitioners [13, 14] can also access this information and treat the patient accordingly, irrespective of the geographical location. Family members can also view these data, and the doctor's review regarding the same remotely. The first CGM was approved in 1999. After that, many more like Eversense and Freestyle Libre have come to the market (Fig. 7.5).

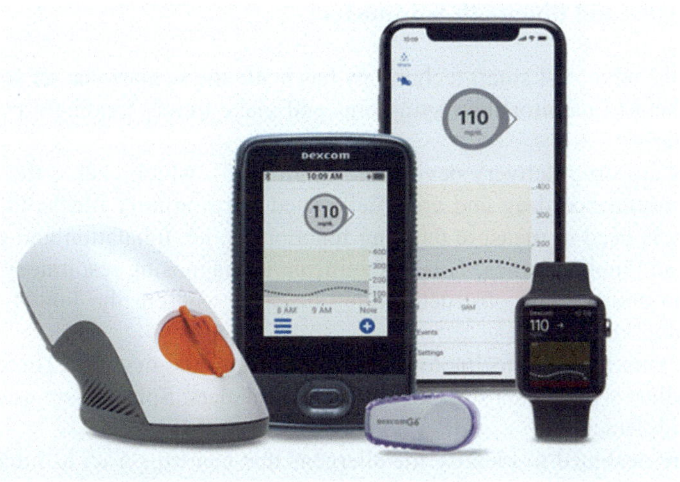

Fig. 7.5 Continuous glucose monitoring (CGM)

Insulin Pen

Another device called Insulin Pen has also proved to be helpful for diabetes patients. An insulin pen can record the amount of insulin injected, the dose's time and the type of insulin injected. The smartpen can suggest the patient of the correct type, time and quantity of insulin injection regularly.

An insulin pen is connected to the smartphone application, where all the data are collected in the store. Patients can also make a note of their meals. This information, along with the insulin dose, can be analysed to determine how eating patterns have affected blood sugar levels. The app can also recommend changes in diet patterns. Long-term data can be stored and interpreted this way, reducing the burden of the caretaker. InPen, Gocap and Esysta are some smart insulin pens in the market.

7.6.2 *Asthma*

Respiratory illnesses like asthma account to significant morbidity amongst people and affect the life quality of millions globally. It is the condition where airways swell and get narrowed, making it difficult to breathe. It is a prevalent chronic, non-communicable disease. It can result in attacks that can be life-threatening.

Smart Inhaler and Bluetooth Spirometer

However, the advent of smart technology has made the scenario better for them by enabling them to monitor their symptoms and make timely treatment possible for them regularly.

Inhalers are drug delivery devices in asthma [15], which enable the patient to inhale the prescribed drug and are chiefly used in respiratory illness like asthma. Spirometry is used to measure the lung functioning, i.e. inhalation and exhalation capacities and lung volumes. This is significant in diagnosing respiratory problems like asthma and chronic obstructive lung diseases wherein the lung functioning might be altered.

Of late, smart inhaler technology has stepped into the markets. These are connected inhalers wherein sensors are attached to inhalers. Spirometers used are also enabled with Bluetooth.

Apps are designed to identify the allergens that can trigger an asthma attack in patients and, thus, issue a prophylactic forecast to the user and prevent an asthmatic attack. Also, these sensors connected to inhalers can monitor the usage of medication in patients. The inhaler reports can be shared with the doctor and check if the correct treatment is being followed or not. Treating doctors can monitor [16] the consistency of medication usage with great ease. Adherence is improved, which in medical terms means that there is more consistency very often. Patients also can use these data to improve their condition by learning how to use the inhaler better.

Propeller Health [17] is one of the biggest producers of smart inhalers. Respimat inhaler and Diskus inhaler are few variants that came into the markets in recent times. These companies collaborate with inhaler and spirometer producing companies and embedded sensors within them. Most sensors work with any inhalers.

Asthma Monitor

Apart from the smart inhalers and Bluetooth spirometers, wearable smart asthma devices are also available. Smart asthma monitors notify the user beforehand of an impending asthmatic attack by either vibration or text message. This device is flexible, small and wearable. So the person wearing it can feel the vibration and get notified before itself. A text message is forwarded to a caretaker or a family member of the patient to draw up a timely action, thus allowing us to manage the episode very early and preventing it from worsening.

The patient can set reminders to maintain regularity of their medications through voice journaling. Also, these smart monitors [18] enable the detection of the inhaler's usage in patients, based on the detected changes. Thus, lots are a boon to asthmatic patients and improve their life quality significantly by helping them set medication reminders. Alert them of an impending asthmatic attack, and also keep a track on their regularity. The app's algorithm is flexible, allowing the device to learn from the changes over time. ADAMM is asthma monitor that has been introduced in the market for consumers. ADANM means Automated Device for Asthma Monitoring and Management.

7.6.3 *Apple in Medical Research*

Apple organization have been working on medical research and healthcare. They have designed medical applications to work along with iPhone and Apple smartwatch [19]. Wearable technology with healthcare benefits has marked a begin of new technology.

Parkinson's Disease

Parkinson's disease leads to stiffening of muscles, resulting in difficulty in walking, body coordination and body balance. This is due to damage of brain or nerve cells. Symptoms begin slowly and worsen over time. It becomes crucial to monitor these patients considering their difficulty in movement and talking.

Doctors or physicians usually conduct physical diagnostic tests regularly to monitor the patient's status, symptoms and condition. Each patient has a diary to record the observations overtime to get a broader idea of symptoms. Researchers at Apple have worked to automate this process. They have designed an app and connected iPhone and Apple smartwatches. The data collected are plotted as a graph, and symptoms fluctuations are monitored every minute. Hourly and daily breakdown analysis reports are generated.

These data are also used for research analysis of different health conditions. A detailed study of the data collected from sensors would help gain an insight into the onset and duration of a specific symptom of seizures if any. In medical terms, it is called epilepsy where the body experiences sudden signal disturbances, leading to unconsciousness and convulsions due to abnormal activity in the brain neuron cells. These epilepsies can be recurrent and sudden episodes. Therefore, it becomes even more crucial to study the information.

Depression

Depression is a mental state where one feels loneliness, stress and grief. Patients often tend to remain silent on their condition. But they must speak out. Therapy sessions are necessary to tackle the symptoms. If worsened, depression can, at times, trigger suicidal thoughts.

Apple smartwatch and applications help in monitoring depression. They have designed an app to assess patients with depressive disorders. Participants used the app to monitor their cognition and mood. Cognition refers to the method of gaining knowledge. Stimulus received is processed by our brain to make a judgement and

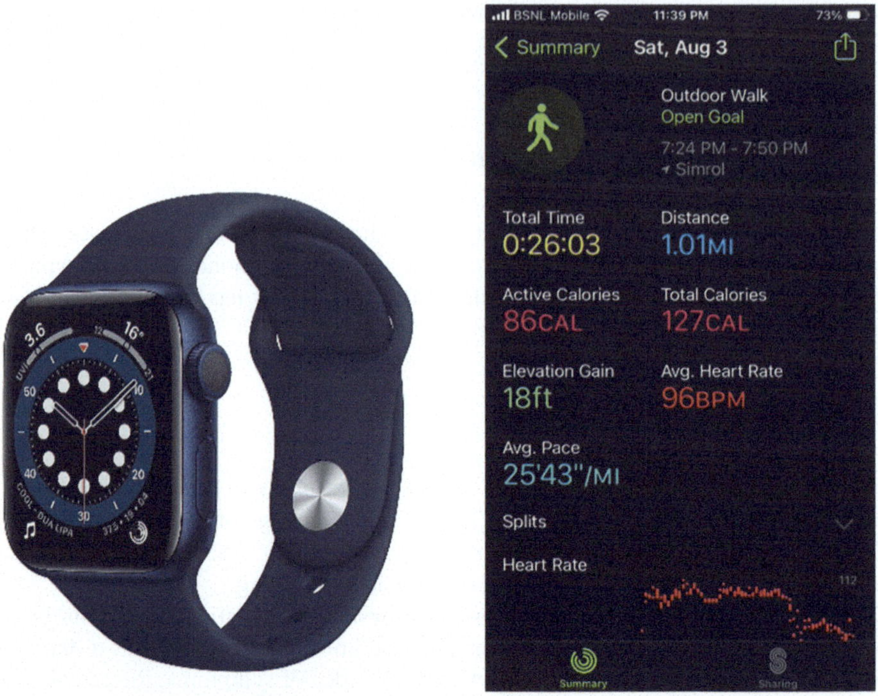
BSNL Mobile
11:39 PM
73%
Summary
Sat, Aug 3
Outdoor Walk
Open Goal
7:24 PM - 7:50 PM
Simrol
Total Time
0:26:03
Distance
1.01MI
Active Calories
86CAL
Total Calories
127CAL
Elevation Gain
18ft
Avg. Heart Rate
96BPM
Avg. Pace
25'43"/MI
Splits
Heart Rate
Summary
Sharing

Apple Watch Apple Application

Fig. 7.6 Apple applications

gain an understanding of events around us. They can be due to conscious or unconscious choices made by our mind.

Daily assessment is done by doing in-depth analysis and cognition tests to derive outcomes. And the results produced are considered to be reliable and robust to a large extent. The collected data have been put to research where the effects of the depression were studied in real time. Like other IoT healthcare devices, Apple apps also share patient information with doctors or professionals to understand the condition.

The app tries to understand the behaviour or pattern in their behaviour, to suggest the person techniques make him feel better. The interactions and conversations with the app help the person understand about emotional well-being (Fig. 7.6).

Fitness and Physical Well-being

Fitness is vital for the muscles and bones in our body. We must give our body regular exercise and physical training sessions. This would improve breathing, the functioning of the heart and lungs. It is necessary to maintain good weight to prevent heart diseases, obesity and a few types of cancers.

There is an application created for the following purpose. GPS is enabled to track the movement of the person. The number of steps taken is recorded along with the distance covered. There are sensors like accelerometer (discussed in earlier Sect. 7.6.3) which is used to estimate the number of calories burned that day. This app is connected with apple smartwatch to track the heartbeat.

The app also analyses sleeping habits by checking phone usage hours and application activities. The app also suggests workout ideas or fitness goals, making it very interactive.

7.6.4 Cancer Treatment

Radiotherapy has emerged as one of the reliable treatment modalities for cancers, mostly around the head and neck region. Despite radiotherapy having the potential to cure most cancers, it comes with its side effects such as extreme dehydration. Radiotherapy is usually given in sessions, i.e. on an outpatient basis. Thus, IoT can play a role here in reducing the symptoms caused both due to cancer and the side effects of radiotherapy. Since most of the time patients are away, they need constant monitoring to address these side effects.

Here, remote sensor technology collects the data from the patient and transmitting it to the treating doctor frequently. Remote sensor technology enables the doctor to have a constant eye on their patients. The doctor can also reschedule the therapies if needed. Bluetooth enabled devices can record any significant fluctuations in parameters like weight or blood pressure of patients and transmit them to the physician.

The patients answer daily questionnaires, and these are assessed by the treating physician who thereby takes a call on the requirement for any intervention in them. Thus, this system can enable the users undergoing radiation therapy for cancer to minimize their side effects and help the treating radiation oncologist to keep a better watch on their patients and their outcomes to the treatment. Overall, IoT is playing a crucial role in improving patients' quality of life by undergoing radiation therapy and improving modality's efficacy. Cyberinfrastructure for Comparative Effectiveness Research (CYCORE) is a platform currently in the market for cancer treatment.

7.6.5 IoT in Pharma Industry

In the pharmaceutical industry, the development of medicines needs to be secure and properly monitored. Safety needs to be maintained when it comes to the distribution of drugs or medicines. If the company fails to meet any other these, it could prove fatal to the patient and lead to a revenue loss if the drugs synthesized have to be discarded.

Therefore, the Pharma industry needs to address these issues and have reasonable control over the facilities and production activities. The company, which would address these concerns, is likely to survive today's competitive markets. Proper shipment of the medicines and in the stipulated time without any delays is very much essential. Few of these operations are outside the facilities and need to be re-looked. The industry's quality and quantity standards need to be higher so that they can reach a larger group of patients in case of emergencies.

IoT has helped these companies to meet the demands in the current day market and improve their connectivity. With the introduction of IoT, everyone involved is connected. People are connected with equipment at lesser costs, making it very economical. The supply chains can be closely monitored. Safety of the structure is ensured in addition to making movements faster.

Pharma industries [20] benefit at three levels: manufacturing, maintenance and delivery. IoT sensors help to determine the apt conditions for working in drug synthesis environment. They handle the weight of chemicals and biomaterials so that the equipment can work properly. This would reduce instances of fraud and danger. Trackers help track the drugs to ensure they reach the supply chain during the demanding hours.

One major drawback in manufacturing the drugs is in equipment. There are many reasons for an asset's failure, such as mechanical damage, excessive voltage, chemical deterioration, unstable environment and a lack of maintenance. Pharmaceutical companies cannot risk unplanned equipment breakdown and supply. If this happens, they will have to discard all the materials. It is hence vital to have a sound monitoring system round the clock throughout the day.

IoT serves this purpose. It helps in tracking the status of the machinery and other facilities continuously. It keeps updating this information on components like sterilizers, vacuum pumps, pressure gauges, heat exchangers, pH probes and multi-media filters air compressors.

This information is used to repair the equipment, assess critical issues and maintain the machinery's regular maintenance. In current times, if a component fails, it would take a considerable amount of time to detect the mishap and then even more time to repair it. This will result in certain facilities' unavailability for a long duration which is referred to as downtime. IoT ensures downtime reduction and maintains safety in the working environment.

Such innovative methods will help in proper planning, ensuring maximum resource utilization with the data collected. If IoT is combined with AI, then the pharma companies can predict the conditions and optimize performance. This would lay the foundation of a perfect modernized system.

Controlling the manufacturing conditions with IoT will make the production activities more transparent. Along with manufacturing, the storage environment needs to be given special attention. Atmospheric indicators such as humidity, radiation, temperature, levels of carbon dioxide and light are to be maintained. This is achieved with several sensors.

There is a screen on which this information is updated continuously. The supervisor or the employee in the lab can keep observing these values and in case of emergencies or odd behaviour take immediate measures. Smart systems can be introduced, predicting this change of conditions and automatically adjusting the parameters to bring back the system to normal conditions. In case there is a disaster, for instance, like machine damage, which can result in leakage of toxic chemicals, the concerned staff member can be alerted. This would help in timely disaster management.

Dutch startup and AntTail developed tiny sensors, which are currently in the market. These sensors are kept in the box while packing the drugs, which help in tracking the packets until their delivery to the consumers. This would help in monitoring the medicines [21] to check if they are delivered correctly and within time (Fig. 7.7).

This tracking is essential unexpected difficulties like vehicle accidents or sudden failure of temperature maintaining units, resulting in fluctuations. Such sudden hard times can have an effect on the customer as well as the pharma company. Therefore, even after production, it becomes more critical to track the supply chain and the delivery route details. If the company becomes aware of the situation, they can ensure specific measures to handle the situation. IoT helps in ensuring that immediate actions are taken to prevent delays or dangers.

Other than sensors, drugs can be packed and marked with batches, tags or smart labels, which can help in identification of the packages. Each batch or QR is unique and helps distinctly track individual delivery until they reach the final destination. Apart from drugs, the vehicles transporting the packages are enabled with GPS to know the geographical location periodically. This will make the shipment process more transparent. The more the number of trackers, the more precise the tracking is as they would serve in case the other breaks down.

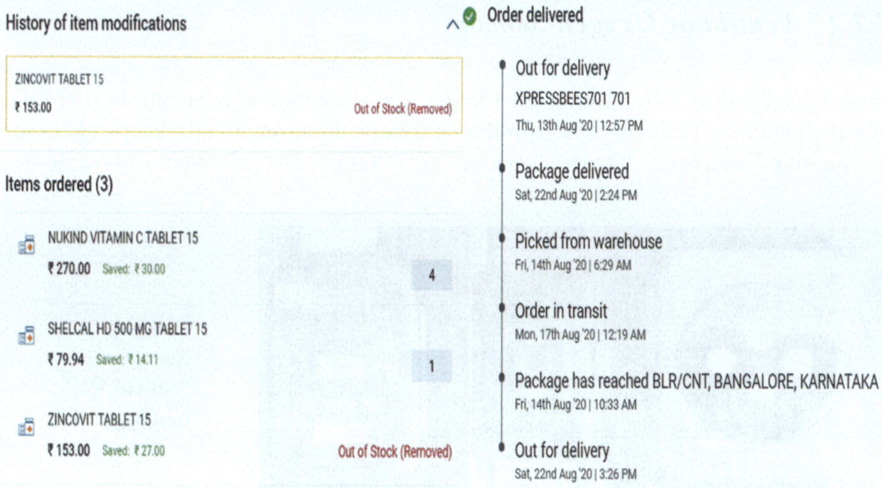

Fig. 7.7 A sample medicine tracking system

The sensors that handle environmental conditions such as temperature, pressure and humidity can alert the driver or the person carrying it, in case of deviation from standards while travelling. The current conditions are compared with the required ones. In case of discrepancy, with such intimidation, timely measures can be taken. If the drugs storage does not meet the storage criteria, they will have to be disposed of. Since all the information has been collected, this can be analysed to predict the frequent mishaps or facilities to be improved. Problems in the delivery route can be worked on to prevent future delays, making the process smoother. Such a report on how the drug was stored will help the caretaker or physician to contribute more to the patient treatment.

7.7 Commonly Used Sensors

7.7.1 Heartbeat

Smartwatches like those of Apple (refer Sect. 7.6.3.3) use a technology called PPG, i.e. photoplethysmography, for measuring heartbeat [22]. Blood absorbs green colour and reflects red colour giving it a red colour. This technology checks the amount of red and green light visible when it looks at the wrist through the skin. The more amount of green light absorption implies a higher heartbeat rate. A similar idea is used in hospitals where pulse measuring devices are connected to tips of fingers (Fig. 7.8).

7.7.2 Ventilator Oxygen Sensor

The oxygen sensor is to monitor the oxygen gas quantity and concentration of oxygen the patient is receiving through the ventilator. It automatically keeps checking at regular intervals. These sensors are made up of electrogalvanic or

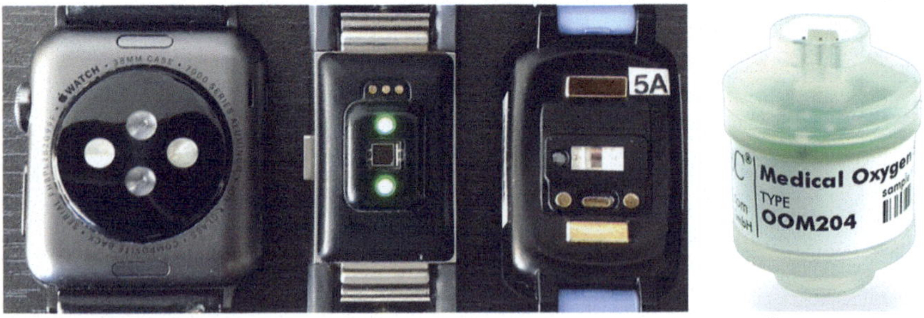

PPG Sensor Ventilator O2 Sensor

Fig. 7.8 PPG sensor ventilator O_2 sensor

electrochemical sensors. They work based on the difference in voltage which varies with difference in oxygen levels.

7.7.3 Temperature Sensors

Temperature sensors measure the surroundings' temperature and convert it into electrical signals that can be recorded and monitored. There are two types of temperatures: contact temperature and non-contact temperature. Contact temperature sensors measure the temperature of the surface they are in contact. Non-contact sensors work by measuring the IR radiations emitted by the object.

7.7.4 Blood Glucose Sensors

Our human body synthesizes enzymes which are proteins. Blood glucose sensors have enzyme-coated strips that react with the blood sample. This meter then calculates the amount of glucose in the blood and sends the output to the monitor. These strips are usually not reusable.

7.8 Conclusion

IoT in healthcare has a bright future. It has a lot of deliverable aim to revolution automation healthcare services. Healthcare facilities across the globe have adopted IoT systems. From top-level hospitals to regular clinics, all are utilizing the real advantages of IoT in healthcare. Upcoming future of IoT in healthcare with being changed with the new IoT innovations will organize business patterns and automate the data monitoring system. IoT can also make healthcare cost-benefit and medically efficient in the future. Many reports say that IoT healthcare will have more customized systems, patient-oriented equipment and doctor-oriented equipment in the next couple of years. With the use of IoT technology, treatment and as well as monitoring will be more precise and proper order. Usually, IoT will also enable patients to access data and personalized care and reduce visits to the hospital.

References

1. Li, X., et al. (November 2011). Smart community: An internet of things applications. *IEEE Communication Magazine, 49*(11), 68–75.
2. Milovanovic, D., Pantovic, V., & Gardasevic, G. (July 2017). Chapter 3: converging technologies for the IoT: Standardization activities and frameworks. In *Emerging trends and applications of the internet of things* (pp. 71–104). IGI Global Publishing.

3. Vasanth, K., & Shert, J. (2012, November). Creating solutions for health through technology innovation. *Texas Instruments*.
4. Viswanathan, H., Lee, E. K., & Pompili, D. (2012, January). Mobile grid computing for data and patient-centric ubiquitous healthcare. In Proc. IEEE workshop ETSIoT.
5. Shahamabadi, M. S., et al. (2013, July). A network mobility solution based on 6LoWPAN hospital wireless sensor network (NEMO-HWSN). In Proc. IMIS.
6. Gravina, R., Ma, C., Pace, P., Aloi, G., Russo, W., Li, W., & Fortino, G. (2017). Cloud-based Activity-aaService cyber–physical framework for human activity monitoring in mobility. *Future Generation Computer Systems, 75*, 158–171.
7. Mainetti, L., Patrono, L., & Vilei, A. (2017). Evolutional wireless sensor networks towards the Internet of Things: A survey. In Milovanovic, D. A., Zoran S. (Eds.). Proc. Soft-Com 2011 (Vol. 2). Bojkovic International Journal of Internet of Things and web services ISSN: 2367–9115 64.
8. Zhon, J., et al. (January 2017). Security and privacy for cloud-based IoT: Challenges, countermeasures, and future directions. *IEEE Communication Magazine, 55*(1), 26–33.
9. Abawaji, J. H., & Hassan, M. M. (May 2017). Federated internet of things and cloud computing pervasive patient health monitoring systems. *IEEE Communication Magazine, 55*(1), 48–53.
10. Sathya, M., Madhan, S., & Jayanthi, K. (2018). Internet of things (IoT) based health monitoring system and challenges. *International Journal of Engineering & Technology*, 175–178.
11. Viswanathan, H., Chen, B., & Pompili, D. (May 2012). Research challenges in computation, communication, and context awareness for ubiquitous healthcare. *IEEE Communication Magazine, 50*(5), 92–99.
12. Ali, Y., Ullah, N., & García-Magariño, I. (2019, November). Internet of Things for healthcare using wireless communications or mobile computing. Wireless communications and mobile computing (Vol. 19).
13. Yin, Y., Zeng, Y., Chen, X., & Fan, Y. (2016). The internet of things in healthcare: An overview. *The Journal of Industrial Information Integration, 1*, 3–13.
14. Fortino, G., Parisi, D., Pirrone, V., & Di Fatta, G. (2014). BodyCloud: A SaaS approach for community body sensor networks. *Future Generation Computer Systems, 35*, 62–79.
15. Jara, A. J. (2010, March/April). A pharmaceutical intelligent information system to detect allergies and adverse drugs reactions based on Internet of Things. In Proc. IEEE PERCOM workshop.
16. Jara, A. J., Zamora-Izguirdo, M. A., & Skarmeta, A. F. (2013). Interconnection framework for mHealth and remote monitoring based on the internet of things. *IEEE Journal on Selected Areas in Communications, 31*(9), 47–65.
17. MehediHassan, M., Gumaei, A., Aloi, G., Fortino, G., & Zhou, M. (2019). A smartphone-enabled fall detection framework for elderly people in connected home healthcare. *IEEE Network, 33*(6), 58–63.
18. Pace, P., Aloi, G., Caliciuri, G., Gravina, R., Savaglio, C., Fortino, G., Ibáñez-Sánchez, G., Fides-Valero, A., Bayo-Monton, J., Uberti, M., Corona, M., Bernini, L., Gulino, M., Costa, A., De Luca, I., & Mortara, M. (2019). INTER-health: An interoperable IoT solution for active and assisted living healthcare services.WF-IoT (pp. 81–86).
19. https://apps.apple.com/in/app/fitness/id1208224953
20. Rasid, M.F.A., et al. (2014). Embedded gateway services for Internet of Things application is ubiquitous healthcare. In Proc. ICoICT.
21. https://www.medlife.com
22. Morak, J., et al. (2012). Design and evolution of a telemonitoring concept based on NFC-enabled mobile phones and sensor devices. *IEEE Transactions on Information Technology in Biomedicine, 16*(1), 17–23.

Part II
Fusion of Internet of Things, Artificial Intelligence, and Cloud Computing in Tackling Pandemic Diseases

Chapter 8
Tele Health Monitoring System in Rural Areas Through Primary Health Center Using IOT for Covid-19

Vijayalaxmi Biradar and G. Durga Sukumar

Abbreviations

BP	Blood pressure
ECG	Electrocardiogram
EMRI	Emergency management and research institute
GPRS	General packet radio service
HAC	Humanitarian activities committee
IEEE	Institute of electrical and electronics engineers
IOT	Internet of things
IT	Information technology
OLED	Organic light emitting diodes
PHC	Primary health center
SARS	Severe acute respiratory syndrome
SIGHT	Special interest group on humanitarian technology
UBA	Unnat bharat abhiyan
USB	Universal serial bus

8.1 Introduction

The surge in the COVID-19 cases in India calls for extensive screening to contain the spread of the deadly virus. The sorry state of affairs in the rural areas of India makes this all the more difficult. Hence Telemedicine comes to the rescue given the existing infrastructural constraints. Spanning over the last decade, telemedicine

V. Biradar (✉)
Department of ECE, Vignan Institute of Technology and Science, Hyderabad, India

G. D. Sukumar
Department of EEE, Vignan Institute of Technology and Science, Hyderabad, India

P. Siarry et al. (eds.), *The Fusion of Internet of Things, Artificial Intelligence, and Cloud Computing in Health Care*, Internet of Things,
https://doi.org/10.1007/978-3-030-75220-0_8

using remote sensing and monitoring has evolved as a dominant alternative enabling combatting the limitations posed by the naïve healthcare system in place in the rural areas of India. With specific reference to COVID-19 pandemic, there is an ever-increasing need for interactions with the people in near real-time instances by providing remote monitoring that provides design efficiency in facilitating feasible operational ease that would best serve our purpose in question by remaining contactless. Moreover the intelligence function can provide us with the much needed data about the pandemic and the resultant clinical interventions. The evolving market of telemedicine has been an asset to all the stakeholders.

The pandemic COVID-19 has again diverted all our energies towards exploring the various avenues provided by this emerging technology for providing a solution to the endless agony faced by the masses in this seemingly never ending crisis by catering to the new challenges posed by the deadly virus and leading to extensive brainstorming about how to use it in the best possible manner during this pressing times.

The field of Telemedicine has been galloping over these years, thanks to the growth of wireless broadband and multifunctional uses of smartphones. There are evidences of using this technology for bringing about a better connect in the rural areas but eventually, it has become a household name with the advent of electronic devices by dint of the use of smart phones, bio peripherals, and 4G and 5G networks and so on. Added to it, the onset of the pandemic Covid-19 has made it a more economical choice in terms of time, effort, and money.

With the popularity of Telemedicine over these years, there has been micro distinction that has been made in terms of (1) access to rural areas, (2) live sharing, and (3) remote monitoring. Thus, this is the most viable tool for the present situation where there is an immense need for going for large-scale screening and subsequent monitoring and catering to the resolution of the illness, not to forget the need for maintaining the safety measures.

Numerous work in this direction can be referred to where there has been use of this technology for detection of symptoms well in time so as to prevent later stage contingencies [1] Minoi (2014) in their study suggested the use of the remote system for blood pressure monitoring that would record, store, and disseminate data to remote server via the wireless network and facilitate retrieving the same by the physician located at different locations via the website [2]. Another study worth mentioning here is that of J Gómez (2016) who propounded that the healthcare amenities can be elevated in the rural areas, having minimal access by promoting health and well-being by use of remote sensing and wireless technology. To cite the contribution of Murthy, the survey thus conducted on mobile-based healthcare systems in various countries around the globe provided the much needed affirmation that this technology would provide a one stop solution for solving the healthcare problems in the rural areas [3]. In their study, Boyi Xu (2014) explained as to how the use of IoT-based system would cater to the needs of collection, analysis, and interpretation of the IoT data and use this flexible method for catering to the need of providing the emergency services as a part of the medical health amenities by disseminating the heterogeneous, thanks to cloud and mobile computing [4]. Not to forget, the work of Hassanalieragh (2015) provided the much needed insight into the art of data acquisition, data transfer, cloud processing, and conception by making use of machine learning approaches to facilitate healthcare systems using remote access [5]. In his work, Kumar (2014) put forth the advantages of Big Data in processing otherwise huge pile of data and would come to the rescue of the medical professionals for realizing the dream of suitable healthcare reforms in rural areas, thus making healthcare amenities available to the masses across the country.

The ultimate objective is to provide for the health and well-being of all the individuals, even those in the remotest part of the country. It works relentlessly on collection, classification, storage, dissemination of the data, and the timely intervention by the doctors.

A lot of milestones have been achieved in these years due to the use of wireless and network capabilities in an ever-growing computing environment. And one such sector that has been benefitted by the same has been the healthcare sector. We have been using telemedicine more often to refer to the employment of communication technology for diagnosis and treatment of the patient in the areas with minimal access by providing remote monitoring and treatment. It is an economical method in terms of time, effort, and money. Moreover, it facilitates personal self-help care of the elderly people at home by providing with simple, easy to use apparatus thereby eliminating the need to visit the physician for routine tests [2]. It is very easy and effective method to monitor and evaluate daily vitals and observe for any deviations from the normal parameters and send the alerts in case of any anomalies observed [6]. The studies that encompasses all these parameters can be classified in terms of type of communication networks used, types of sensors used, the devices for monitoring that have been used, and the algorithms developed therein [7]. This section provides with the details of these determinants. As is evident from the figure above, the components included have been bio signal sensors, units for processing, communication networks, and medical center.

Figure 8.1: Main components of Telemedicine system.

This emerging technology has come to the rescue of the healthcare centers in providing a cost-effective solution for catering to the needs of the patients and the ease of functioning for the physicians alike. With the growth of Internet of Things (IoT) technologies, there has been a paradigm shift from in-person consultation to telemedicine.

This paper proposes a Telehealth Monitoring System in rural areas by using IoT in the Primary Health Center during these Covid-19 times to facilitate monitoring of the preliminary vitals of the patient along with the room condition in which the patient resides in real-time. This system has made use of five sensors for capturing the data from the Primary Health Center in questioning with regards to the heart beat, body temperature, Pulse rate, Blood Pressure, Blood Glucose monitoring. The reports are disseminated using a website www.sfpieee.in designed for the same to the registered medical professionals deployed for and trained for the same so as to get an idea about the condition of the patient. The prototype has been tested and has been found to satisfy the criteria of suitability, feasibility, and acceptability, thereby making the system plausible.

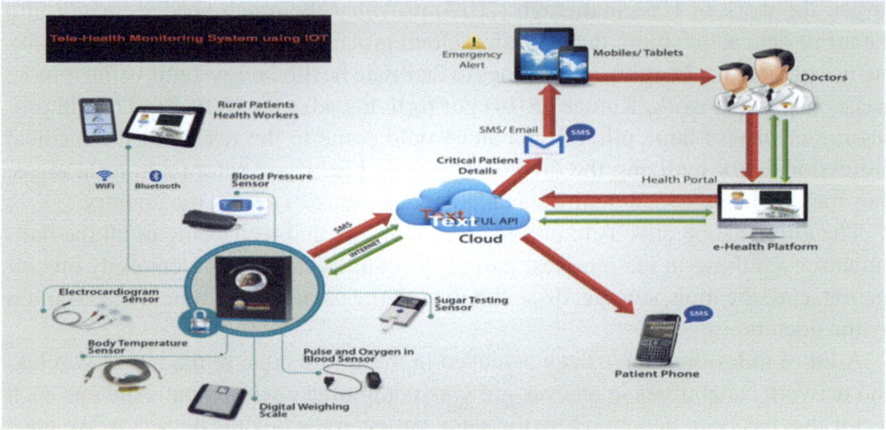

Fig. 8.1 Model of telehealth monitoring system using IOT

8.2 System Design and Description

The hardware components that were put to use have been enumerated as follows:

8.2.1 Noncontact Temperature Sensor

Despite of availability of noncontact temperature in online sources, it was decided to develop the same to make it cost-effective using **Arduino and an Infrared temperature sensor** using noncontact temperature sensor **MLX90614.**

Components Used

- Arduino Pro Mini
- MLX90614 Infrared Temperature Sensor
- OLED Display—SSD1306
- Laser Diode
- 9 V Battery
- Push button
- Battery Clip
- Connecting wires

There are many temperature sensors available in the market and we have been using the DHT11 Sensor and LM35 extensively for many applications where atmospheric humidity or temperature has to be measured. But here, for a thermal gun we need a sensor that could sense the temperature of a particular object (not ambient) without directly getting in contact with the object. For this purpose, we have

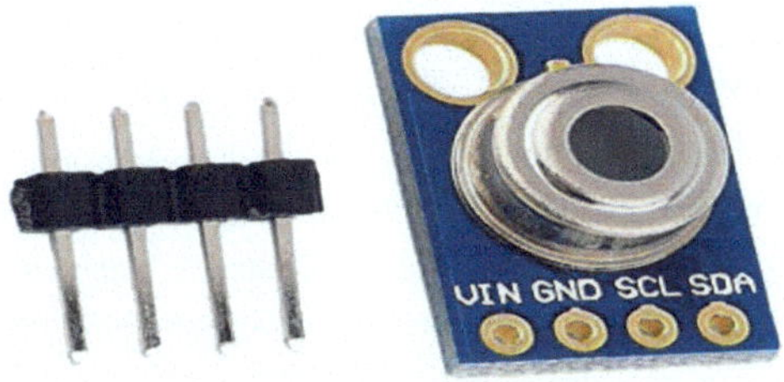

Fig. 8.2 MLX90614 noncontact temperature sensor

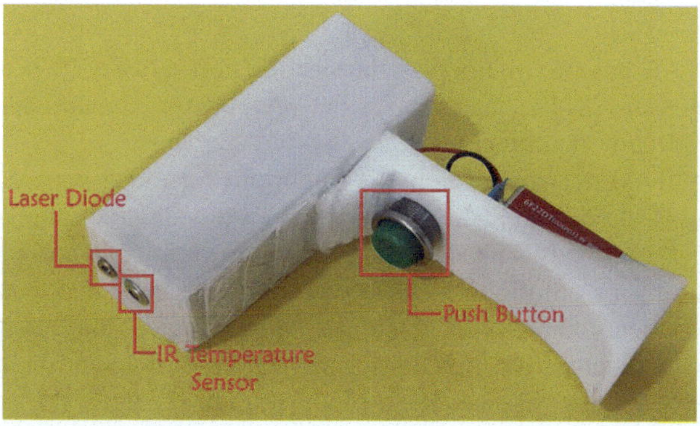

Fig. 8.3 Temperature sensor gun using Arduino

contact less temperature sensors which utilize Laser or IR to calculate the temperature of an object. The MLX90614 is one such sensor that uses IR energy to detect the temperature of an object (Fig. 8.2).

The sensing range to be in a conical shape from the point of sensor is shown. So, as we go far from the measuring object, the sensing area increases by twofolds. Meaning for every 1 cm we move away from the object the sensing area grows by 2 cm. In our thermal gun **we have placed a laser diode on top of the sensor** to know where the sensing area of the sensor is currently pointing at. I found that the values were reliable if the gun is pointed at 2 cm away from the object and the accuracy goes down as we move away. The entire circuit is powered by the 9 V battery through a push button. When the push button is pressed, the 9 V battery is connected to the RAW pin of Arduino which is then regulated to 5 V using the on-board voltage regulator. This 5 V is then used to power the OLED module, Sensor, and Laser diode (Fig. 8.3).

8.2.2 Blood Pressure Sensor

Blood pressure is the pressure of the blood in the arteries as it is pumped around the body by the heart. When your heart beats, it contracts and pushes blood through the arteries to the rest of your body. This force creates pressure on the arteries. Blood

Table 8.1 Classification of blood pressure for adults (18 years and older)

	Systolic (mmHg)	Diastolic (mmHg)
Hypotension	<90	<60
Desired	90–119	60–79
Prehypertension	120–139	80–89
Stage 1 hypertension	140–159	90–99
Stage 2 hypertension	160–179	100–109
Hypertensive crisis	≥180	≥110

pressure is recorded as two numbers— the systolic pressure (as the heart beats) over the diastolic pressure (as the heart relaxes between beats). The unit which measures this is called Sphygmomanometer.

Monitoring blood pressure at home is important for many people, especially if you have high blood pressure. Blood pressure does not stay the same all the time. It changes to meet your body's needs. It is affected by various factors including body position, breathing or emotional state, exercise, and sleep. It is best to measure blood pressure when you are relaxed and sitting or lying down (Table 8.1).

High blood pressure (hypertension) can lead to serious problems like heart attack, stroke, or kidney disease. High blood pressure usually does not have any symptoms, so you need to have your blood pressure checked regularly.

Blood Pressure Sensor Procedure

Step 1: Connect Blood Pressure on the wrist as shown in figure.
Step 2: Press ON button (2) as shown in figure.
Step 3: Wait for few seconds, Note down the Blood Pressure value from the screen and upload on website (Fig. 8.4).

8.2.3 Pulse Oximeter Sensor

COVID-19 is a disease caused by the SARS-CoV-2 virus that primarily attacks a person's respiratory system. Some milder symptoms can include fever, aches, and chills, but it can also lead to more serious conditions such as pneumonia. A person who has pneumonia or even slight shortness of breath might not know when to go to a hospital, especially as they start to get even more overwhelmed. This is why I created this open source pulse oximeter, which can assist in getting people the help they need and get accurate information about their current condition (Fig. 8.5).

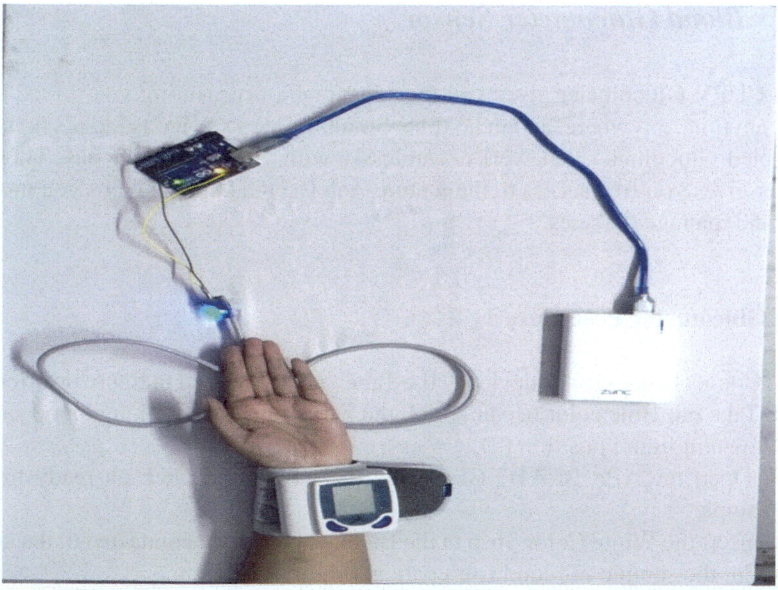

Fig. 8.4 Blood pressure sensor

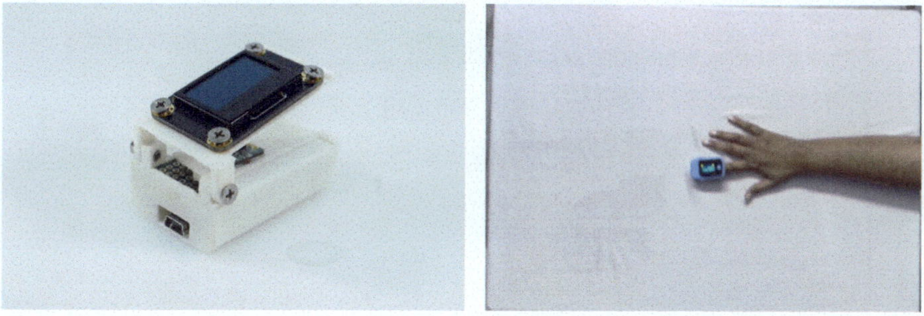

Fig. 8.5 Pulse oximeter sensor

Pulse Oximeter Sensor Procedure

Step 1: Open the Pulse Oximeter sensor.
Step 2: Place the Finger as shown in the figure.
Step 3: Press the ON button (1) as shown in figure.
Step 4: Note down the reading of Oxygen level and Pulse Heart Rate and upload in the website.

8.2.4 Blood Glucometer Sensor

BeatO CURV Glucometer gives you the advantage of measuring your blood sugar levels, anytime, anywhere, and in no time. Small in size – CURV is India's first USB Connected Glucometer that works seamlessly with all Android phones. This glucometer gives you free access to the feature-rich BeatO App that helps you monitor better and manage diabetes.

Blood Glucometer Procedure

Step 1: Connect Black color device to the Tablet port as shown in figure position (1).
Step 2: Take out Blue color needle, prick the patient finger for taking blood sample as shown in figure position (2).
Step 3: Open the APP BEATO Care from the tablet, and click on ready to take the sample.
Step 4: Insert the White Color Strip in the Black color device connected to the tablet.
Step 5: Put the sample of blood from patient finger to the strip.
Step 6: Wait for 5 s, observe in the APP and note down the reading. Upload in the website (Fig. 8.6).

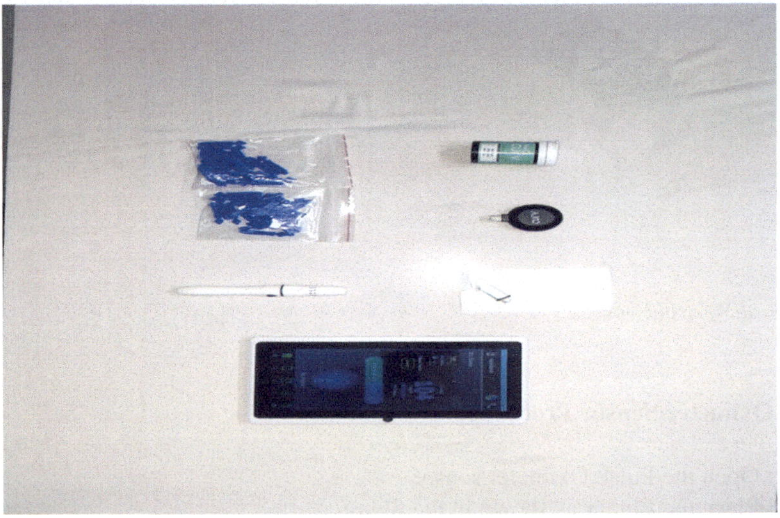

Fig. 8.6 Blood glucometer sensor

8.2.5 ECG Sensor

An ECG Sensor with disposable electrodes attaches directly to the chest to detect every heart beat. The electrodes of ECG sensor will convert heart beat to electric signal. ECG Sensor is very light weight, slim, and accurately measures continuous heart beat and gives rate data of heart beat. This device is always used by trained doctor and medical assistances.

Electrodes of ECG Sensor have three pins and connected by cable with 30 in. in length. It is make ECG sensor easy to connect with controller and placed at the waist or pocket. In additional, the plug-in for the cable is a male sound plug which will make the cable to be easily removed or inserted into the amplifier board. The sensor assembled on an arm pulse and a leg pulse. All of every sensor electrodes have methods to assemble in body. So, training and tutorials are needed for user. You can choose the type of electrode to measure heart beat.

ECG records the electrical activity generated by heart muscle depolarizations, which propagate in pulsating electrical waves towards the skin. Although the electricity amount is in fact very small, it can be picked up reliably with ECG electrodes attached to the skin. The full ECG setup comprises at least four electrodes which are placed on the chest or at the four extremities according to standard nomenclature (RA = right arm; LA = left arm; RL = right leg; LL = left leg). Of course, variations of this setup exist to allow more flexible and less intrusive recordings, for example, by attaching the electrodes to the forearms and legs. ECG electrodes are typically wet sensors, requiring the use of a conductive gel to increase conductivity between skin and electrodes.

ECG Procedure

Step 1: Connect Probes and ECG modules as given in.
Connection of ECG with Arduino:

Arduino 3.3 V --------- 3.3 V pin
Arduino pin 10 -------- L0+
Arduino Pin 11 -------- L0-
Arduino Analog 1 (A1) ------- Output
Arduino Gnd ----------- Gnd

Electrode pad location shown in Fig. 8.7a

Step 2: Power ON the Arduino Board using Power hub
Step 3: Open Arduino IDE

GoTo → Tools → Serial Plotter
Step 4: Download the data
Step 5: Upload

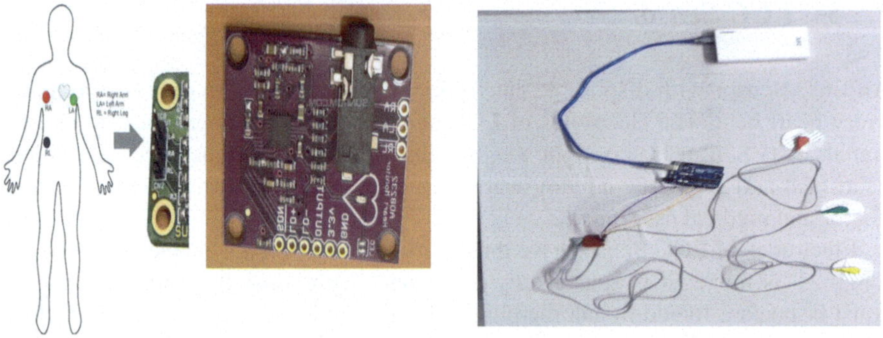

(a) (b)

Fig. 8.7 ECG sensor (**a**) Electrode pad location (**b**) ECG probes interfacing with Arduino

8.2.6 Website

Health of citizens is a serious area of concern for countries around the world, as the reach of healthcare services remains limited due to variety of constraints. Benefits of advancements in medical sciences and related technologies as a result are not available at all. At present, good hospitals are available only in urban areas. It is very much required to transform the healthcare with IT. Various aspects of Telemedicine are required to provide the health services in the country to bridge the gaps. They will become essential in rural areas where there is a scarcity of doctors and the hospitals.

Telehealth monitoring system is an innovative system for improving healthcare system from long distance using IOT. This system creates communication among patients healthcare professionals. In rural areas, there are Public Health Center (PHC) in few areas not even one PHC is also not available. Hence it is really difficult to get the treatment of huge number of villagers in rural areas and gather the data. Hence, this system monitors and measures different parameters like pulse, breath rate, oxygen in blood, ECG signals, glucose levels, BP, lung capacity, snore waves, body temperature, etc. using this system. This data is collected and sent to the cloud database in PHC where doctors will monitor the data and provide necessary treatment to the needy and also able to call for an ambulance in emergency. Telehealth monitoring is an innovative system of improving healthcare delivery from long distance using the telecommunication and modern information technologies. This system creates communication among patients and healthcare professionals maintaining convenience and commitment. The data are kept confidential and safely transferred from one place to another. In rural areas, patients go to PHC for their treatment. It is proposed to develop an automated Telehealth monitoring system and establish a communication between doctor and patient.

The website www.spfieee.in is developed to establish the connection between village PHC and doctors in the urban areas. The recognized PHC from the village

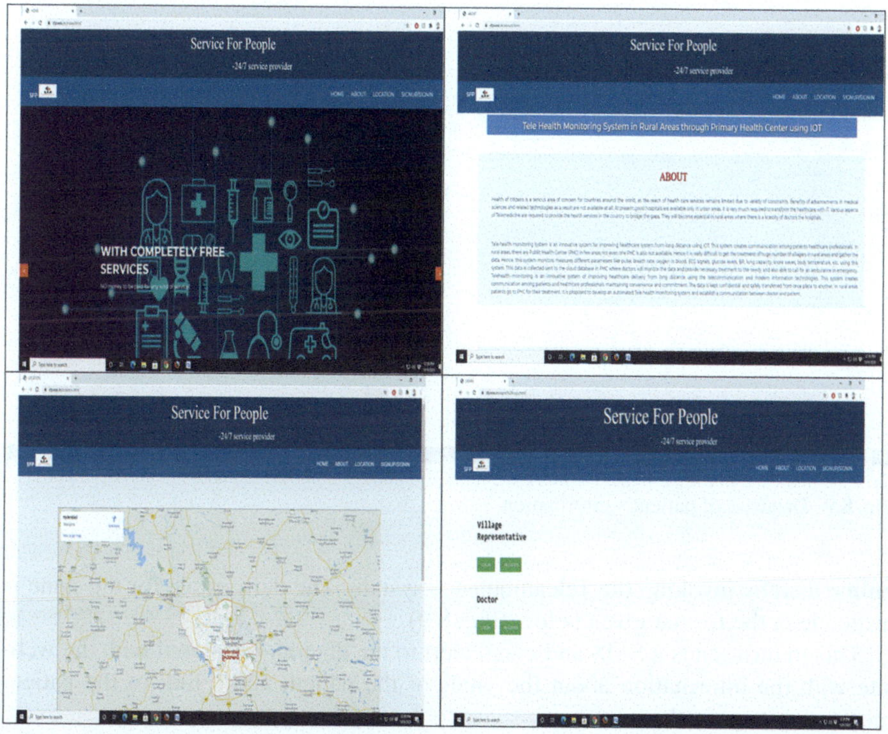

Fig. 8.8 Website developed for interaction

has to register in the website by giving all correct credentials, to avoid problems. Also the doctor who is willing to serve the people at no cost should register through this website with all credentials. Once the PHC is registered, then they are responsible for uploading the data to the website of the patient which they can send to any specific doctor based on specialization and problem of the patient by selecting the doctor from the list of registered doctors from the website. After selecting the doctor, the PHC will send the data to doctor through SMS and also E-mail. The screen shots of the website are shown in Fig. 8.8.

8.3 Implementation and Results

The T-health Monitoring System in the question has been designed by using numerous IoT components and machine learning algorithms. The working of the same ensures the retrieval of the case sheet of the patient in a predetermined format to be used for future references. Further, in case of an emergency or contingency, the cloud process of the PHC responds and in no time, there is a sharing of information

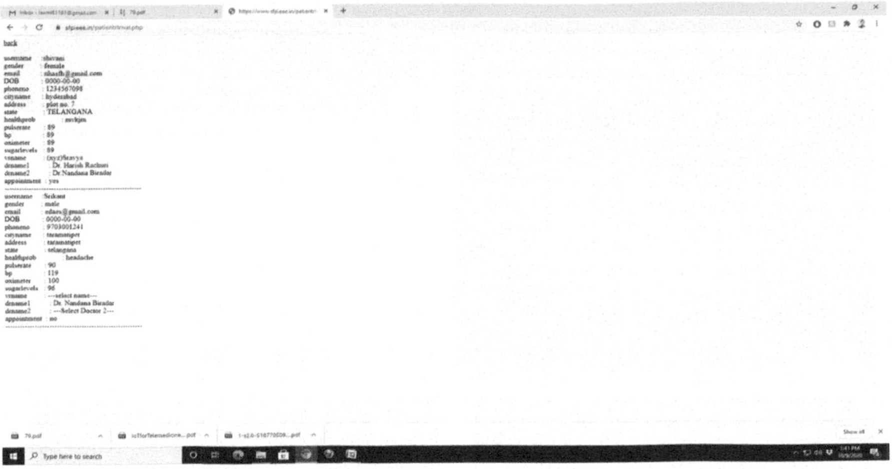
back
username :shivani
gender : female
DOB : 0000-00-00
phoneno : 1234567098
cityname : hyderabad
address : plot no. 7
state : TELANGANA
pulserate : 89
bp : 89
sugarlevels : 89
dname1 : Dr. Harish Rachuri
dname2 : Dr Nandana Biradar
appointment : yes
username :Srikant
gender : male
email : edaes@gmail.com
DOB : 0000-00-00
phoneno : 9703001241
cityname : taramatipet
address : taramatipet
state : telangana
healthprob : headache
pulserate : 90
bp : 119
oximeter : 100
sugarlevels : 96
vtname : ---select name---
dname1 : Dr. Nandana Biradar
dname2 : ---Select Doctor 2---
appointment : no

Fig. 8.9 Database of patient's information

online thereby invoking the Teleambulance system. The deliverable for the same is available in the format given below (Fig. 8.9).

This in turn sends a SMS and email alert to the doctors registered with the website with the information about the vitals of the patient and a link of the patient monitoring page is shared.

The doctor or the care taker in the question could track the location of the patient by the link provided in the index page which provides the information based on live location sharing on Google Maps. However in case of GPRS failure, alternatively the last known location of the patient would be available (Figs. 8.10 and 8.11).

As can be seen in the image below, the all-inclusive IOT kit comprising of non-contact temperature sensor, blood pressure sensor, glucometer, ECG sensor, power backup for the same, and an android tablet for accessing the website and uploading the necessary information was handed over to the PHC of Taramatipet village of Telangana State. The staff deployed at the PHC were provided with training to use the same, i.e., checking the vitals with the sensors and uploading the same in the website along with selection of the registered doctors using the unique IDs assigned to each of them (Fig. 8.12).

8.4 Conclusion

Health of citizens is a serious area of concern for countries around the world, as the reach of healthcare services remains limited due to variety of constraints. Benefits of advancements in medical sciences and related technologies as a result are not available at all. The older population is growing faster in almost all regions of the world. Rural divide in India:

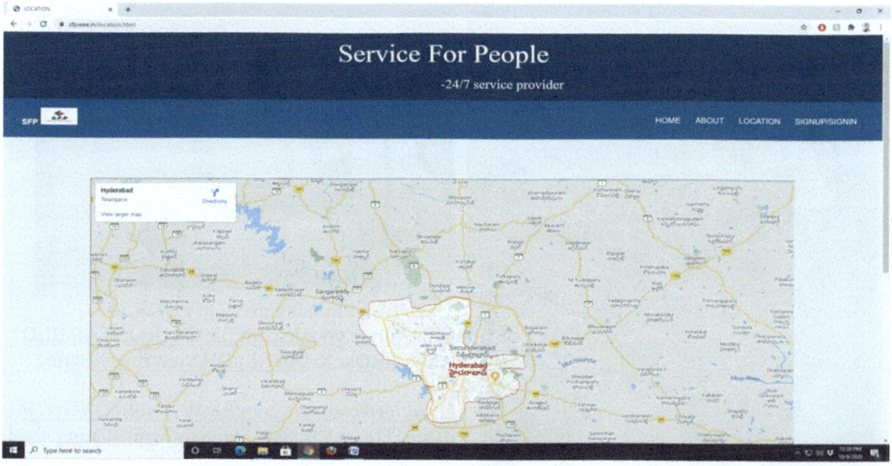

Fig. 8.10 Google maps location during emergency

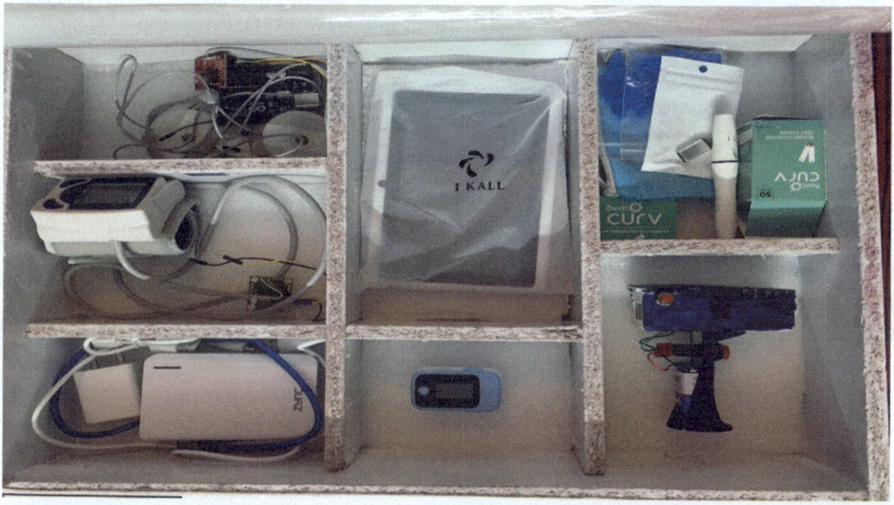

Fig. 8.11 Complete IOT medical kit

- Rural population is spread over 6,40,000 villages.
- About 11% of all episodes in rural areas do not receive healthcare.
- About 12% of people living in rural areas have no access to health facility.

As we are aware about the situation of Covid-19 worldwide, extensive screening is going on worldwide but still we are not able to reach every corner of the world. The situation is still worst in countries with highly populated areas like China, India. At present, good hospitals are available only in urban areas. It is very much required to transform the healthcare with IT. Various aspects of Telemedicine are

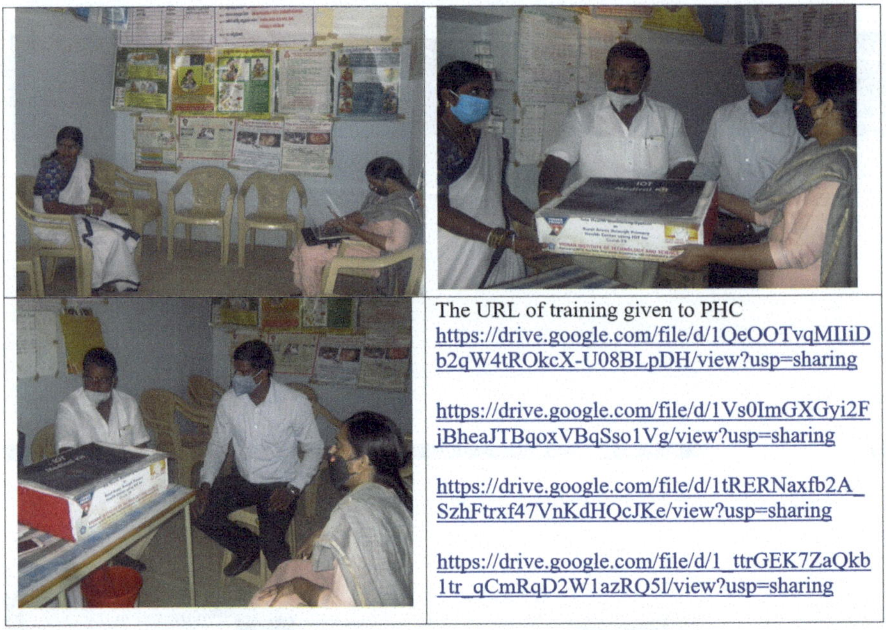

Fig. 8.12 Handing over of IOT medical kit to Taramatipet village PHC

required to provide the health services in the country to bridge the gaps. They will become essential in rural areas where there is a scarcity of doctors and the hospitals. Telehealth monitoring system is an innovative system for improving healthcare system from long distance using IOT. This system creates communication among patients and healthcare professionals. In rural areas, there is Public Health Center (PHC) and in few areas not even one PHC is also not available. Hence it is really difficult to get the treatment of huge number of villagers in rural areas and gather the data. Hence, this system monitors and measures different parameters like pulse, breath rate, oxygen in blood, ECG signals, glucose levels, BP, lung capacity, snore waves, body temperature, etc. using this system. This data is collected and sent to the cloud database in PHC where doctors will monitor the data and able to call for an ambulance in emergency. The project was successfully implemented in Abdullapurmet village of Telangana State. A small handbook is also created in local language Telugu with proper explanation about operation of all devices.

Website Developed: www.sfpieee.in

Bibliography

1. Dimitrov, D. V. (2016). Medical internet of things and big data in healthcare. *Healthcare Informatics Research, 22*(3), 156–163.
2. Kamilaris, A., & Pitsillides, A. (2016). Mobile phone computing and the internet of things: A survey. *IEEE Internet of Things Journal, 3*(6), 885–898.

3. Yu, L., Lu, Y., & Zhu, X. (2012). Smart hospital based on internet of things. *Journal of Networks, 7*(10), 1654–1661.
4. Brown, M. J., Subramanian, A., Curry, T. B., Kor, D. J., Moran, S. L., & Rohleder, T. R. (2014). Improving operating room productivity via parallel anesthesia processing. *International Journal of Health Care Quality Assurance, 27*(8), 697–706.
5. Shini, S., Thomas, T., & Chithraranjan, K. (2012). Cloud-based medical image exchange-security challenges. *Procedia Engineering, 38*, 3454–3461.
6. Alami, H., Gagnon, M.-P., & Fortin, J.-P. (2015). Telehealth in light of cloud computing: Clinical, technological, regulatory and policy issues. *Journal of the International Society for Telemedicine and eHealth, 4*, 5–1.
7. Alamri, A. (2012). Cloud-based e-health multimedia framework for heterogeneous network. In Multimedia and expo workshops (ICMEW), 2012 IEEE international conference on (pp. 447–452). IEEE.
8. Matlani, P., & Londhe, N. D.. (2013). A cloud computing-based telemedicine service. In Point-of-care healthcare technologies (PHT), 2013 IEEE (pp. 326–330). IEEE.
9. Thilakanathan, D., Chen, S., Nepal, S., Calvo, R., & Alem, L. (2014). A platform for secure monitoring and sharing of generic health data in the cloud. *Future Generation Computer Systems, 35*, 102–113.
10. Hossain, M. S., & Muhammad, G. (2016). Cloud-assisted industrial internet of things (IIoT)–enabled framework for health monitoring. *Computer Networks, 101*, 192–202.
11. Stradolini, F., Lavalle, E., De Micheli, G., Ros, P. M., Demarchi, D., & Carrara, S. (2016). Paradigm-shifting players for IoT: Smart-watches for intensive care monitoring. In *International Conference on Wireless Mobile Communication and Healthcare* (pp. 71–78). Springer.
12. Banos, O., Villalonga, C., Damas, M., Gloesekoetter, P., Pomares, H., & Rojas, I. (2014). Physiodroid: Combining wearable health sensors and mobile devices for a ubiquitous, continuous, and personal monitoring. *The Scientific World Journal, 2014.*
13. Rolim, C. O., Koch, F. L., Westphall, C. B., Werner, J., Fracalossi, A., & Salvador, G. S. (2010). A cloud computing solution for patient's data collection in healthcare institutions. In eHealth, telemedicine, and social medicine, 2010. ETELEMED'10. Second international conference on (pp. 95–99). IEEE.
14. Stradolini, F., Riario, S., Boero, C., Baj-Rossi, C., Taurino, I., Surrel, G., De Micheli, G., & Carrara, S. (2015). Wireless monitoring of endogenous and exogenous biomolecules on an android interface. *IEEE Sensors Journal, 16*(9), 3163–3170.
15. Stradolini, F., Tuoheti, A., Ros, P. M., Demarchi, D., & Carrara, S. (2017). Raspberry pi based system for portable and simultaneous monitoring of anesthetics and therapeutic compounds. In CAS (NGCAS), 2017 new generation of (pp. 101–104). IEEE.
16. Seim, A. R., Meyer, M., & Sandberg, W. S. (2005). Does parallel workflow impact anesthesia quality? In AMIA annual symposium proceedings (Vol. 2005, p. 1053). American Medical Informatics Association.
17. Pryv. (2017). e-health data middleware. http://pryv.com/. Accessed 20 November 2017.
18. Sofia Lydia, N., Francesca, S., Abuduwaili, T., Danilo, D., Alkis H.A., & Sandro, C. (2017). Architecture and procedures for ph and temperature monitoring in medical applications. IEEE Sensors Conference.
19. Gutte, A., & Vadali, R. (2018). IoT-based health monitoring system using raspberry Pi. IEEE fourth international conference on computing communication control and automation (ICCUBEA).
20. Chowdary, K. C., Krishna, K. L., Prasad, K. L., & Thejesh, K. (2018). An efficient wireless health monitoring system. Proceedings of the IEEE second international conference on I-SMAC (IoT in social, mobile, analytics and cloud) (I-SMAC).
21. Lavanya, Nivetha, M., Revasree, K., & Sandhiya, K. (2018). Smart chair-a telemedicine-based health monitoring system. In Proceedings of the 2nd international conference on electronics, communication and aerospace technology (ICECA 2018). IEEE conference record.

22. Irmansyah, M., Sution, A. N., Madona, E., & Putra, R. (2018). Low-cost heart rate portable device for risk patients with loT and warning system. International conference on applied information technology and innovation (ICAITI).
23. Patti, E., Donatelli, M., Macii, E., & Acquaviva, A. (2018). IoT software infrastructure for remote monitoring of patients with chronic metabolic disorders. IEEE Computer Society.
24. Pawar, A., & Ghumbre, S. (2017). A survey on IoT applications, security challenges and counter measures. In Proceedings of IEEE international conference on computing, analytics and security trends (CAST).
25. Al-Hamadi, H., & Chen, I. (2017). Trust-based decision making for health IoT systems. *IEEE Internet of Things Journal*, (99).
26. Thakar, A. T., & Pandya, S. (2017). Survey of IoT enables healthcare devices. Proceedings of the IEEE 2017 international conference on computing methodologies and communication (ICCMC).
27. Attila, A., Garai, Á., & Péntek, I. (2016). Common open telemedicine hub and infrastructure with Interface recommendation. 11th IEEE international symposium on applied computational intelligence and informatics.
28. Arduino Architecture. https://www.engineersgarage.com/what-is-gsm-gprs-module
29. Systems design. https://en.wikipedia.org/wiki/Systems_design
30. UML - Standard Diagrams https://www.tutorialspoint.com/uml/uml_standard_diagrams.htm
31. The Internet of Things in healthcare: an overview. https://scholar.google.com/citations?user=Y4opLB8AAAAJ&hl=en
32. Envisioning inclusive futures: technology-based assistive sensory and action substitution. https://www.infona.pl/resource/bwmeta1.element.elsevier-3d45bfdd-fe55-359f-84e4-674a21cae024.
33. A multiple communication standards compatible IoT system for medical usage. http://ieeexplore.ieee.org/document/6577775/?reload=true
34. Ubiquitous data accessing method in IoT-based information system for emergency medical services. https://www.deepdyve.com/lp/institute-of-electrical-and-electronics-engineers/ubiquitousdata-accessing-method-in-iot-based-information-system-for-YCZzyY5W9g
35. Implementation of a medical support system considering P2P and IoT technologies. https://www.computer.org/csdl/proceedings/cisis/2014/4325/00/4325a101-abs.html
36. Acquisition and management of biomedical data using Internet of Things concepts. http://ieeexplore.ieee.org/document/7050625/
37. Secure end-to-end communication for constrained devices in IoT-enabled ambient assisted living systems. https://www.computer.org/csdl/proceedings/wf-iot/2015/0366/00/07389141-abs.html
38. Software Testing. https://en.wikipedia.org/wiki/Software_testing
39. Sensors. https://tkkrlab.nl/wiki/Arduino_37_sensors
40. Amini, A., Chen, W., Fortino, G., Li, Y., Pan, Y, & Wang, M. D. (2020). Editorial Special Issue on AI-driven informatics, sensing, imaging and big data analytics for fighting the COVID-19 pandemic. *IEEE Journal of Biomedical and Health Informatics, 24*(10), 2731–2732.
41. Sameerlyengar, F. T. B., Gravina, R., Guerrieri, A., Fortino, G., & Sangiovanni-Vincentelli, A. L. (2008). A framework for creating healthcare monitoring applications using wireless body sensor networks. *BODYNETS, 2008*, 8.
42. Piccialli, F., Somma, V. D., Giampaolo, F., Cuomo, S., & Fortino, G. (2021). A survey on deep learning in medicine: Why, how and when? *Information Fusion, 66*, 111–137.

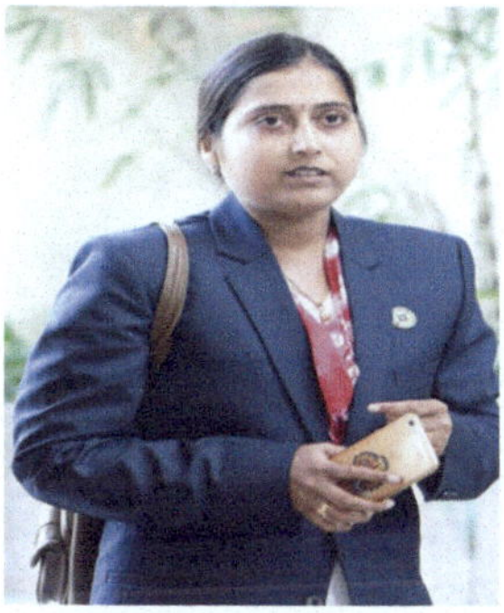

Vijayalaxmi Biradar completed her Doctorate from GITAM Institute of Technology, GITAM University, Vishakapatnam, Andhra Pradesh, India. She received her B.E (E&CE) degree from GNDEC, Visveswaraiah Technological University, Belgaum, Karnataka, India in 2003 and M.Tech (DE&CS) from JNT University, Hyderabad, Telangana, India in 2008. Her area of research is Digital Image Processing. She has published 25 Journal papers, 12 International Conference papers, and 13 National Conference papers. She received Best Paper award in August 2013 in IEEE International conference organized by Saveetha University, Chennai, India. She also received Best Paper Award in Springer Conference ICICSE, 2016 at Hyderabad. She is the Life Member of ISTE and Member of IEEE. She is Past Vice Chair of IEEE WIE AG Hyderabad Section, 2015 and Present Chair of IEEE WIE AG Hyderabad Section, 2016 -17. She received Early Career Research (ECR) grant from Science & Engineering Research Board (SERB), Govt. of India of 26.68 Lakhs, and $3,000 from EPICS in IEEE for the Project Titled "Smart Security System for an Orphanage". Project Investigator for the project selected for final presentation at R10 IEEE HTC 2019 at Depok Indonesia on 12th–14th November, 2019, USD 7,500, "IOT based online Telemedicine system for old age home". Two patent to her credit. She is currently, Senior Member of IEEE, also a member of Control System Society, CIS & GRSS, and also a member of Special Interest Group on Humanitarian Technology (SIGHT). Also member of IEI, PI-Coordinator of Unnat Bharat Abhiyaan (UBA).

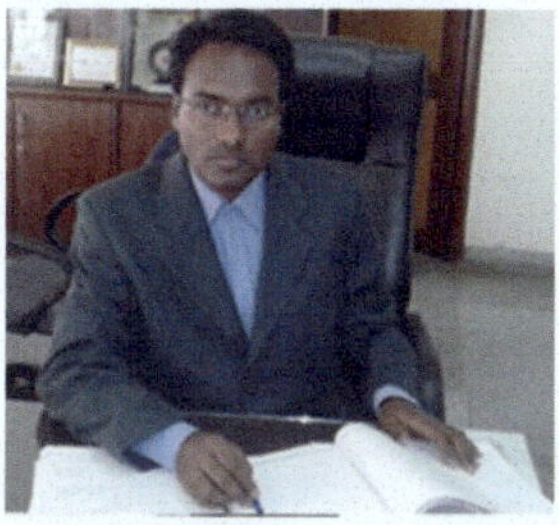

G. Durga Sukumar completed Doctorate in the year 2013 from Indian Institute of Technology (IIT), Roorkee and received 'A' Grade for his thesis from thesis evaluators. He served in various positions during his career as Software Engineer in Complete object solutions, Assistant Professor, and Associate Professor in reputed Engineering colleges. Presently he is working as Principal and Professor at Vignan Institute of Technology and Science, Hyderabad. Currently, he is a Senior Member of IEEE. He is also a member of Power & Energy Society (PES) and also a member of Special Interest Group on Humanitarian Technology (SIGHT). His research areas are Renewable Energy, Solar Energy, Power Electronics & Industrial Drives, Energy Management, and Controller Design. He received research projects from Department of Science and Technology (DST), Govt. of India, titled "Development of Photo Voltaic Solar Panel with Neuro-Fuzzy Control", worth 27.94 L, MNRE Project titled "Development of Energy Management controller-based Inverter with improved PV system fed Organization", worth 74.56 L, and Fund for Improvement of S&T Infrastructure (FIST), worth 50 L.It is worth to mention that there are 25 Publications in Scopus/SCI Indexed Journals, 12 IEEE, and other International/National Conference papers during his career. Presently he is guiding six Research Scholars, of which two students have completed their Doctorates. He actively engages research scholars in scholarly work and mentoring has resulted in publications at various International/National conferences and Journals. One patent to his credit titled **"Intelligent Embedded Priority based Energy Management System and method" in April 2018.**

Chapter 9
Artificial Intelligence for Disease Identification and Diagnosis

A. Lakshmi Muddana, Krishna Keerthi Chennam, and V. Revathi

9.1 Introduction to Medical Data Processing

Data is crucial in finding a solution to any problem. It plays a fundamental role in identifying diseases, finding causes of diseases, and treatment. Increased computational power, low storage costs, and availability of internet have driven the health center to maintain electronic health records. Advancements in medical devices and advances in data analytics led to the application of AI techniques in healthcare in detection and prognosis of diseases. Different types of cancer, heart-related diseases, and epidemics like Covid-19 [1], are leading causes of patient suffering and death. Early diagnosis and detection are crucial to prevent deterioration of patient health and mortality.

AI has driven advances in many fields including finance, agriculture, computer vision, e-commerce, driver less cars, voice-activated personal assistants, and healthcare. Medical data are in the form of medical notes, electronic health records, data from medical devices, lab test results, and images [2]. Data are available in both structured form like images, gene expression, and unstructured form like clinical notes. Application of AI techniques on medical data processing can (1) Uncover clinically relevant information hidden in massive amounts of data that can give health risk alerts and health outcome predictions, (2) Can reduce errors that are inevitable in human clinical practice, (3) More accurate and reliable information to doctors in disease identification and treatment, (4) Reduces manual work and subjectiveness,

A. L. Muddana (✉) · V. Revathi (✉)
GITAM University, Hyderabad, India
e-mail: amuddana@gitam.edu; rvankaya@gitam.edu

K. K. Chennam
Muffakham Jah College of Engineering and Technology, Hyderabad, India
e-mail: krishna.keerthi@mjcollege.ac.in

P. Siarry et al. (eds.), *The Fusion of Internet of Things, Artificial Intelligence, and Cloud Computing in Health Care*, Internet of Things,
https://doi.org/10.1007/978-3-030-75220-0_9

(5) Can find patterns from large scale data to predict the outbreak of pandemics, and (6) AI can combine data from different sources like medical records, radiology images, genome sequence, fitness band data to create personalized treatment plans.

Challenges of medical data processing include (1) Small datasets because data are not stored or due to privacy reasons, (2) Unbalanced datasets in case of cancer and rare diseases, (3) Unavailability of labeled data as labeling is time-consuming and requires doctors with a specialized skill set, (4) Subjectivity in identifying the diseases that hinders decision making, (5) Variability in patients environment and genes.

Medical data can use:

1. Supervised learning methods for building predictive models.
2. Unsupervised learning methods as preprocessing steps for feature extraction, dimensionality reduction, and to identify subgroups before sending to predictive models.
3. Deep learning methods require large amounts of labeled data [3]. But unlabeled data are available in abundance. Semisupervised approach uses a combination of supervised and unsupervised methods when labels or outcomes are missing in the instances of the datasets [4].

AI techniques for medical data processing can be categorized into

1. Machine learning methods like Support vector machines, K-Nearest Neighbors, Ensemble methods that take patients disease history, gene expressions, diagnostic results, clinical symptoms, medication, disease indicators in building the models for disease identification, and diagnosis [5].
2. Deep learning methods that build neural networks to capture nonlinear relationships. It can uncover nonlinear patterns in the data. Popular neural networks are Convolution neural networks for medical Images analysis and LSTM models for sequence data processing.

AI in healthcare is used to support decision making in disease prevention, control, and personalized treatment. It is critical in ensuring that doctors focus on cases that truly matters and leaving the routine ones to the machine. Physicians cannot be replaced by machines but can assist them to make better clinical decisions with more accuracy.

Some of the popular healthcare solutions using AI are IBM Watson Health, Google DeepMind that help in cancer diagnosis, predicting patient outcomes, averting blindness, etc. Ancora Medical that helps in cancer treatment, CloudMedx Health to extract data from electronic health records and outputs clinical insights for healthcare professionals [6].

9.2 Preprocessing Techniques

The dataset needs some sort of initial processing before giving as input to the model, called preprocessing. It is a crucial step in model building so that meaningful insights are drawn from the data. Different preprocessing methods are normalizing data, handling categorical features, handling missing data, handling label noise, elimination of outliers, etc.

Feature scaling: Some of the machine learning methods use gradient descent algorithm as an optimization technique. This algorithm requires the feature ranges to be on a similar scale for fast convergence. Also distance-based methods like K-Nearest Neighbors, K-Means use distance between the data points to measure the similarity. Hence, feature values are to be brought to similar scale. Popular feature scaling techniques are:

Normalization: Feature values are scaled down to the range of 0–1. This is a preferred method if the machine learning algorithm makes no assumption about the data distribution.

Standardization: Feature values are scaled such that the mean is 0 and standard deviation is 1. This method is helpful when the underlying data is normally distributed and also not affected by outliers.

Feature clipping: Sometimes dataset may have outliers. Specify, minimum and maximum values for the features so that values outside minimum and maximum specified are clipped to specified minimum and maximum. Another preprocessing step required in neural networks is to convert categorical data into numerical data since strings will not be converted to float by neural network and may generate error during model fitting.

Batch normalization normalizes inputs to each layer of the neural network.

This results in faster convergence and also provides a bit of regularization.

9.2.1 Handling Missing Data

Some values of the features may not be available in the dataset called missing data or null values. Missing data arise due to data corruption, communication errors, malfunctioning of devices, accidental clicks, and in some cases, data may not be specified deliberately like religion or age of a person [7].

Missing data can be categorized into [8, 9].

1. Missing Completely At Random (MCAR): Where missingness is not related to any characteristics of the dataset like material loss.
2. Missing At Random (MAR): The data are dependent on another feature, which is missing, e.g., Creatine value is dependent on a urine sample, which was missing.
3. Missing Not At Random (MNAR): Data value is missing and is related to the reason for its missing intentionally, e.g., age of female, income of person deliberately not specified.

Missing values will weaken the model by introducing bias. Handling missing data plays an important role in medical datasets since complete datasets produce robust models. Hence, missing values are handled as a preprocessing step before giving the dataset as input to the model.

Methods for handling missing data are [10].

1. **Deletion:** Remove the data based on the proportion of missing values. Deletion can be applied on a row or column, or both. Applying on row deletes the entire observation that has one or more missing values. This may be done when missing data is limited to a small number of observations but may result in producing biased estimates. Dropping the variable or attribute is preferred when more than 60% of values are missing, and the variable is insignificant.
2. **Imputation:**Imputation is estimating the missing value. This can be done by
   (a) Using a measure of central tendency like mean, median for continuous data, and mode for categorical data.
   (b) Use machine learning algorithms like KNN, XGBoost, Random forests to impute the missing values. KNN is widely used which can predict both discrete and continuous values.

9.2.2 Handling Noisy Labels

Data labeling is expensive and time-consuming as knowledge experts are required for labeling. In real-world scenarios, labels may also go wrong sometimes and the reasons may be.

1. The available information is insufficient due to poor quality data.
2. Experts often make mistakes during labeling.
3. Incorrect labels may come from communication or encoding problems. Real-world databases are estimated to contain around 5% of encoding errors.
4. Mistakes made during data entry.
5. Annotators may give incorrect labels when part of disease symptoms are given.
6. Variability in interpretation by experts.

   Label noise is different from outliers and feature noise. Label noise in training data decreases performance and increases complexity in learning.

   Methods to handle label noise are:

1. Use label noise-robust models like AdaBoost, naive Bayes, and random forest rather than decision tress and support vector machine.
2. Use data cleansing methods to remove mislabeled samples by outlier detection, anomaly detection, and voting filtering.
3. Use Label noise-tolerant learning algorithms that use prior information to detect like Bayesian prior, beta priors, Hidden Markov, Graphical methods, and probabilistic models.
4. Reduce the label noise in training data. Instead of giving large data with label noise for training, select small data with correct labels, and then apply predictions on it. Then voting of ensemble classifiers can be applied.

Carla E. Brodley [11] used filtering of data for wrong label identification before training the model. Aritra Ghosh [12] introduced noise tolerance risk minimization procedures with different loss functions like sigmoid loss, ramp loss, etc. to deal with label noise. Identification of mislabeled samples is done by Jeremy Speth [13], introducing multilabel identification. Wang et al [14] introduced an iterative learning framework for addressing the label noise issue by three steps including iterative label noise detection, discriminative feature learning and reweighting. Nithika Nigam [15] conducted a survey on different methods to deal with label noise in deep learning algorithms and statistical methods used in nondeep learning methods like bagging and voting mechanism.

Perona et al. [16] discussed Image denoising methods related to partial differential equations (PDEs), Rudin et al. [17] proposed variation-based image restoration with free local constraints, Domain transformations such as wavelets by Coifman [18], DCT method by Yaroslavsky [19], BLS-GSM by Portilla [20]. L Gondara [21] discussed nonlocal techniques including NL-means [22] reviewed different denoising algorithms. Dabov [23] proposed different domain transformations like BM3D. Models exploiting sparse coding techniques are mentioned in [24–26]. Vincent [27] discussed different ways for Extracting and composing robust features with denoising autoencoders.

9.3 Methods to Handle Unbalanced Datasets

The majority of medical datasets are unbalanced. Most of the Machine learning algorithms are designed to perform well when the number of samples in each class are nearly equal. Popular algorithms for balancing numerical datasets are SMOTE, MSMOTE.

SMOTE algorithm is applied on two cancer datasets [28] having features characterizing cell nuclei of the tumor. Dataset1 (Wisconsin) has 30 features computed from digitized image of fine needle aspirate of a breast mass, Dataset2 with 9 features describing the breast tumor characteristics and labels that indicate benign or malignancy of the tumor. Both the datasets have imbalanced classes. Datasets contained 16 null values in bare. Nuclei feature and was replaced by mean value of that feature. As the range of values of the features varies, the features were normalized in both the datasets. Datasets also exhibit class imbalance as shown in Table 9.1. Different methods are available for balancing the imbalanced datasets like Up-sampling and Down-sampling. As the dataset size is small, up-sampling is applied using the SMOTE algorithm. The algorithm synthesizes the samples by taking k-nearest neighbors of the randomly picked minority samples. The resultant datasets after applying SMOTE algorithm are shown in Table 9.2.

Table 9.1 Breast cancer datasets

DataSets	No of features	No. of samples with malignancy	No. of normal samples	Total number of samples
DataSet1	30	212	357	569
DataSet2	9	241	458	699

Table 9.2 Dataset after up-sampling

DataSets	No. of samples with malignancy	No. of normal samples	Total number of samples
DataSet1	357	357	714
DataSet2	458	458	916

9.4 Handling Small Datasets

Typically, real-world medical datasets are small in size and may have a large number of features. This could be due to the nonrecording of patient information, few instances in rare diseases, privacy issues, etc [29, 30]. This challenge needs to be addressed for the model to be accurate and robust. This challenge can be handled using different machine learning techniques like regularization, data augmentation, transfer learning, etc.

9.4.1 Regularization Techniques

One of the factors for poor model performance overfitting. It occurs when the model performs well on training data but performs poorly on the unseen test data.

Methods to combat the overfitting problem are

[font = red!50!black] Reduce the features of the dataset. But it may not be the right choice as it may result in the loss of useful information. Collect more data to increase the dataset size to train the model. But it may not always be possible to collect more data. Perform **Data Augmentation** to create new examples from existing examples of the dataset so as to in increasing dataset size. During the training process, as the number of iterations in training increase, train loss and validation loss decrease. But after some point, validation performance decreases. Stop training the model at this point called **Early stopping**.

Regularization penalizes the parameters taking large values and avoids overfitting. Different regularization techniques are

[font = red!50!black] **L1 regularization** is also called Lasso regression, where the sum of absolute values of a coefficient is added as a penalty term to the loss function. It shrinks the coefficient towards zero and discourages learning complex models to avoid overfitting. **L2** regularization is also called ridge regression, where sum of squares of the coefficient is added to the loss function. **Dropout**

regularization is used in deep learning. In each iteration of training, some nodes of the neural network are randomly made inactive. This results in having a different set of nodes in each iteration giving different outputs. It penalizes the weight matrices of nodes. Smaller weight matrices lead to simpler models and reduce overfitting.

9.4.2 Data Augmentation

In deep learning models, the neural network contains many layers to model complex relations in the data. Deep networks have more neurons in hidden layers creating a large number of trainable parameters, which require large datasets. Medical datasets are small in size due to the unavailability of recorded information. To handle the small size datasets, apply transformations on the available data to synthesize new data points, called data augmentation.

For the model to generalize well, the dataset size should be big enough and have variations in the data. Train the model with synthetically modified data to get better performance. Data augmentation can address the issues of diversity of data, amount of data, and also solve class imbalance issues. It is applied as a preprocessing step before applying the learning algorithm called off-line data augmentation, which is preferred for small datasets. Online data augmentation performs translation on a mini-batch, which is preferred for large datasets.

Data augmentation can be applied to different data forms like numerical, image, and text. Popular numerical data augmentation techniques are SMOTE and MSMOTE, which are already discussed in Sect. 9.3.

Image data augmentation: In real-world scenarios, images might have been taken under different conditions like different locations, orientations, scale, and brightness. Image data augmentation can be done by applying transformations on images like geometric transformations, color space transformations. Geometric transformations include rotation, flipping, scaling, and cropping. Flipping should be done carefully on medical data sets. For example, in chest X-ray if we perform a flip, then heart position will change from left to right which can yield to the case of dextrocardia. Rotation of image may result in a change of dimensions and need to be resized. Color space transformations like color casting, varying brightness, noise injection, etc. used when challenges are connected to the lighting of images [31, 32]. Image data augmentation is useful in computer vision tasks like object detection, image classification, image segmentation, etc. (Figs. 9.1, 9.2, 9.3, and 9.4).

These transformations may lead to changes in the image geometry and the image may lose its original features. This can be overcome with modern techniques like Generative Adversarial networks (GAN), neural style transfer that perform more realistic transformations.

GAN is a deep learning-based generative modeling approach to generate new images from available images. The model consists of two submodels. Generators submodel learns patterns in input and generate new images. A random vector is

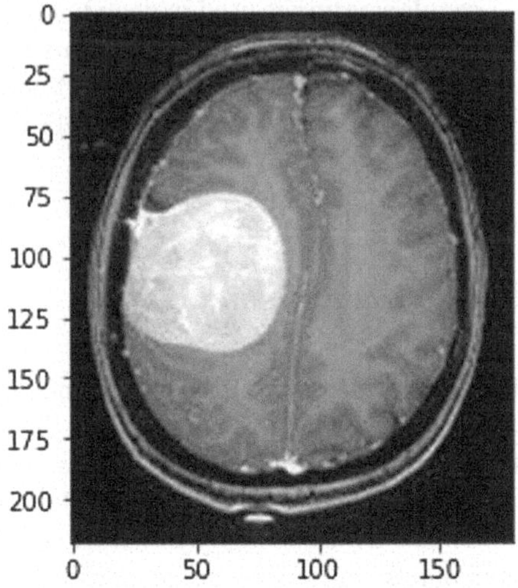

Fig. 9.1 BrainTumor sample image

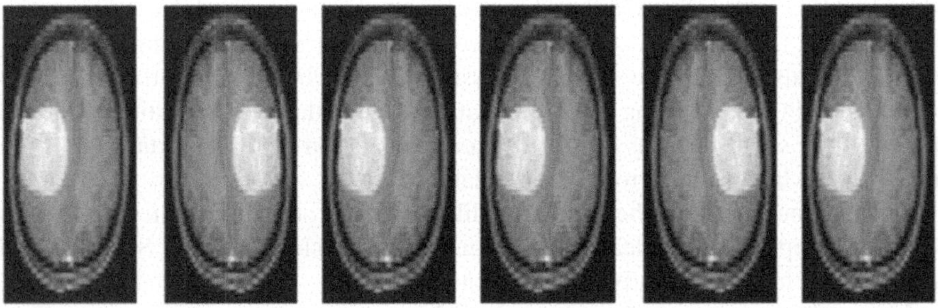

Fig. 9.2 After horizontal shift

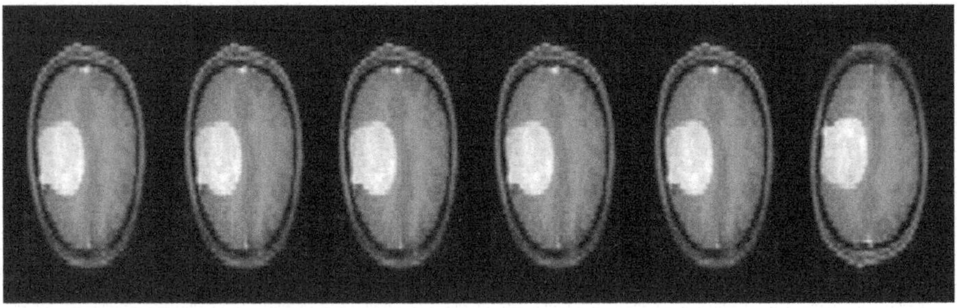

Fig. 9.3 After vertical shift

drawn from Gaussian distribution and is used as a seed in the generative process. The generated images look very similar to real images from the domain. The discriminative submodel classifies whether a given image is a real or generated one [33–35]. Popular use cases of GAN are filling images from the outline, converting

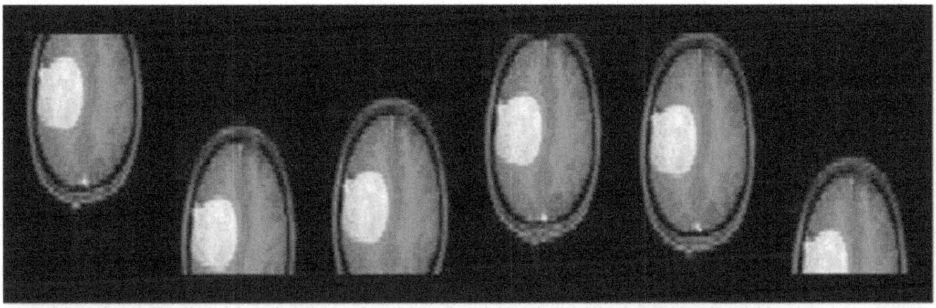

Fig. 9.4 After height shift

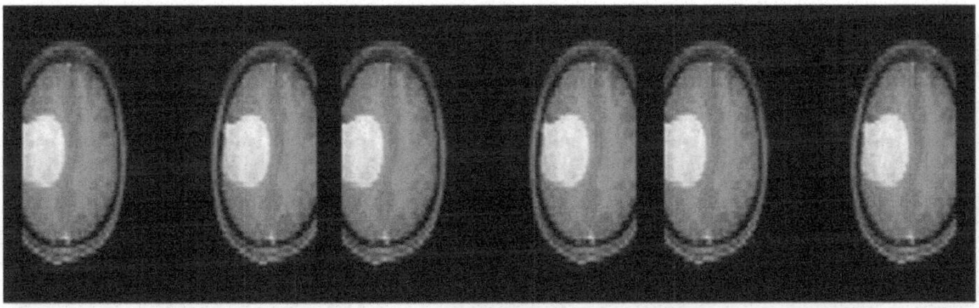

Fig. 9.5 After width shift

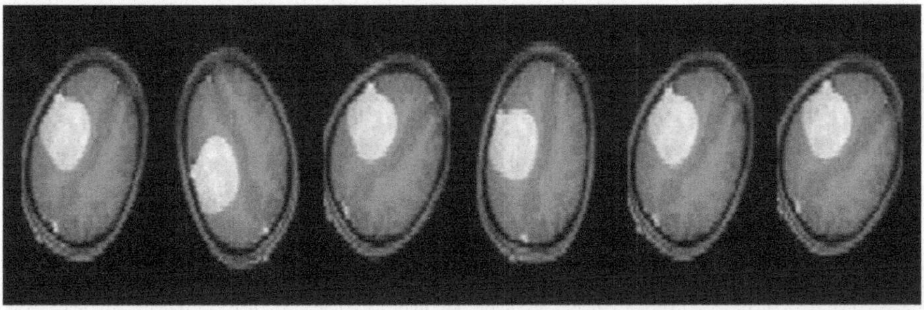

Fig. 9.6 After rotation

black and white images to color, and photo realistic depictions of product prototypes. In medical images, discriminator is used as regularizer or discriminator for abnormal images.

Neural Style Transfer (NST): New image is generated by taking the content of one image (content image) and style of another image (style image). The generated image looks like a new image. The image looks more artistic than realistic (Figs. 9.5, 9.6, 9.7, and 9.8).

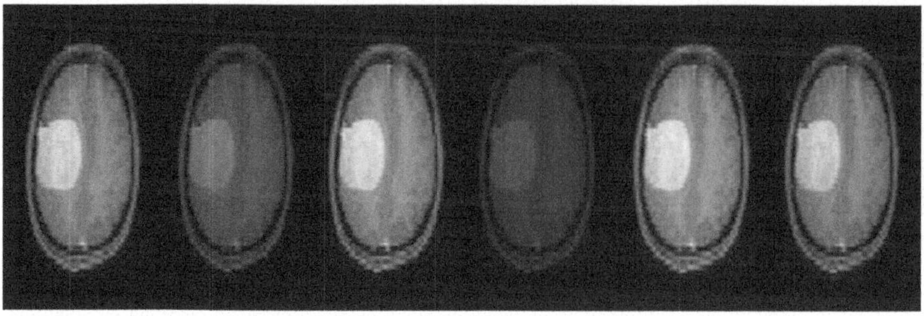

Fig. 9.7 After brightness effect

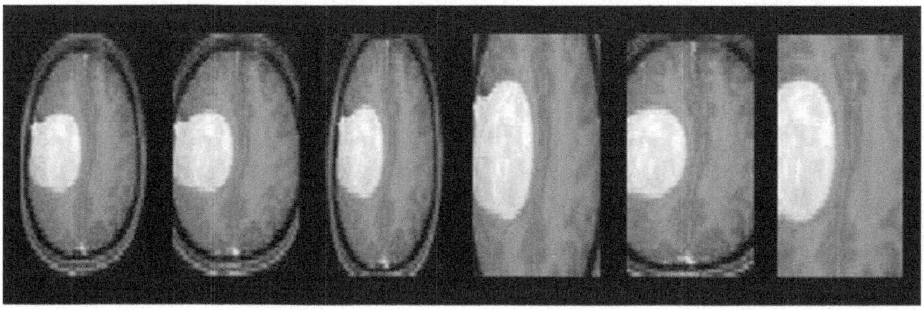

Fig. 9.8 After applying zoom effect

9.4.3 Transfer Learning

CNN can learn complex mappings when trained on enough data. Medical datasets are typically small in size. Training deep neural networks on small datasets results in overfitting. When we train deep neural networks on an image dataset, the first few layers of convnet recognize horizontal and vertical lines and colors. The next few layers learn simple shapes and colors using the features learned in previous layers. Subsequent layers try to learn parts of an object. The last layers recognize whole objects and perform classification. In any convolutional neural networks, other than the last few layers, the layers learn basic features. Using the pretrained model and replacing only the last few layers result in saving training time and computational power required. Deep learning networks take long training time on large datasets. Models like VGG, ResNet, InceptionNet are trained on benchmark datasets with millions of examples and thousands of classes. These top-performing models are made available and platforms like Keras provide libraries to reuse them [36]. Goal of Transfer Learning is to learn from related classification tasks for relevant data by identifying various types of abnormalities [37]. Transfer learning in Medical Imaging can be done by using two types (1) Same domain different task: The easiest method is to use learning from various tasks in similar domains. (2) Different

Table 9.3 Model performance using transfer learning

DataSet	Model	Train accuracy	Validation accuracy	Train loss	Validation loss
Covid-19 Chest X-ray with transfer learning	VGG16 (classifier)	1	1	0.0042	0.0013
Covid-19 Chest X-ray with transfer learning	VGG16 (freez 10 layers)	0.9889	1	0.022	0.0018
Brain tumor with transfer learning	VGG16 (classifier)	0.9802	0.9841	0.1003	0.0924
Brain tumor with transfer learning	VGG16 (freez 10 layers)	0.8063	0.8181	0.4213	0.4047

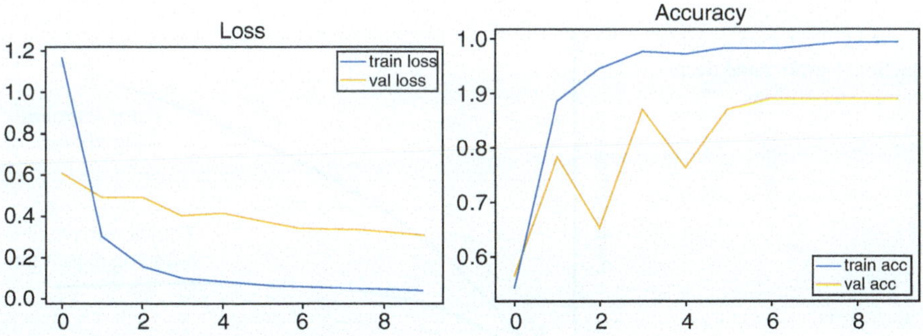

Fig. 9.9 Loss and accuracy curves for Covid−19 chest x-ray

domains same task: Initial start point is identified and then network tuned for the final task [38, 39]. Using pretrained models brings the benefit of decreased training time and results in lower generalization error.

Transfer learning can be used as:

(a) Classifier where pretrained model is downloaded and new image is input to predict the class.
(b) Can be used as a feature extractor. Layers prior to the output layer can be used as input to the layers of the new model. Take layers of pretrained models, freeze them and add new layers on top of these to train on the new small dataset. Pretrained weights are used as initial weights to the new model and continue learning on the new dataset.

Table 9.3 shows the model performance after applying transfer learning (a) as a classifier, (b) freezing 10 layers of VGG16 model, on two datasets Covid-19 chest X-ray images and Brain tumor images. Figures 9.9 and 9.10 show Loss and Accuracy curves, on Covid-19 Chest X-ray dataset, before and after transfer learning.

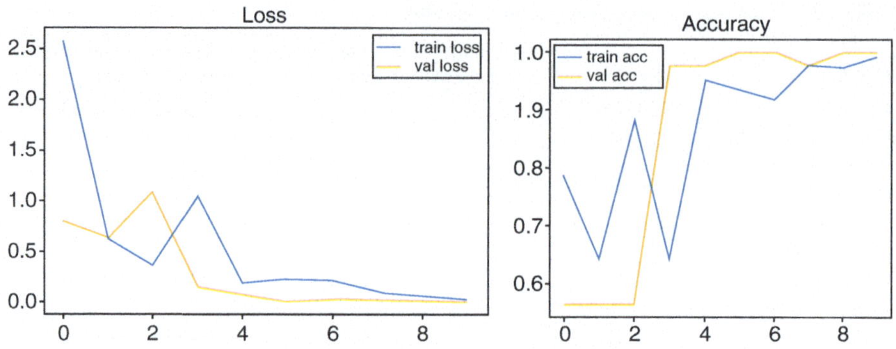

Fig. 9.10 Loss and accuracy curves for Covid−19 chest X-ray after transfer learning

Fig. 9.11 Performance of machine learning and deep learning algorithms

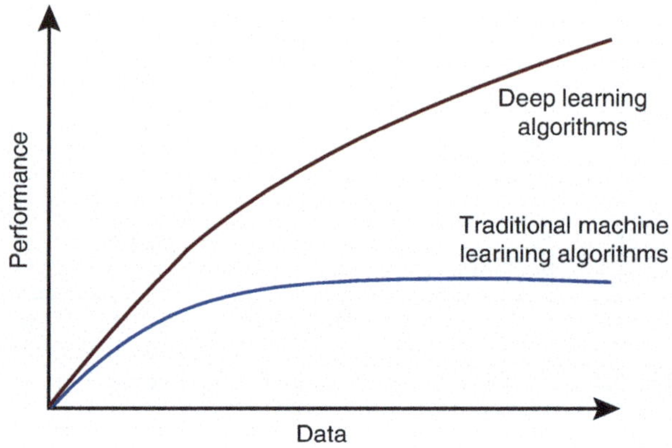

9.5 Deep Learning Techniques

Traditional machine learning algorithms like Logistic Regression, Decision Trees, K-NN, and SVM can make use of the volume of data to some extent. Their performance will not improve further even if more data are available, as depicted in Fig. 9.11.

Deep learning techniques can make use of voluminous data by building complex model to learn nonlinear relationship among data. With lot of activities being digitized, like electronic health records, data are recorded and made available. This large amount of data can be utilized using deep learning methods to give more accuracy compared to machine learning methods. Deep learning algorithms are inspired by the structure and functioning of the human brain called artificial neural networks. Different Deep learning applications in healthcare are, detecting and diagnosing cancer cells, disease prediction and treatment, drug discovery, precision medicine, identifying health insurance fraud, etc [40].

Different neural network architectures are

[font = red!50!black]Feed forward neural networks (FNN), Convolutional neural networks (CNN), for image input like MRI images, X-rays, CT-scans. Recurrent neural networks (RNN), for sequence data like text, audio, time series data.

9.5.1 Autoencoders

Autoencoder is a type of neural network used for unsupervised learning where the dataset contains few labels or no labels. It encodes input data to some hidden representation and then decodes backward to original form. Autoencoder consists of three parts:

[font = red!50!black]**Encoder** that maps input data to hidden or compressed representation. **Bottleneck** layer represents compressed representation of input. Decoder that maps hidden representation back to original data as losslessly as possible by minimizing Reconstruction loss function.
Autoencoder performs nonlinear transformation to learn abstract features using neural networks. Classification or regression can then be applied on latent features.

Autoencoder architectures may include:

[font = red!50!black]Simple Feed Forward Networks Convolutional autoencoders that contain convolutional encoding and decoding layers to process image input. It is better suited for image processing for Image reconstruction, Image colorization, Latent space clustering, and Generating high resolution images. LSTM networks for sequence data.

Use cases of autoencoders are data compression, image denoising, dimensionality reduction and feature selection, and extraction ignoring noise. So it works well for correlated input features.

Autoencoders are built, with the following architecture, on Covid-19 chest X-ray dataset having 181 train images and 56 test images as shown in Table 9.4.

Table 9.4 Covid-19 chest X-ray dataset having 181 train images and 56 test images

Layer (type)	Outshape	Param
input5(*InputLayer*)	[(None, 240, 240, 3)]	0
conv2d18(*Conv2D*)	(None, 240, 240, 32)	896
max*pooling2d8*(*MaxPooling*2)	(None, 120, 120, 32)	0
(Conv2D)19	(None, 120, 120, 32)	9248
up*sampling2d8*(*UpSampling*2)	(None, 120, 120, 32)	0
conv2d21(*Conv2D*)	(None, 120, 120, 32)	9248
up*sampling2d9*(*UpSampling*2)	(None, 240, 240, 32)	0
conv2d22(*Conv2D*)	(None, 240, 240, 3)	867

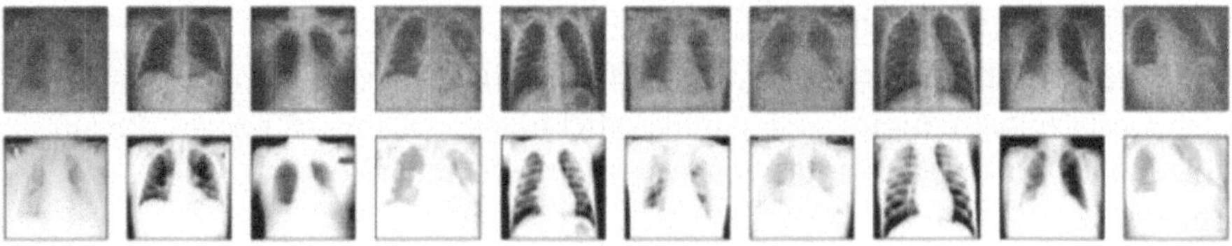

Fig. 9.12 Eliminated denoised output image of autoencoder

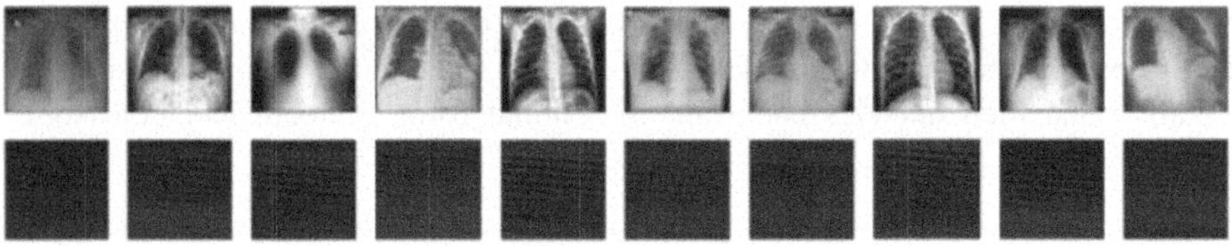

Fig. 9.13 Latent feature learning using autoencoder

Table 9.5 Model performance on breast cancer datasets using Machine learning algorithms

DataSets	Logistic regression	Logistic regression	SVM	SVM
	Train accuracy	Test accuracy	Train accuracy	Test accuracy
DataSet1	97.51	98.39	97.89	98.39
DataSet2	96.96	97.29	98.15	97.34

Total params: 29,507
Trainable params: 29,507
Nontrainable params: 0

Following is the output when autoencoder is used for denoising in Fig. 9.12 and latent feature learning using autoencoder as shown in Fig. 9.13

9.5.2 Neural Networks for Medical Datasets

Logistic regression and SVM models are rebuilt on the two up-sampled Breast cancer datasets described in Sect. 9.3, which shows the performance of the machine learning algorithms as shown in Table 9.5.

To improve the performance, a semisupervised learning technique can be adopted. Feature learning was applied using autoencoders to determine latent features. Autoencoder was tuned with different optimizers and mini batch sizes. Low loss was obtained with RMSPROP optimizer with batch size of 16 and trained for 100 epochs.

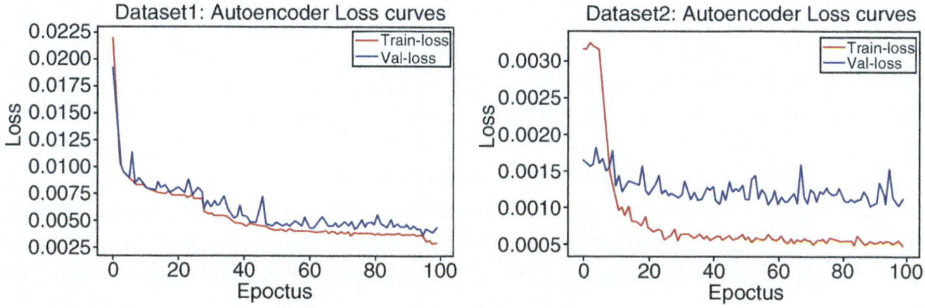

Fig. 9.14 Loss curves of autoencoder on breast cancer datasets

Table 9.6 Model performance on breast cancer using neural networks

DataSets	Feed forward neural network	Feed forward neural network
DataSets	Train accuracy	Test accuracy
DataSet1	99.81	98.88
DataSet2	98.98	99.12

Loss curves as depicted in Fig. 9.14, show good performance of the autoencoder. On the learned features of up-sampled data, the Feed forward Neural network classifier model was built. Neural network was tuned with different optimizers, batch sizes and number of hidden layers. Good train accuracy, test accuracy, and low variance were achieved with ADAM optimizer, nine hidden layers, and mini batch size of 16. The accuracy measures on train and test data are shown in Table 9.6.

Semisupervised learning using autoencoders for latent feature learning on Up-sampled data and neural network model for binary classifier has shown good performance. This gives good train, test accuracy, and could reduce the variance to less than 1% in both the datasets.

9.5.3 Convolutional Neural Networks (CNN)

Deep learning architectures are popular for image tasks. CNN is a type of deep neural network used for image input to perform feature extraction, classification, finding patterns, and in other computer vision tasks [37]. Applications include object detection, object classification, driverless vehicles, etc. Convolutional networks eliminate manual feature extraction and automatically detect important features of an image. CNN has a sequence of layers where each layer of the network detects different features of the image. The output of each layer is input to the next layer. It performs a series of convolution and pooling operations followed by fully connected layers. Convolution layer performs convolution operation that merges two sets of information like image and convolution filter, which produces a feature map. The input image is put through filters that activate certain features of images. The convolution operation is followed by pooling to reduce the dimension and number of parameters. This reduces training time and avoids overfitting. Commonly used pooling methods are maximum or average pooling.

Each neuron in the network takes inputs from previous layer neurons, applies activation function to produce output, which then becomes an input to next layer neurons. The activation function introduces nonlinearity into the output of neurons. Nonlinear activations perform transformations on an input to learn complex relationships. Popular Activation functions are Relu, Sigmoid, Tanh. Visualizing intermediate layers output on Covid-19 Chest X-Ray dataset is shown in Fig. 9.15.

Two Convolutional networks were built to classify Covid-19 Chest X-Ray dataset. Model 1 is a simple network with one convolution and max pooling layer. Model 2 is a deep network with three blocks of convolution and pooling layers. The model was fine-tuned on different optimizers. SGD / RMSProp found to be performing well with less variance is shown in Table 9.7. Loss and accuracy curves are shown in Figs. 9.16 and 9.17.

9.6 Open Research Problems

Methods to integrate complete data of patients like clinical notes, test values, disease indicators of patients, gene expression data, and medical images are required, to develop a comprehensive model. Such models can accurately predict diseases and help in personalized treatment.

Not many datasets are available on various diseases. There is a need for developing datasets on different diseases and make them available for research. Researchers need to build Generative models to perform more realistic transformations on medical images to increase the dataset size than simple data augmentation methods. This helps in developing complex models on small datasets and to avoid overfitting.

Many medical datasets are small in size. Use of pretrained models helps when the dataset size is small and new models can be built on these for faster training on new problems. Open source high-performing models like VGG, InceptionNet, ResNet on medical image datasets are needed which can be used for transfer learning.

Label noise in medical datasets significantly impacts the predictions and in supporting decision making. Focus is required in developing the methods to identify and handle label noise in medical datasets.

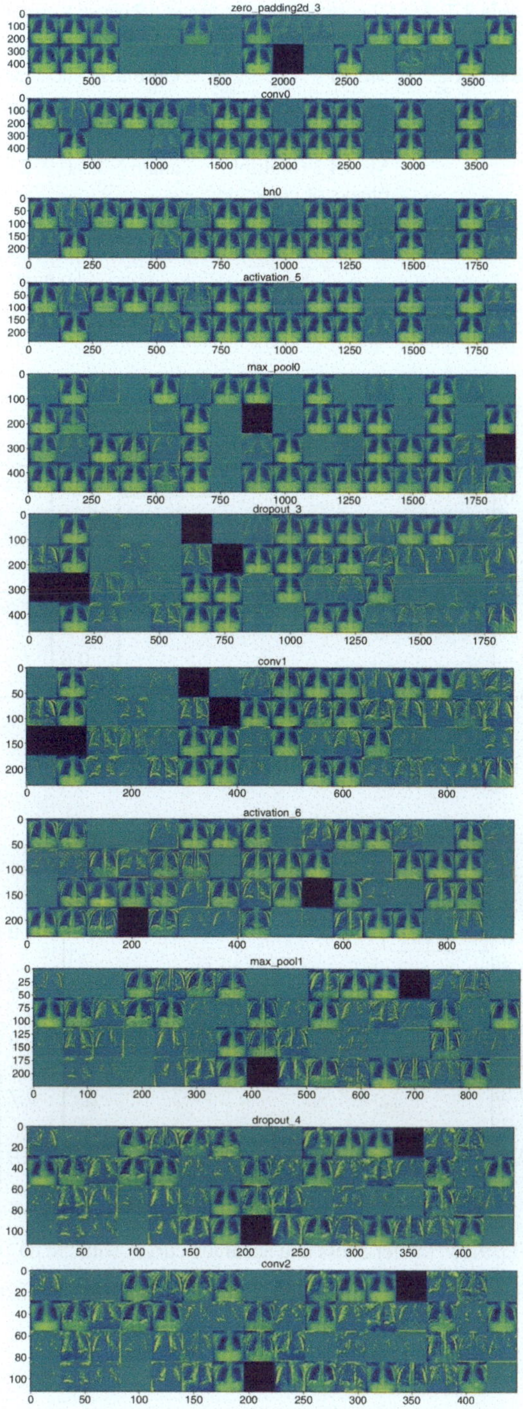

Fig. 9.15 Visualization of intermediate layers of covid-19 chest X-ray

Table 9.7 Model performance on covid-19 chest X-ray using CNN

DataSet	Model	Optimizer	Train accuracy	Validation accuracy	Train loss	Validation loss
Covid-19 Chest X-ray	Model 1 (one layer)	adam	0.9944	0.8913	0.0357	0.3068
	Model 2 (multiple blocks of conv and pooling layers)	adam	0.9723	0.913	0.1121	0.245
		sgd	0.9889	0.9782	0.0629	0.1791
		sgd	0.9889	0.9782	0.0629	0.1791
		adagrad	0.9944	0.8478	0.032	0.30144

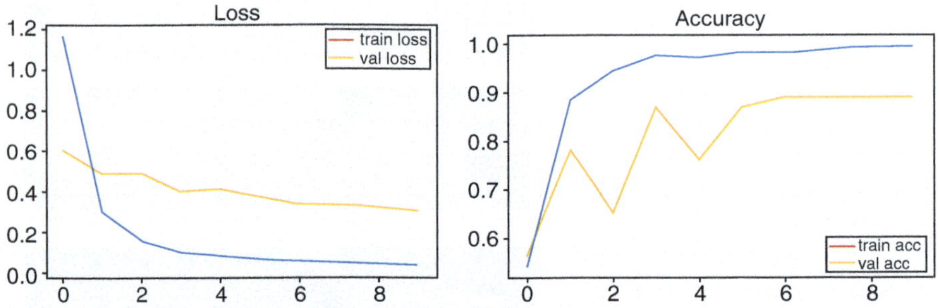

Fig. 9.16 Loss and accuracy curves of model 1

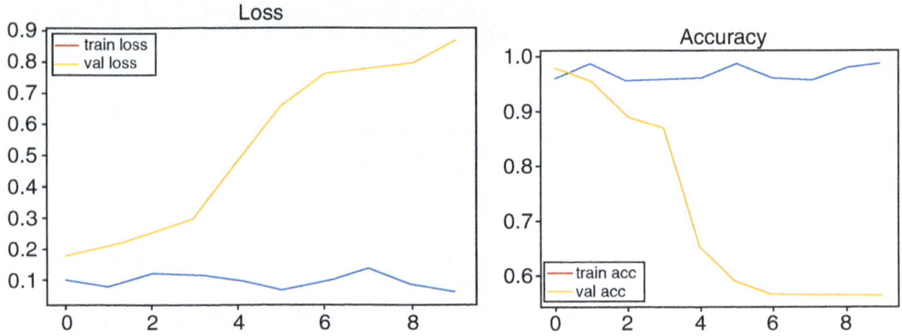

Fig. 9.17 Model 2 loss and accuracy curves with "SGD" optimizer

9.7 Future Scope

Deep learning models results in more accuracy when trained on large datasets. As real-world medical datasets are typically small, datasets can be augmented with more realistic images using generative models. GAN architecture and its performance on medical datasets can be discussed in the future work. Reinforcement learning techniques can be explored on medical datasets, in progressive decision making of disease diagnosis.

9.8 Conclusion

The chapter discusses the challenges in medical data processing for detecting and diagnosing diseases. The challenges include small datasets, missing data, and unbalanced datasets. Various methods to deal with the challenges like imputing missing data, increasing the dataset size using data augmentation techniques, Transfer learning using predefined models like VGG, ResNet, InceptioNet, and regularization methods are discussed. These methods are applied on medical datasets and the results are presented. Neural network models on two cancer datasets are built and the results are presented. Convolution network architectures for classifying medical image datasets to predict diseases like Covid-19 and Brain Tumor are presented. Autoencoders are built for image denoising, dimensionality reduction, and feature extractions to improve the model performance are presented on cancer datasets. The chapter concludes with open research problems and future scope to be explored in utilizing AI to provide robust healthcare solutions.

References

1. Amini, A., Chen, W., Fortino, G., Li, Y., Pan, Y. & Wang, M. D. (2020). Editorial: Special issue on AI-driven informatics, sensing, imaging and big data analytics for fighting the covid-19 pandemic. *IEEE Journal of Biomedical and Health Informatics, 24*(10).
2. Iyengar, S., Bonda, F. T., Gravina, R., Guerrieri, A., Fortino, G., & Sangiovanni Vincentelli, A., 2008, March. A framework for creating healthcare monitoring applications using wireless body sensor networks. In Proceedings of the ICST 3rd international conference on body area networks (pp. 1–2).
3. Piccialli, F., Di Somma, V., Giampaolo, F., Cuomo, S., & Fortino, G. (2021). A survey on deep learning in medicine: Why, how and when? *Information Fusion, 66*, 111–137.
4. Wang, Z., Wu, D., Gravina, R., Fortino, G., Jiang, Y., & Tang, K. (2017). Kernel fusion-based extreme learning machine for cross-location activity recognition. *Information Fusion, 37*, 1–9.
5. Chatterjee, R., Maitra, T., Islam, S. H., Hassan, M. M., Alamri, A., & Fortino, G. (2019). A novel machine learning-based feature selection for motor imagery EEG signal classification in internet of medical things environment. *Future Generation Computer Systems, 98*, 419–434.

6. Aluvalu, R., & Muddana, L. (2016). A dynamic attribute-based risk aware access control model (DA-RAAC) for cloud computing. 2016 IEEE international conference on computational intelligence and computing research (ICCIC). IEEE.
7. Köse, T., Özgür, S., Coşgun, E., Keskinoğlu, A., & Keskinoğlu, P. (2013). The prevention and handling of the missing data. *Korean Journal of Anesthesiology, 64*(5), 402–406.
8. Leke, C. A., & Marwala, T. (2019). Introduction to missing data estimation. In *Deep learning and missing data in engineering systems of studies in big data* (Vol. 48, pp. 1–20). Springer.
9. Sterne, J. A. C., White, I. R., Carlin, J. B., et al. (2009). Multiple imputation for missing data in epidemiological and clinical research: Potential and pitfalls. *BMJ, 338*(1), b2393.
10. Wells, B. J., Nowacki, A. S., Chagin, K., & Kattan, M. W. (2017). Strategies for handling missing data in electronic health record derived data. *eGEMs (Generating Evidence & Methods to Improve Patient Outcomes), 1*(3).
11. Brodley, C. E., & Fried, M. A. (1999). Identifying mislabeled training data. *Journal of Artificial Intelligence Research, 11*, 131–167.
12. Ghosh, A., Manwani, N., & Sastry, P. S. (2015). Making risk minimization tolerant to label noise. *Elsevier Neurocomputing, 160*, 93–107.
13. Speth, J., & Hand, E. M. (2019). Automated label noise identification for facial attribute recognition. Proceedings of the IEEE/CVF conference on computer vision and pattern recognition (CVPR) workshops (pp. 25–28).
14. Wang, Y., & Liu, W., et al. (2018). Iterative learning with open-set noisy labels. 2018 IEEE/CVF conference on computer vision and pattern recognition. https://doi.org/10.1109/CVPR.2018.00906.
15. Nigam, N., Dutta, T., & Hari, P. G. (2019). Impact of noisy labels in learning techniques: A survey. In Conference: Advances in data and information sciences.
16. Perona, P., & Malik, J. (1990). Scale-space and edge detection using anisotropic diffusion. *IEEE Transactions on Pattern Analysis and Machine Intelligence, 12*(7), 629–639.
17. Rudin, L. I., & Osher, S.. Total variation-based image restoration with free local constraints. Image Processing, 1994. Proceedings. ICIP-94. IEEE international conference (Vol. 1). IEEE.
18. Coifman, R. R., & Donoho, D. L. (1995). *Translation-invariant denoising*. Springer.
19. Yaroslavsky, L. P., Egiazarian, K. O., & Astola, J. T.. (2001). Transform domain image restoration methods: Review, comparison, and interpretation. Photonics west 2001-electronic imaging. *International Society for Optics and Photonics.*
20. Portilla, J., et al. (2003). Image denoising using scale mixtures of Gaussians in the wavelet domain. *IEEE Transactions on Image Processing, 12*(11), 1338–1351.
21. Gondara, L. (2016). Medical image denoising using convolutional denoising autoencoders. In 2016 IEEE 16th international conference on data mining workshops (ICDMW), Barcelona, Spain (pp. 241–246).
22. Buades, A., Coll, B., & Morel, J.-M. (2005). A review of image denoising algorithms, with a new one. *Multiscale Modeling and Simulation, 4*(2), 490–530.
23. Dabov, K., et al. (2007). Image denoising by sparse 3-D transform domain collaborative filtering. *IEEE Transactions on Image Processing, 16*(8), 2080–2095.
24. Olshausen, B. A., & Field, D. J. (1997). Sparse coding with an overcomplete basis set: A strategy employed by V1? *Vision Research, 37*(23), 3311–3325.
25. Elad, M., & Aharon, M. (2006). Image denoising via sparse and redundant representations over learned dictionaries. *IEEE Transactions on Image Processing, 15*(12), 3736–3745.
26. Mairal, J., et al. (2009). Online dictionary learning for sparse coding. Proceedings of the 26th annual international conference on machine learning. ACM.
27. Vincent, P., et al. (2008). Extracting and composing robust features with denoising autoencoders. Proceedings of the 25th international conference on machine learning. ACM.
28. Akkalakshmi, M., Riyazuddin, Y. M., Revathi, V., & Pal, A. (2020). Autoencoder-based feature learning and up-sampling to enhance cancer prediction. *International Journal of Future Generation Communication and Networking, 13*(1), 1453–1459.
29. Payan, A., & Montana, G. (2015). Predicting Alzheimer's disease: A neuroimaging study with 3D convolutional neural networks. arXiv preprint arXiv:1502.02506.

30. Mansoor, A., Cerrolaza, J., Idrees, R., Biggs, E., Alsharid, M., Avery, R., & Linguraru, M. G. (2016). Deep learning-guided partitioned shape model for anterior visual pathway segmentation. *IEEE Transactions on Medical Imaging, 35*(8), 1856–1865. https://doi.org/10.1109/TMI.2016.2535222
31. Wong, K. K., Fortino, G., & Abbott, D. (2020). Deep learning-based cardiovascular image diagnosis: A promising challenge. *Future Generation Computer Systems, 110*, 802–811.
32. Khan, S. R., Sikandar, M., Almogren, A., Din, I. U., Guerrieri, A., & Fortino, G. (2020). IoMT-based computational approach for detecting brain tumor. *Future Generation Computer Systems, 109*, 360–367.
33. Jabbar, M. A., Aluvalu, R., & Reddy, S. (2017). Cluster-based ensemble classification for intrusion detection system. In Proceedings of the 9th international conference on machine learning and computing (pp. 253–257). ACM.
34. Xu, J., Xiang, L., Liu, Q., Gilmore, H., Wu, J., Tang, J., & Madabhushi, A. (2016). Stacked sparse autoencoder (SSAE) for nuclei detection on breast cancer histopathology images. *IEEE Transactions on Medical Imaging, 35*, 119–130.
35. Cheng, J.-Z., Ni, D., Chou, Y.-H., et al. (2016). Computer-aided diagnosis with deep learning architecture: Applications to breast lesions in US images and pulmonary nodules in CT scans. *Scientific Reports, 6*, 24454. https://doi.org/10.1038/srep24454
36. Ismail, W. N., Hassan, M. M., Alsalamah, H. A., & Fortino, G. (2020). CNN-based health model for regular health factors analysis in internet-of-medical things environment. *IEEE Access, 8*, 52541–52549.
37. Pan, S. J., & Yang, Q. (2010). A survey on transfer learning. *IEEE Transactions on Knowledge and Data Engineering, 22*(10), 1345–1359.
38. Zhang, R., Zheng, Y., Mak, T. W. C., Yu, R., Wong, S. H., Lau, J. Y., & Poon, C. C. (2017). Automatic detection and classification of colorectal polyps by transferring low-level CNN features from nonmedical domain. *IEEE Journal of Biomedical and Health Informatics, 21*(1), 41–47.
39. Menegola, A., Fornaciali, M., Pires, R., Bittencourt, F. V., Avila, S., & Valle, E. (2017). Knowledge transfer for melanoma screening with deep learning. In International symposium on biomedical imaging (ISBI) (pp. 297–300). IEEE.
40. Litjens, G., Kooi, T., Bejnordi, B. E., Setio, A. A. A., Ciompi, F., Ghafoorian, M., van der Laak, J. A., Van Ginneken, B., & Sánchez, C. I. (2017). A survey on deep learning in medical image analysis. *Medical Image Analysis, 42*, 60–88.

Chapter 10
Predicting Epidemic Outbreaks Using IOT, Artificial Intelligence and Cloud

S. Shitharth, Gouse Baig Mohammad, and K. Sangeetha

10.1 Introduction

After celebrating a new year 2020, no one knows is sick. As usual, it feels like a very fine day. A few people around you are sick and suddenly, you get that everyone is sick and it sounds very threatening. It was happening very rapidly. This is the paradox of pandemic. In this article, we are going to analyze the outbreak of COVID-19 using Machine Learning.

At very end of the year December 2019 outbreak in China, the WHO organization had foundSARS-CoV-2 as a new type of coronavirus and at the drop of the hat outbreak spread around the world. Novel Coronavirus also known as COVID-19 is caused by SARS-CoV-2. This coronavirus is enough capable to infect dozens of people around it. The virus starts showing it's symptoms after 10 to 12 days, which is most worried thing. COVID-19 thread is not the first and last viral pandemic. However, like never before this virus killing people and spreading very massively.

On 30 January 2020, a very first report is generated by Kerala-based laboratory who confirmed case of COVID-19. The patient is student by profession who returns earlier from Wuhan. After some days, a 65-year-old man from Mumbai who had travel history to the UAE is reported as 10th victim found in India. The PMO and the MoHFW have close eyes on 2019-nCoV situation. When ministry saw things

S. Shitharth (✉) · G. B. Mohammad
Department of Computer Science and Engineering, Vardhaman College of Engineering, Hyderabad, India
e-mail: gousebaig@vardhaman.org

K. Sangeetha
Department of Computer Science and Engineering, KG Reddy College of Engineering and Technology, Hyderabad, India
e-mail: sangeetha@kgr.ac.in

P. Siarry et al. (eds.), *The Fusion of Internet of Things, Artificial Intelligence, and Cloud Computing in Health Care*, Internet of Things,
https://doi.org/10.1007/978-3-030-75220-0_10

are going worst, then the Prime minister of India came up with a decision and addressed on same day of 24th march 2020. He clarified real situation and requested to be self-quarantine.

Now it became extremely important and essential to control the novel corona virus not only in India but also throughout the world. Without getting late WHO announces COVID-19 outbreak as a pandemic. Now ministry needs to control the spread of virus and predict its risks of infection. The major priority is to identify the infected patient and collect as much as data by testing individual ones.

Here is main role of Healthcare services. They can able to collect the reports by doing testing, researching vaccines for this virus, curing patients. They are also able to provide death reports, confirm reports, bed requirements and all [1].

IT sector also having their own challenges in this pandemic, like collecting massive volume of data generated by clinics, medicals. These reports are essential to analyze outbreak, tracking virus, identifying risk, understanding virus better, diagnose current patients, predict the spreading of virus, predict further pandemics and most important securing our future [2].

All these magic could happen by using Machine Learning, Big Data, Deep learning and Artificial Intelligence and those techie words will be proven soon as a trump card in this war.

Therefore, what is CoronaVirus, how it infects and how pandemic works we have to understand it first. In addition, how can we take help from ML, AI, Deep Learning and Big Data to fight with COVID-19.

10.1.1 What Is COVID-19? (the Problem)

Coronavirus is an infectious disease emerged in Wuhan, China. The new coronavirus spread through person to person. This virus spreads primary through droplets of saliva or by coughing and sneezing. It is diagnosed with a laboratory test. There is no vaccine available for this virus till date.

10.1.2 How Can We Detect? (the Symptoms)

Coronavirus works on different people in a different way. Most of the people have good immunity to fight with this virus. So, they will recover naturally, without hospitalization. This type of people gets only mild to moderate level of Illinois.

Here are some common symptoms:

1. Fever
2. Dry Cough
3. Weakness

Here are some major symptoms:

1. Breathing problem
2. Chest pain
3. Loss of speech or movement

10.1.3 How Can We Break the Virus? (the Solution)

This virus can infect bodies, if it cannot find bodies to infect it will end automatically. Social distancing, self-quarantine, sanitizing are the effective ways to stop infecting people and spreading the virus.

10.1.4 What Is Outbreak, Epidemic and Pandemic?

COVID-19 has a unique property which makes this virus most dangerous. This virus grows **exponentially**. That means, it become double day-by-day and unfortunately there is no vaccine available to cure the patients.

However, it cannot go on last. The virus will eventually stop finding people to infect and ultimate will go slow down the count. This is called **logistic growth.**

An **outbreak** is when the disease happens in unpredicted multitude. It may stick in one zone or expand more extensively. An outbreak can last for few days or some years. Sometimes, authority reviews a single case of a contagious disease to be an outbreak. This could happen when if it is disclosed disease or virus, if it is latest to a community or if it is been missing from a community for a long-term [3].

An **epidemic** is when transmissible disease expands rapidly in regional community than experts/authority would expect. It usually infects a larger region than an outbreak [4].

A **pandemic** is when an epidemic occurs across countries or continents. It infects in large amount and takes more lives than an epidemic. The WHO announces COVID-19 as a pandemic when it became clear that the disease was severe and that it was growing rapidly over a large region [5].

10.2 Environment and Tools

10.2.1 Machine Learning

Overview

ML is an emerging technology day by day in different sectors. Now-a-days ‘health care’ is the area where ML applications are in high demand. But the question is that, **what is machine learning?**

ML is a form of AI (artificial intelligence) that enables s/w applications to become more precise in predicting systems results without being explicitly programmed. ML is an approach of data analysis that robotizes analytical model building [6]. It is an arm of AI based on the goal that machines should be able to grasp and self-adjust through previous experience. To fight the COVID-19 Pandemic AI-Driven Informatics, Sensing, Imaging and Big Data Analytics are highly useful and its results are so authentic [7].

The process of grasping and learning starts with analyzing on data. The primary focus is giving access to the systems to learn automates without user interference and changes actions accordingly.

Why Is Machine Learning Important?

ML can help to enhance 'health related data management and exchange of health statistics' with the aim of technologize updated workflows, ease access to clinical data and upgrading the precision and flow of health details [8].

It also help to pathologists make faster and more precise diagnose further more to identify patients who might sake of new types of treatments and therapies.

Methods of Machine Learning

Two main trendy methods of ML are supervised learning and unsupervised learning. Supervised learning is about 70% of ML, although unsupervised learning is about 10–20% of ML. Reinforcement learning and semi-supervised learning methods are less used. Gaming, finance sector and manufacturing sector lie under reinforcement learning [9].

Supervised Machine Learning Algorithms

Supervised learning is all about 'Classification' and 'Regression'. This algorithm enables fraud detection, e-mail spam detection, diagnostics and image classification. It also helps in risk assessment and scores prediction. The technic is able to issue targets for any new input after sufficient training. The machine learning algorithm further compares its output with the right results, intended output and search errors to modify and customize the model accordingly [10, 11].

Unsupervised Machine Learning Algorithms

Unsupervised ML supports 'Dimensionality Reduction' and 'Clustering'. Dimensionality includes text mining, face recognition, big data visualization and image recognition. It also helps in biology, city-planning sectors. Unsupervised learning does study and analyze in order to systems could derive a function to set out a hidden structure from unlabelled data [12]. The system is not able to check correct output, but it can able to analyze the data and can draw inferences from provided datasets to describe hidden structures from unlabelled data. These algorithms do not need any pre-requirements like training with desired outcome data. Instead, they use an iterative approach called Deep Learning to review data and arrive at wind-up [13, 14].

Semi-Supervised Machine Learning Algorithms

This is a sort of combination of supervised and unsupervised learning and use both labelled and unlabelled data for analyzing. This type of ML can be used for methods like classification, regression and prediction. In semi-supervised learning, it would be like face and voice recognition techniques. In a typical situation, the algorithm will use a small amount of labelled data with a large amount of unlabelled data [15].

Reinforcement Machine Learning Algorithms

Reinforcement ML again uses same methods such as classification, regression and prediction. Reinforcement learning is very different from supervised learning. This ML algorithm is all about sequential decisions, in other hand in supervised learning decision made under starting inputs [16] (Table 10.1).

The Machine Learning Process (Fig. 10.1)

10.2.2 Deep Learning

Overview

A survey on deep learning in medicine: Why, how and when? [19] shows the impact of the algorithm in the medicine field. It is an arm of machine learning. Alike ML, deep learning also has supervised, unsupervised and reinforcement learning in it.

Table 10.1 Difference between supervised learning and unsupervised learning [17, 18]

Factors	Supervised learning	Unsupervised learning
Input	Well-known and labelled data	Unspecified data
Complexity	Very complicated	Less complicated
Number of classes	Known	Undisclosed
Accuracy	Precise and authentic	Average in accuracy and reliable

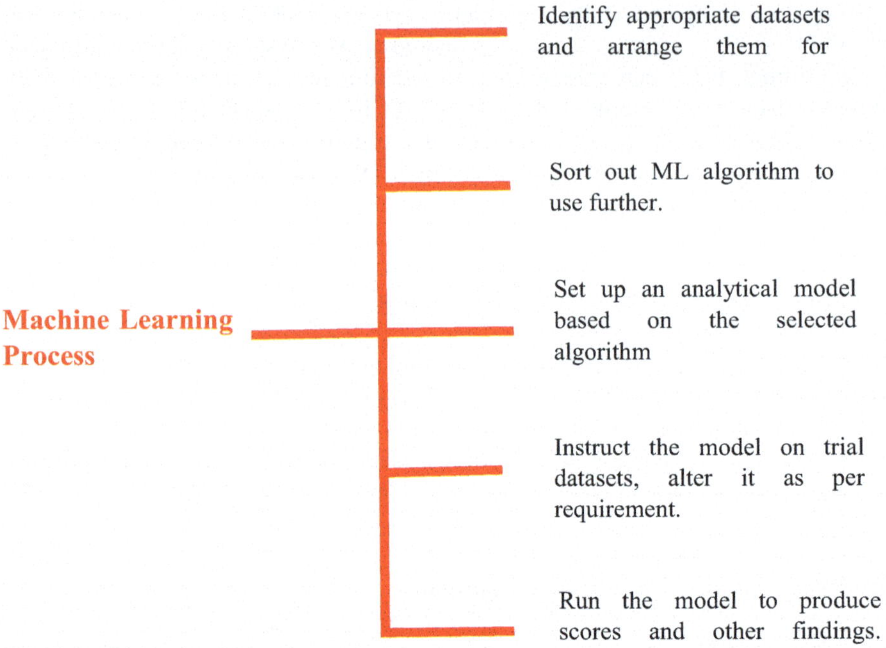

Fig. 10.1 Machine learning process [3]

The word 'deep' in deep learning indicates use of multiple layers in network. Most of the latest models are built on artificial neural network, CNN, although they also have propositional formulas sorted in layer-wise (Fig. 10.2).

Deep Learning is all about integrating such unseen layers between the initial and the final layer. Even Deep learning-based cardiovascular image diagnosis also been in research to show the versatility of the algorithm [20].

Methods of Deep Learning

There are some different methods implemented in deep learning. Every suggested method has a certain use case like the sort of data we have, so it is either supervised or unsupervised learning, what kind of task you would want to solve [21]. Therefore, it is all about on these factors, you choose one of the methods that can best solve your problem (Fig. 10.3) (Table 10.2).

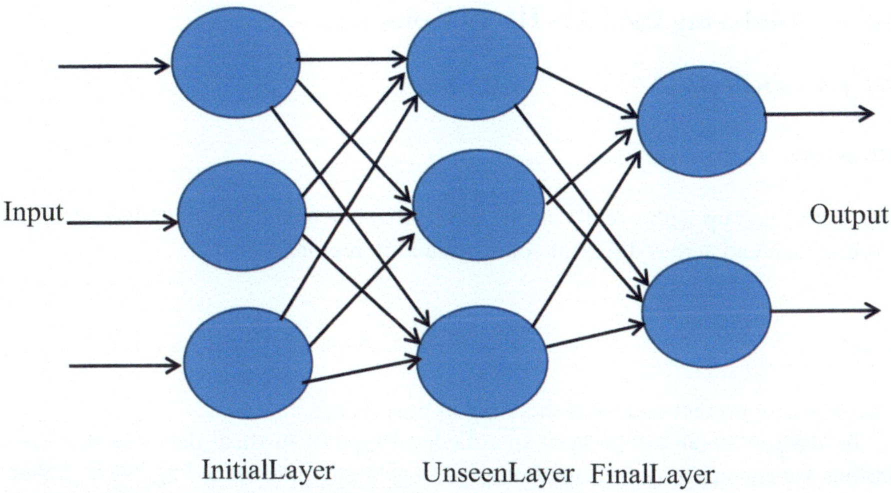

Fig. 10.2 Shallow neural network [5]

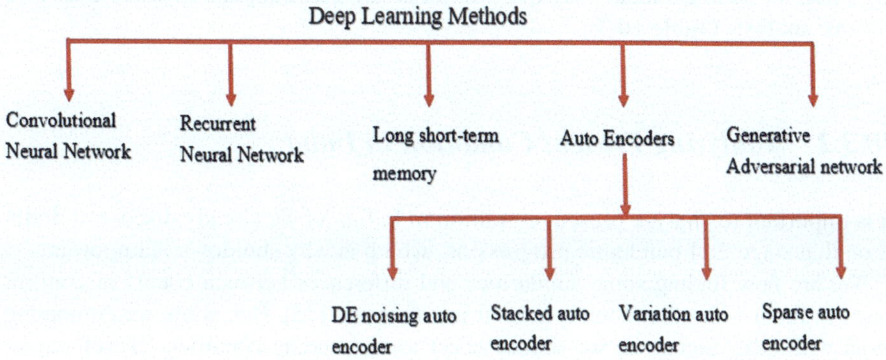

Fig. 10.3 Deep learning method [5]

Table 10.2 Deep learning versus machine learning [5]

Factors	Deep learning	Machine learning
Data requirement	Requires large data.	Can train on less data.
Accuracy	Provides high accuracy	Gives less accuracy.
Training time	Takes longer to train.	Take lesser time to train.
Hardware dependency	Requires GPU.	Trains on CPU.
Hyper parameter tuning	Can be tuned in various different ways.	Limited tuning capabilities.

10.3 Analyzing the COVID-19 Epidemic

10.3.1 Overview

Objective

Idea is to come up with a really strong model that can able to predict how coronavirus could spread across different countries and in regions.

Goal

The task is to predict spread of the virus in next 7 days.

To analyze situation, we need to collect all type of medical data. On that data further, we can apply various methods and to get better understanding, we visualize this data graphically (pie chart, bar graphs, etc.) [22].

Here, we are using **python,** a scripting language. This programming language is very effective when it comes to analyzing on big data.

(a) First, let us understand why these libraries are essential and how we use it, in our analysis (Table 10.3).

10.3.2 Analyzing Present Condition in India

It is important to analyze present condition in India. As we already discussed, India is on that stage 2 of pandemic progression, which is why shutdown is important.

We are now finding some similarities and differences between counts of confirm cases in India with other country's confirmation cases [25]. But, while we comparing India with other countries, we should select same trending countries. Therefore, we could analyze future domestic losses and we will be preparing for any other unknown risk.

We are also exploring worldwide data and keep updating to our healthcare sector and the dataset. We already have a dataset in form of excel file. Using that same data, we are creating a frame using ***Pandas.*** This library helps us to read tabular form of data.

Table 10.3 Libraries [9]

Libraries	Description
Pandas	It is mainly used for data analysis and manipulation.
Matplotlib	It is a graph plot library. It gives an OOP-based API for insert plots into applications by using GUI [23].
Seaborn	This library based on matplotlib. It is mainly used for statistical data visualization [24].
Folium	We used this library to populate a geographical map.

Track Cases in Indian States/Territories

Now, we have name of states in India (Fig. 10.4).

Find Total Confirm Cases

Now, we are finding Total No. of confirm cases (National + International) (Fig. 10.5).

So, as per statistics, as of 22nd March 2020 India has total **562** confirmed cases.

Graphical Representation (Total Cases) (Fig. 10.6)

As per figure, the darker the red is in each of these cells the more the number of fatalities are. Actually here, we coloured each cell according to the fatality rate. As we can see, 'Karnataka', 'Kerala' and 'Maharashtra' have largest number of cases 41, 109, 101, respectively. Least Number of cases are in 'Chhattisgarh', 'Manipur' and 'Mizoram' with only one case each, as per 25th March statistics [26].

	S. No.	Name of State / UT	Total Confirmed cases (Indian National)	Total Confirmed cases (Foreign National)	Cured	Death
0	1	Andhra Pradesh	9	0	0	0
1	2	Bihar	3	0	0	1
2	3	Chhattisgarh	1	0	0	0
3	4	Delhi	30	1	6	1
4	5	Gujarat	32	1	0	1
5	6	Haryana	14	14	11	0
6	7	Himachal Pradesh	3	0	0	1
7	8	Karnataka	41	0	3	1
8	9	Kerala	101	8	4	0
9	10	Madhya Pradesh	9	0	0	0
10	11	Maharashtra	98	3	0	2
11	12	Manipur	1	0	0	0
12	13	Mizoram	1	0	0	0
13	14	Odisha	2	0	0	0
14	15	Puducherry	1	0	0	0
15	16	Punjab	29	0	0	1

Fig. 10.4 COVID cases in India [2]. Total confirm cases (Indian National), Total confirm cases (Foreign National), cured cases and death cases

```
total_cases=df['Total cases'].sum()
print('Total No. of confirmed covid-19 cases till date[22/03/2020]:',total_cases)

Total No. of confirmed covid-19 cases till date[22/03/2020]: 562
```

Fig. 10.5 Confirmed cases in India [2]

	Name of State / UT	Total Confirmed cases (Indian National)	Total Confirmed cases (Foreign National)	Cured	Death	Total cases
0	Andhra Pradesh	9	0	0	0	9
1	Bihar	3	0	0	1	3
2	Chhattisgarh	1	0	0	0	1
3	Delhi	30	1	6	1	31
4	Gujarat	32	1	0	1	33
5	Haryana	14	14	11	0	28
6	Himachal Pradesh	3	0	0	1	3
7	Karnataka	41	0	3	1	41
8	Kerala	101	8	4	0	109
9	Madhya Pradesh	9	0	0	0	9
10	Maharashtra	98	3	0	2	101
11	Manipur	1	0	0	0	1
12	Mizoram	1	0	0	0	1
13	Odisha	2	0	0	0	2
14	Puducherry	1	0	0	0	1
15	Punjab	29	0	0	1	29
16	Rajasthan	30	2	3	0	32
17	Tamil Nadu	16	2	1	0	18
18	Telengana	25	10	1	0	35
19	Chandigarh	7	0	0	0	7
20	Jammu and Kashmir	7	0	1	0	7
21	Ladakh	13	0	0	0	13
22	Uttar Pradesh	34	1	11	0	35
23	Uttarakhand	3	1	0	0	4
24	West Bengal	9	0	0	1	9

Fig. 10.6 Graphical representation of confirmed cases in India [6]

Find Total Active Cases

Now we have total death cases, total cured patients and sum of all. However, these data are not more relevant for our analysis.

What actually we are seeking is ***Active cases***. We only want to know the number of people that have been hospitalized at that moment (Fig. 10.7).

```
#Toatl cases= Number of death + Cured
df['Total Active'] = df['Total cases'] - (df['Death'] + df['Cured'])
total_active=df['Total Active'].sum()
print('Total number of active COVID-19 cases across India:', total_active)
Tot_Cases = df.groupby('Name of State / UT')['Total Active'].sum().sort_values(ascending=False).to_frame()
Tot_Cases.style.background_gradient(cmap='Reds')

Total number of active COVID-19 cases across India: 512
```

$$\text{Total Active Cases} = \text{Total cases} - \left(\text{Total Death} + \text{Total Cured}\right)$$

We can clearly see that, 'Kerala' and 'Maharashtra' have highest number of Active cases and combined cases in India have 512 of count [27].

Here, we have grouped states and union territories and further we sorted them by the value of their total active cases. Again, here we used same red-coloured gradient to visualize it better.

Name of State / UT	Total Active
Kerala	105
Maharashtra	99
Karnataka	37
Telengana	34
Gujarat	32
Rajasthan	29
Punjab	28
Uttar Pradesh	24
Delhi	24
Tamil Nadu	17
Haryana	17
Ladakh	13
Madhya Pradesh	9
Andhra Pradesh	9
West Bengal	8
Chandigarh	7
Jammu and Kashmir	6
Uttarakhand	4
Himachal Pradesh	2
Odisha	2
Bihar	2
Manipur	1
Mizoram	1
Puducherry	1
Chhattisgarh	1

Fig. 10.7 Active cases in India

groupby():
This is a pivot function mostly we use in excel sheets. It actually turns wide table format into long table format.

Location-based Tracking *(Total Cases)* (Fig. 10.8)

Here, we used ***Folium*** library as *folium.map()* and we specified the location (Longitude and Latitude). We also use a red circle marker whose size depends on the number of cases in their particular region [28].

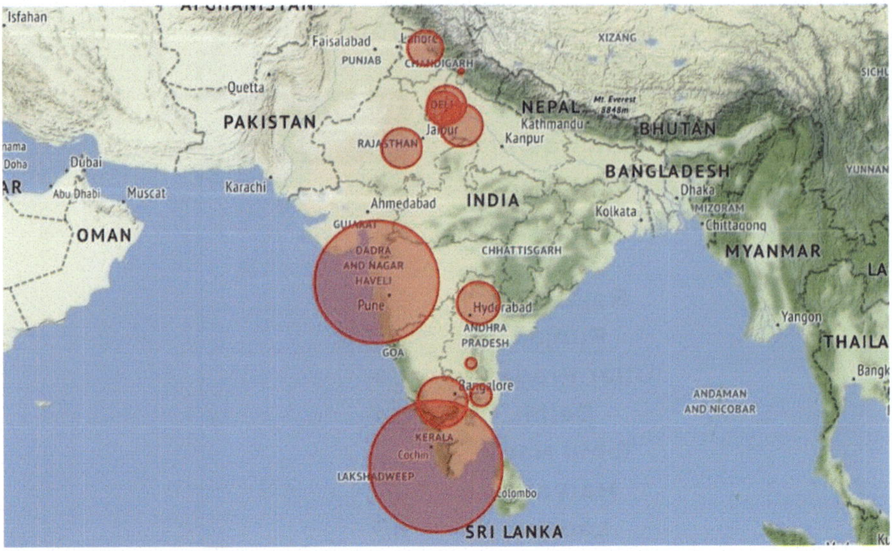

Fig. 10.8 Visualizing the spread geographically

As we can see, 'Kerala' immediately followed by 'Maharashtra' both have very big red circles. In addition, north Indian side has some couple of circles and east side of India is less affected region.

Confirmed Versus Recovered Cases (Fig. 10.9)

Here, we are basically using ***seaborn*** library for visualization where we are plotting a couple of bar graphs to showing and comprising total number of sure cases and total number of cured cases in Indian territories. Pink represents total number of cases similarly, cured cases are in green colour [29, 30].

As we can see, again 'Kerala', 'Karnataka' and 'Maharashtra' have highest number of cases and also, 'Haryana' and 'Uttar Pradesh' have good recovery.

If we compare 'Kerala' with 'Maharashtra', Kerala despites maximum number of cases and also maximum number of recovery than Maharashtra [31]. So, conclusion from above graph is that, the net percentage of affected people in Kerala is much lesser than Maharashtra.

Rise of Coronavirus Cases (Fig. 10.10)

Here, we use a scatter plot and a line plus marker for a better understanding and visualization. This graph shows an actual rise of coronavirus cases in India.

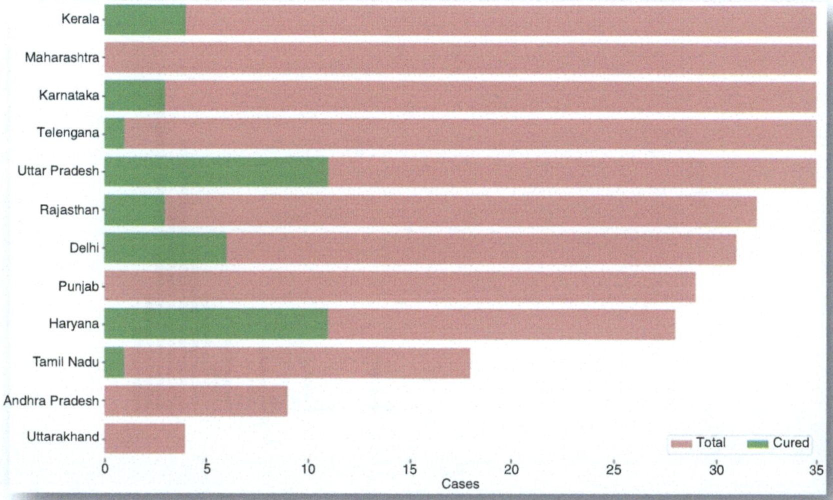

Fig. 10.9 Total cases and recovered cases

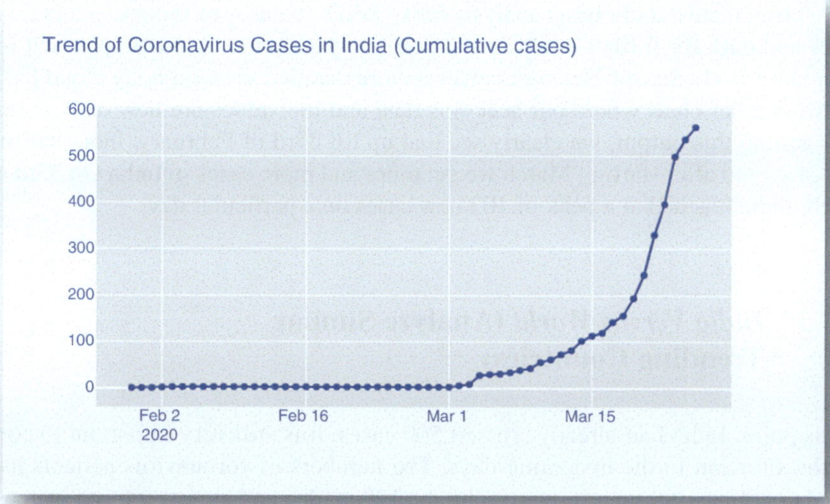

Fig. 10.10 Trend of coronavirus cases in India [32]

In that above graph, X-axis intended to months similarly, Y-axis intended the cases rise in India. We can easily see how the graph takes a jump in March (Fig. 10.11).

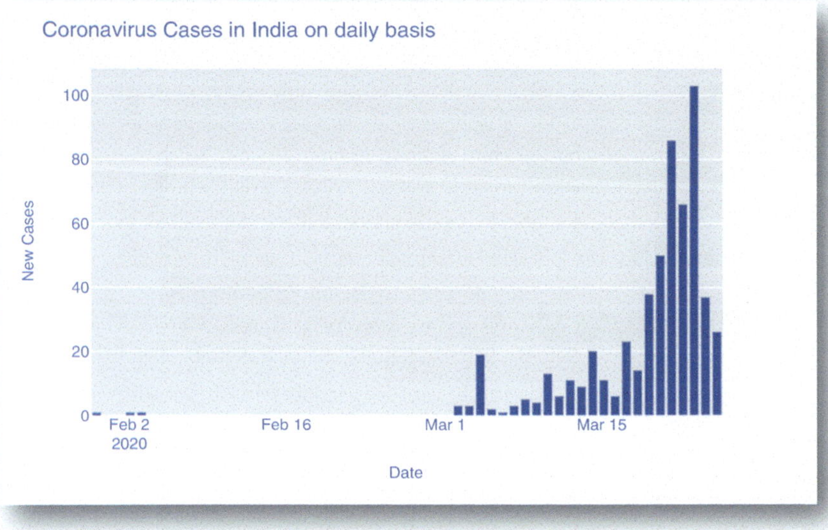

Fig. 10.11 Daily basis analysis [33]

We also create a daily basis analysis for COVID-19 cases in India to get precise values and data for further analysis and accurate prediction. A SaaS approach for community Body Sensor Networks gives a more detailed view on body cloud [34].

This is a bar chart where our access is date and the values are new daily cases. After getting this output, we clearly see that up till 23rd of February, India has too little cases and after starting March we get more and more cases in India.On 23rd of March, India reached at a peak of 103 new cases on a particular day.

10.3.3 *India Versus World* (Analyze Similar Trending Countries)

At this point, India had already crossed 500 cases. It is still very important to contain the situation in the upcoming days. The numbers of coronavirus patients had started doubling after many countries hit the 100 marks, and almost starting increasing exponentially.

Now, we have, all confirmed, recovered and death cases report and monthly-daily analysis. Up till here, we analyze about India only. Its time to compare and analyze India with few similar trending cases countries [35].

It is more important to analyze present condition of world. So, we are now finding some similar situations in other countries. These data will help us for better prediction and preparation [36].

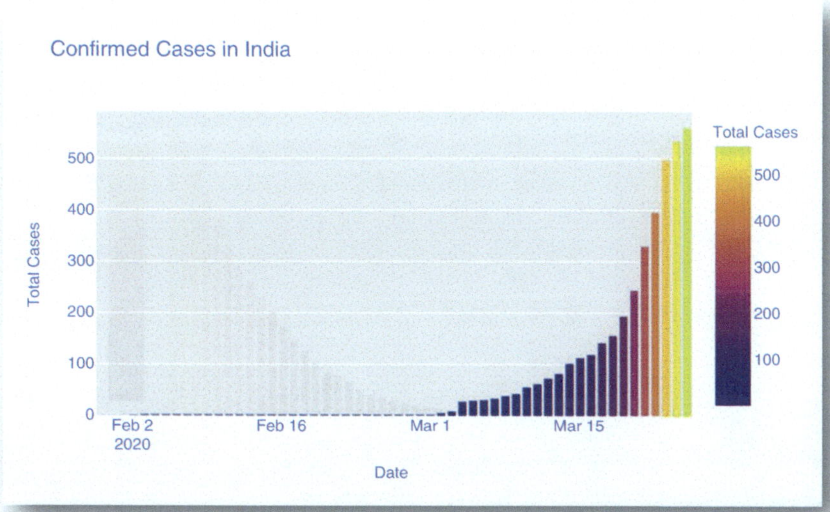

Fig. 10.12 India

India ***(Confirmed Cases)*** **(Fig. 10.12)**

For this type of graph, we imported column graph using plot Li and some colour gradient. The more dense the colour, the higher the confirm rate. As per our title, we are comparing India with world [37]. This is the graph for India. India has exponential growth in confirm cases and it has taken a hit since 3rd–4th of March.

Italy ***(Confirmed Cases)***

If we talk about Italy's condition, we can see a sharp and exponential increase in confirm case reports after the 3rd–4th of March. But, this graph looks so even and in flow, there are no breaks and kinks unlike India. At the end of March, it shows 69k cases from Italy that is much more than India (Figs. 10.13 and 10.14).

South Korea ***(Confirmed Cases)***

South Korea's graph has started to completely become a sigmoid curve since the 7th of March, the actual story behind is, South Korea had started the extensive testing. The government took very strong decision that anyone who got even mildest infection has been quarantined in this country [38].

This idea really works so that the curve is almost flattened in last few days of March. On 22nd–24th of March, the confirm cases seem so minimal (Fig. 10.15).

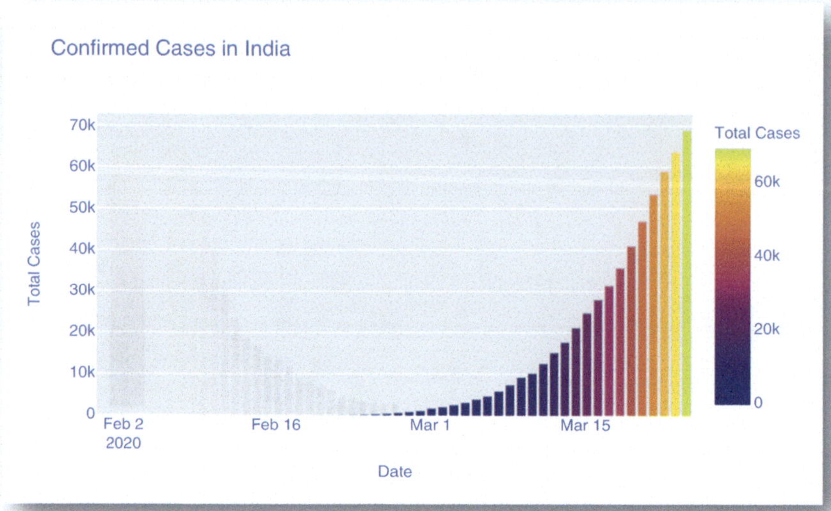

Fig. 10.13 Confirmed cases in Italy

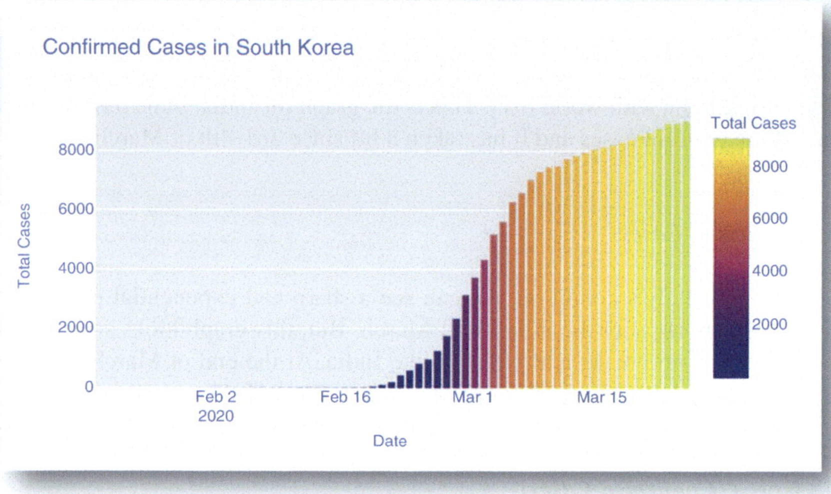

Fig. 10.14 Confirmed cases in South Korea

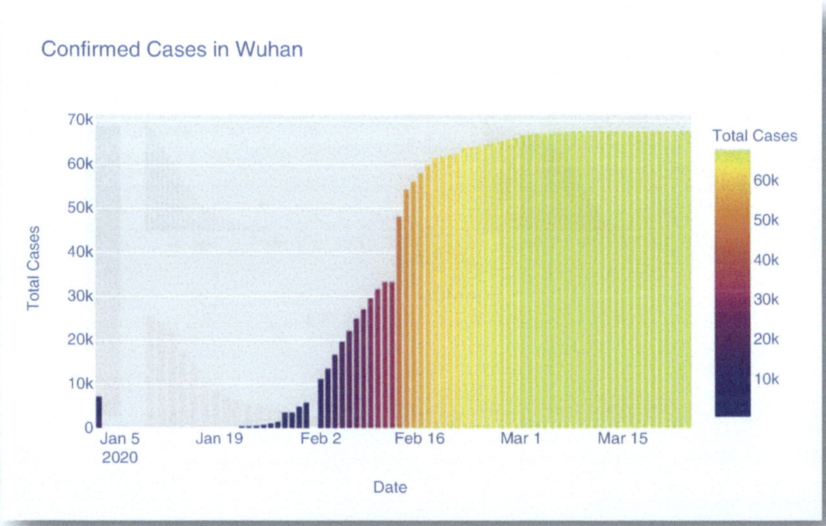

Fig. 10.15 Confirm cases in Wuhan

Wuhan

Wuhan's graph is also following sigmoid pattern. On 12th–13th February, there is steep rise. But it is successfully started to flatten out just after 66k–67k on 3rd of March.

China also has their own unique story; China has started to get help from some *artificial intelligent* models, which have helped them to diagnose people with flu on a very extensive scale. They used to scan bodies with heat mapping sensors, these sensors are much able to pick out people with even mild temperatures, which will help to quarantine and diagnose people and this project at its best in machine learning [39].

From the above visualization, one can infer the following:

- Confirmed cases in India are rising exponentially with no fixed pattern (Very less test in India).
- Confirmed cases in Italy are rising exponentially with a certain fixed pattern.
- Confirmed cases in South Korea are rising gradually.
- There have been almost negligible numbers of confirmed cases in Wuhan a week.

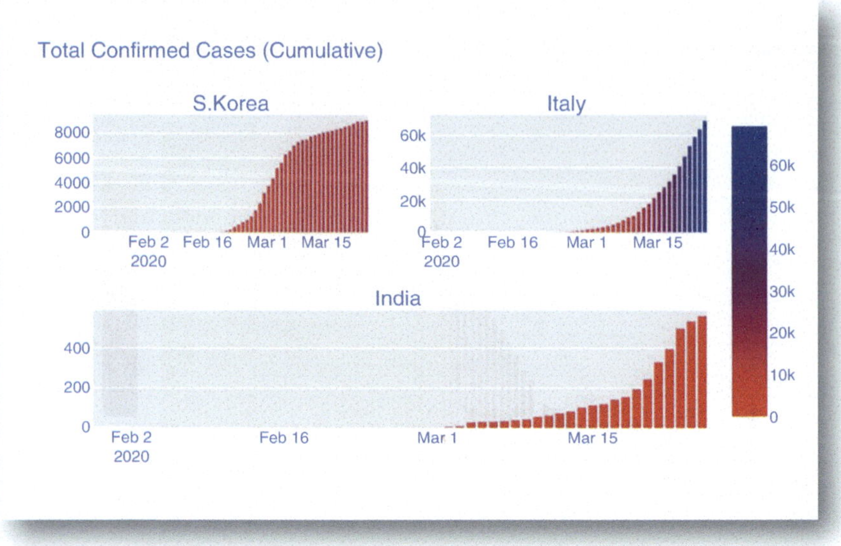

Fig. 10.16 India: 562 Italy: 69 k South Korea: 9 k

Overall Comparison (Fig. 10.16)

The more number of cumulative cases per day the bluer the graph becomes. So, we take some countries South Korea, Italy to compare. We put all graphs into a single canvas to differentiate them properly. This type of visualization will contribute more than the previous one [40].

We can see that, India has comparatively fewer cases than South Korea and Italy on the same date. At the same time, if we campier India with these countries, India has large population. What is the reason behind India has less cases? Let us figure it out.

Trend after Crossing 100 Cases *(India, South Korea, Italy)* (Fig. 10.17)

As we can see, after crossing 100 cases the graph shows India has minimum number of cases and other both countries cross the mark of 5,600.

If we compare India with Italy and South Korea, India has low number in cases when it comes to in this pandemic. Why this is happening?

According to CNN reports, India is actually not testing people enough to find out whether the total number of reported cases are genuine or not and why is a highly populated country with billions of people testing so in less count [41].

By the experts, India has testing below scale because of being under resourced and an uneven public-health system.

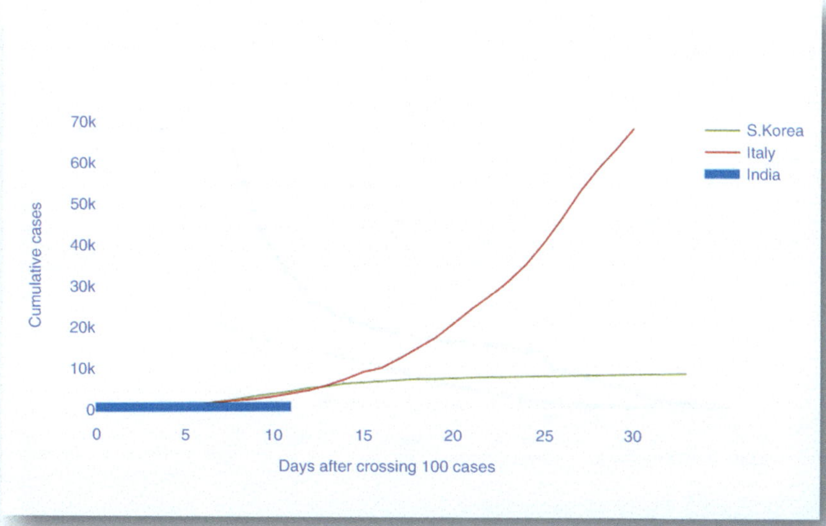

Fig. 10.17 RED: Italy; Green: South Korea; Blue: India

10.3.4 Visualize Worldwide Data (Fig. 10.18)

Here we are using coloured lines with markers. Blue lines show total number of confirmed cases around the world, Green lines show recovered patients and similarly red line intended to total number of death cases due to the coronavirus in world.

As we can see, between point A and B there is sudden rise in graph and not a perfect curve. Actually, in that particular day 12th of February, an organization came up with a unique method of counting affected people, but by the end of the day they realize that this is not a proper method to count fatalities. Hence, they came back to the original method of counting.

10.4 Forecasting/Prediction

10.4.1 Forecasting Total Number of Cases Worldwide

For Forecasting and prediction here, we use an open source software called 'Prophet' which is developed by Facebook core data science team.

We actually use Prophet for forecasting in sort of time series results based data on an additive model where non-linear trends are suitable with yearly, weekly and daily basis.

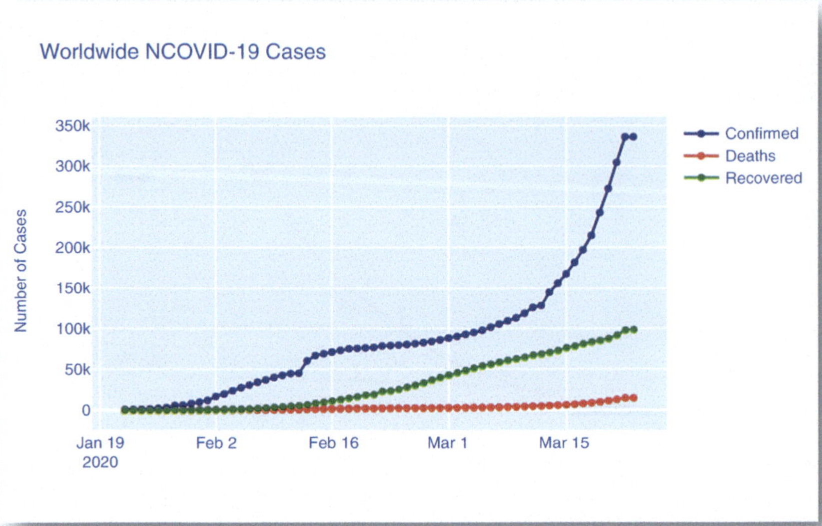

Fig. 10.18 Worldwide graph

Why Prophet?

- **Precise and quick:** Prophet is mainly utilized in different applications in Facebook for building authenticate and valid forecasts for goal setting. It is enough quick that you may get forecasts in a bit by using Stan module. Facebook finds it to execute better than any other approach.
- **Automated:** Get a reasonable forecast on messy data with no manual effort. Prophet is robust to outliers, missing data and dramatic changes in your time series.
- **Availability:** Facebook has introduced the Prophet Module procedure with support of Python and R programming language. Both languages share the Stan code. You can use any language that you are comfortable.

Confirm Cases Forecast

Now, it is time to predict upcoming coronavirus cases in the world. Here we are trying to find out a range within which the prediction is going to occur and in an addition to that we are finding upper limit and lower limit so that our prediction and values will not deflect so much (Fig. 10.19).

- yhat:- values which are predicted.
- yhat_lower:- It shows lower limit which is predicted.
- yhat_upper:- It shows how much high cases could go.

	ds	yhat	yhat_lower	yhat_upper
64	2020-03-26	355136.872975	334546.613119	374775.244231
65	2020-03-27	372235.326938	352367.910827	391712.469992
66	2020-03-28	388674.964143	367586.464833	410613.983488
67	2020-03-29	405307.954675	382990.550208	427082.101462
68	2020-03-30	418529.648466	394208.184567	439971.819186

Fig. 10.19 Confirm cases prediction

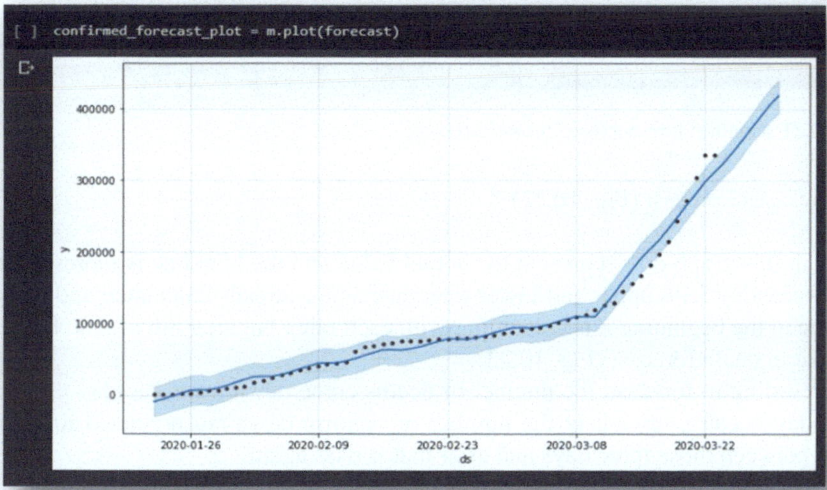

Fig. 10.20 Confirm forecast

Tolerance lies between yhat_lower to yhat_upper (Fig. 10.20).

Here we visualize the data in graph by putting some plots. We use *prophet plot* Method to plot forecast by passing forecast frame.

As per graph, we can see the graph's line goes beyond 24th of March. Graph is raising constantly day by day (Fig. 10.21).

This graph actually focusses on a particular days of a week. As we can see, there is a dip on Tuesday to Wednesday [42]. These are because there is huge dip in the cases in the china in that particular day.

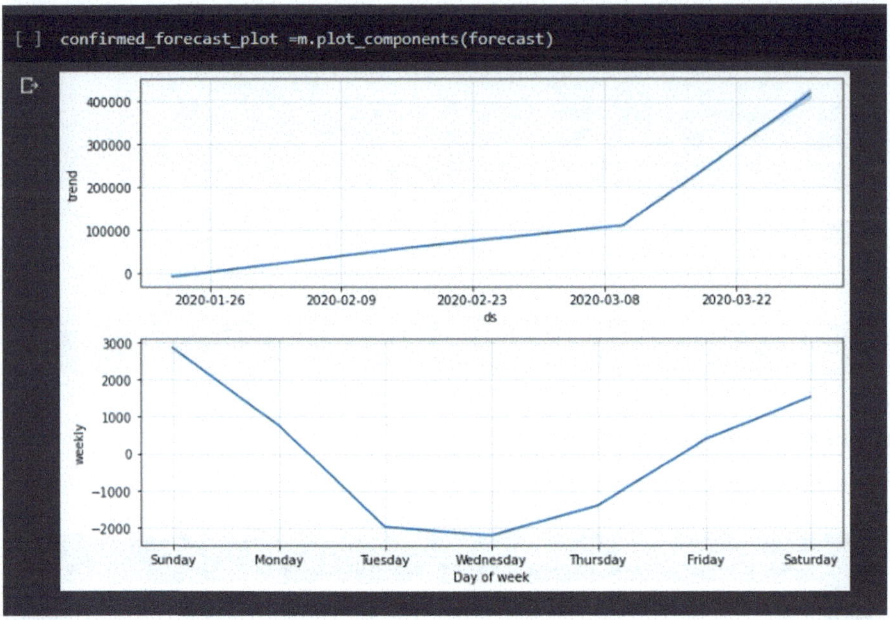

Fig. 10.21 Confirm forecast *(weekly analysis)*

Death Cases Forecast (Fig. 10.22)

Here, in this graph dots represent the actual value and the blue line is representing the forecasting with upper and lower tolerance as we already calculated and as we can see in the beginning it is coinciding with each other but after 8th of march there is spike in death forecast (Fig. 10.23).

According to forecast, the number of deaths come down from Tuesday through Thursday because obviously the number of confirm cases are predicted to come down between those three days and after that it rises again.

10.5 Conclusion

Do not take your cough and cold lightly as you would. If you look at the data, the number of cases in India are rising just like in Italy, Wuhan, South Korea, Spain and the USA. We have crossed 100,000 cases already. Do not let lower awareness and fewer test numbers ruin the health of our world. Currently, India is a deadly and risky zone as there are very few COVID- 19 test centres available. Imagine how many infected people are still around you and are infecting others unknowingly. If the spread of coronavirus goes along with the forecast and as per our model then it would come up with big loss of lives as it presents the exponential growth of the transmission worldwide.

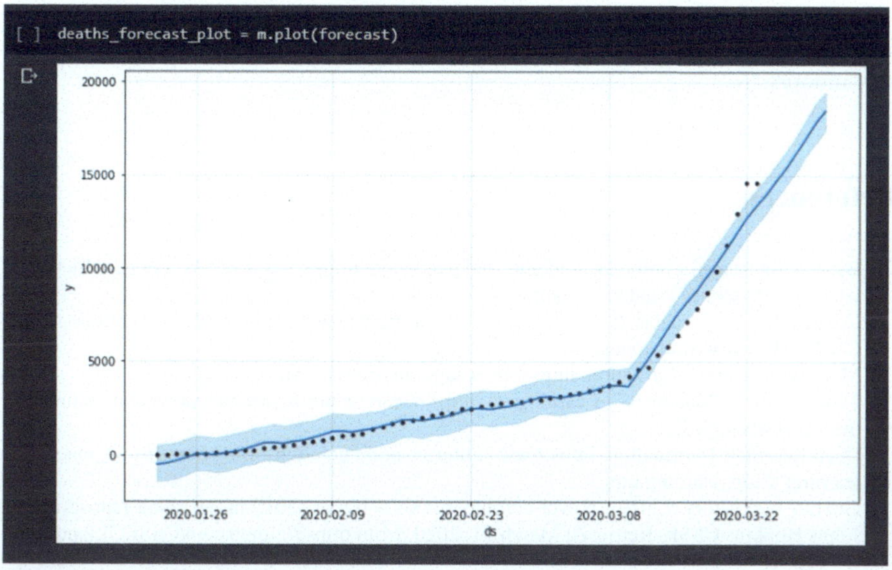

Fig. 10.22 Death forecast

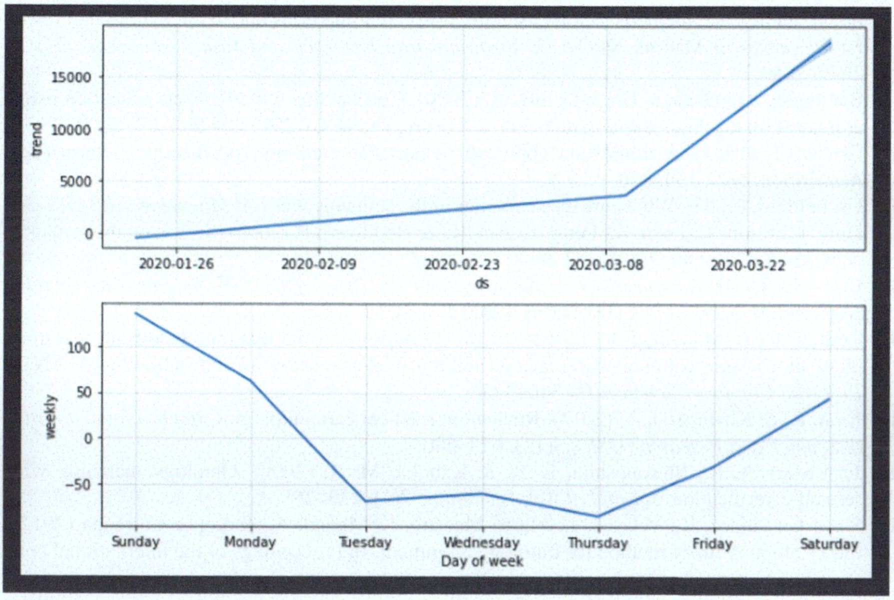

Fig. 10.23 Death forecast *(weekly analysis)*

Let us give a hand in fighting this pandemic at least by quarantining ourselves by staying indoors and protecting others and ourselves around us. Take precautions, stay indoors.

References

1. Basic definitions for outbreak epidemic and pandemic. https://www.webmd.com/cold-and-flu/what-are-epidemics-pandemics-outbreaks
2. Covid-2019 datasets from https://www.kaggle.com/allen-institute-for-ai/CORD-19-research-challenge
3. Machine learning information. https://en.wikipedia.org/wiki/Machine_learning
4. Types of Machine Learning. https://searchenterpriseai.techtarget.com/definition/machinelearningML
5. Deep Learning Information. https://www.tutorialspoint.com/tensorflow/tensorflow_machine_learning_deep_learning.htm
6. GitHub Repository. (2019). Novel coronavirus COVID-19 (2019-nCoV) data repository by Johns Hopkins CSSE. Retrieved March 31, 2020, from https://github.com/CSSEGISandData/COVID-19
7. Amini, A., Chen, W., Fortino, G., Li, Y., Pan, Y., & Wang, M. D. (2020). AI-driven informatics, sensing, imaging and big data analytics for fighting the COVID-19 pandemic. *IEEE Journal of Biomedical and Health Informatics, 24*(10), 2731–2732.
8. Navares, R., Díaz, J., Linares, C., & Aznarte, J. L. (2018). Comparing ARIMA and computational intelligence methods to forecast daily hospital admissions due to circulatory and respiratory causes in Madrid. *Stochastic Environmental Research and Risk Assessment, 32*(10), 2849–2859.
9. Barstugan, M., Ozkaya, U., & Ozturk, S. (2020). Coronavirus (covid-19) classification using ct images by machine learning methods. arXiv preprint arXiv:2003.09424.
10. Gruber, T. (1993). A translation approach to portable ontology specifications. *Knowledge Acquisition, 5*(2), 199–220.
11. Uschold, M. (2003). Where are the semantics in the semantic web? *AI Magazine, 24*(3), 25–36.
12. Ding, L., Finin, T., Joshi, A., Peng, Y., Pan, R., & Reddivari, P. (2005). Search on the semantic web. *IEEE Computer, 10*(38), 62–69.
13. Horrocks, I. (2007). Semantic web: the story so far. In *Proc. of the 2007 int. cross- disciplinary conf. on web accessibility (W4A)* (pp. 120–125). ACM.
14. Zeshan, F., & Mohamad, R. (2012). Medical ontology in the dynamic healthcare environment, the 3rd international conference on ambient systems, networks and technologies (ANT). *Procedia Computer Science, 10*, 340–348.
15. Kaur, P., & Khamparia, A. (2014). Review on medical care ontologies. *International Journal of Science and Research (IJSR), 3*(12), 677–680.
16. Jean-Mary, Y. R., Shironoshita, E. P., & Kabuka, M. R. (2009). Ontology matching with semantic verification. *Journal of Web Semantics, 7*(3), 235–251.
17. Susel Fernández, R., Velasco, J., Marsa-Maestre, I., Miguel, A., & Lopez-Carmona (2012). Fuzzy align: A fuzzy method for ontology alignment. In Proceedings of the international conference on knowledge engineering and ontology development.
18. Shitharth, S., Sangeetha, & Kumar, P. (2019). Integrated probability relevancy classification (IPRC) for IDS in SCADA. *Design Framework for wireless network, Lecture notes in network and systems, Springer, 82*(1), 41–64.
19. Piccialli, F., Somma, V. D., Giampaolo, F., Cuomo, S., & Fortino, G. (2021). A survey on deep learning in medicine: Why, how and when? *Information Fusion, 66*, 111–137.

20. Wong, K. K. L., Fortino, G., & Abbott, D. (2021). Deep learning-based cardiovascular image diagnosis: A promising challenge. *Future Generation Computer Systems, 110*, 802–811.
21. Ngo, D., & Bellahsene, Z. (2012). YAM++: A multi-strategy based approach for ontology matching task. In *Lecture notes in computer science (including subseries lecture notes in artificial intelligence and lecture notes in bioinformatics) LNAI* (Vol. 7603, pp. 421–425).
22. Bodenreider, O. (2013). *Disease ontology, encyclopedia of systems biology* (pp. 578–581). Springer.
23. Ibrahim, A. M., Hashi, H. A., & Mohamed, A. A. (2013). Ontology driven information retrieval for healthcare information system: A case study. *International Journal of Network Security & Its Applications (IJNSA), 5*(1).
24. Babcock, S., Lindsay, G., Cowell, J. B., & Smith, B. (2020). The infectious disease ontology in the age of COVID-19. In OSF preprints. Center for Open Science.
25. He, Y., et al. (2020). CIDO-a community-based ontology for coronavirus disease knowledge and data integration, sharing, and analysis. http://www.nature.com/scientificdata.
26. Oyelade, O. N., & Ezugwu, A. E. (2020). COVID19: A natural language processing and ontology-oriented temporal case-based framework for early detection and diagnosis of novel coronavirus. Preprint www.preprints.org.
27. Shitharth, S., Shaik, M., Sirajudeen, & Sangeetha. (2019). Mining of intrusion attack in SCADA network using clustering and genetically seeded flora-based optimal classification algorithm. *Information Security, IET, 14*(1), 1–11.
28. Pirouz, B., Shaffiee Haghshenas, S., Shaffiee Haghshenas, S., & Piro, P. (2020). Investigating a serious challenge in the sustainable development process: Analysis of confirmed cases of COVID-19 (new type of coronavirus) through a binary classification using artificial intelligence and regression analysis. *Sustainability, 12*(6), 2427.
29. Mohammed, A., Al-qaness, Ewees, A. A., Fan, H., & El Aziz, M. A. (2020). Optimization method for forecasting confirmed cases of COVID-19 in China. *Journal of Clinical Medicine, 9*(3), 674.
30. Gruninger, M., & Lee, J. (2002). Ontology – Applications and Design. *Communications of the ACM, 45*(2), 39–41.
31. Uschold, M., & Jasper, R. (1999). A framework for understanding and classifying ontology applications. In Proceedings of the IJCAI-99 workshop on ontologies and problem- solving methods (KRR5) (pp. 1–11). Stockholm, Sweden.
32. Maedche, A., & Staab, S. (2001). Ontology learning for the Semantic Web. *IEEE Intelligent Systems, 16*(2), 72–79.
33. Mao, M. (2008). Ontology mapping: Towards semantic interoperability in distributed and heterogeneous environments. Ph.D. dissertation, Pittsburgh University, Pittsburgh, PA.
34. Fortino, G., Parisi, D., Pirrone, V., & Di Fatta, G. (2014). BodyCloud: A SaaS approach for community body sensor networks. *Future Generation Computer Systems, 35*, 62–79.
35. Shvaiko, P., & Euzenat, J. (2013). Ontology matching: State of the art and future challenges. *IEEE Trans on Knowledge and Data Engineering, 25*(1), 158–176.
36. Niles, I., & Pease, A. (2001). Towards a standard upper ontology. In Proceedings of the 2nd international conference on formal ontology in information systems (FOIS- 2001) (Vol. 2001, pp. 2–9).
37. El-Sappagh, S., Franda, F., Ali, F., & Kwak, K.-S. (2018). SNOMED CT standard ontology based on the ontology for general medical science. *BMC Medical Informatics and Decision Making*. Article number: 76.
38. Buitelaar, P., Cimiano, P., Grobelnik, M., & Sintek, M. (2005, October). Ontology learning from text, tutorial at ECML/PKDD, Porto.
39. Aleksovski, Z., Klein, M., Ten Kate, W., & van Harmelen, F. (2006). Matching unstructured vocabularies using a background Ontology. In Proceedings of knowledge engineering and knowledge management (EKAW) (pp. 182–197).

40. Lopez, V., Uren, V., Motta, E., & Pasin, M. (2007). Aqua Log: An ontology-driven question answering system for organizational semantic intranets. *Web Semantics: Science, Services and Agents on the World Wide Web, 5*(2), 72–105.
41. Tablan, V., Damljanovi, D., & Bontcheva, K. (2008). A natural language query interface to structured information. In *The semantic web: Research and applications, LNCS 5021* (pp. 361–375). Springer.
42. Dasgupta, S., Patel, R., Padia, A., & Shah, K. (2013). Description logics-based formalization of Wh- queries, CoRRabs. 1312.6948.

Chapter 11
A Review of Computational Intelligence Technologies for Tackling Covid-19 Pandemic

Anamika Rana and Sushma Malik

11.1 Introduction

Several epidemics invaded the world in world history until now. The World Health Organization (WHO) and a number of national agencies of the countries fight against these epidemics to date. The first case of COVID-19 was confirmed in Wuhan city of China in December 2019. Coronavirus spread in more than 185 countries infecting more than 7,145,800 persons and also causing 407,067 deaths by June 09, 2020 [1]. The novel coronavirus, Covid-19, was initiated from Wuhan and has stretched speedily across the world. WHO declared Covid-19 as a pandemic in the world [2]. The new infection spread by the virus of the corona family and at present time the globe is a threat from the Covid-19. Till now, many countries around the globe have observed huge cases of Covid-19. The main target of this virus is those people who have less immunity, old age, and have any medical problems especially linked with lungs. Till now no vaccine is available for Covid-19.

The variety of inflamed humans is growing daily with the aid of using day with inside the world due to the transmittable nature of coronavirus. The transmission of coronavirus is spread person to person contacts and also occurred in community transmission. Coronavirus can spread a range of illnesses wherein respiratory is one of them. COVID-19 symptoms may become up within 2 weeks after the infection. The only prevention is the main concern to manage the Covid-19. Covid-19 affects the daily life of human beings. It mainly affects the health, economic, and social life of human beings [3].

A. Rana (✉)
Maharaja Surajmal Institute, New Delhi, India

S. Malik
Institute of Innovation in Technology and Management, New Delhi, India

P. Siarry et al. (eds.), *The Fusion of Internet of Things, Artificial Intelligence, and Cloud Computing in Health Care*, Internet of Things,
https://doi.org/10.1007/978-3-030-75220-0_11

The life of human beings is mostly influenced by COVID-19 and also slows down the growth of activities in the world. The detection of coronavirus near the beginning stage is very essential to control the increase of the virus because of its transmittable nature. Some characteristics of this virus are listed as [4]:

- **High spread rate:** In a few months, coronavirus spread in the world and become a pandemic globally. The movements of people globally by crossing international borders are the main reason for its spread and from human to human contact.
- **Specific Target:** Old age people are the main target because they have low immunity and other respiratory problems. People with other medical issues like diabetes, heart problem; blood pressure are also the targets of this virus.
- **Recovery Rate:** The recovery rate of coronavirus infected patients is low globally and differs from country to country.

This pandemic has affected all the domains and also modifies the way of life. Due to COVID-19, countries have a huge loss which cannot be estimated both in the economy and life of citizens. To recover this economic loss and save a life, deployment of emerging technologies is used to battle this invisible enemy. AI domain is used to pick out the COVID-19 symptoms with the usage of CT images. The high speed of the internet is needed for teleconferencing and telemedicine which is provided by 5G network technology and additionally assist to ship and receive heavy length pictures very fast. IoT tool is used to connect all the devices of hospitals with the internet and help to provide updated information to health workers. Data may be shared remotely with the help of blockchain technology in a secure manner and assist to streamline the supply chains of various types of medical equipment like face masks, PPE kits, sanitizer, etc., and many more technologies are used during this pandemic time. Section 11.2 of this chapter is clearing up the role of CI technologies in this pandemic environment and how it saves life globally. Section 11.3 summarizes the literature review of research papers written by academic researchers in the COVID-19 pandemic time on a number of CI technologies like AI, IoT, and other technologies including, blockchain, including Cloud computing, Drones, Big data, and 5G network technology.

11.2 Role of Computational Intelligence (CI) to Quash Covid-19

Pandemics have been frightening human beings again and again. The various pandemics like SARS, H1N1, Ebola, and many more have shown their teeth in the precedent but from every pandemic, human beings learn a new way to battle and save their life from these kinds of outbreaks with the help of technologies [5]. Technology refers to techniques, frameworks, and developed the many devices which are designed by the use of scientific information are useful for a practical purpose.

To combat coronavirus, various technologies play an essential role like AI technology helps to spot the patients and virus, disease tracking, and prediction [6]. IoT technology connects all the medical equipments with the internet and helps the healthcare workers to provide the treatment remotely and diminish the physical contacts. The amalgamation of AI with medical imaging can modify the way of diagnosis. Machine learning develops algorithms that improve the decision-making process. Technology plays a critical role to deal with the COVID-19 situation by using robotics to supply food packets and medicines to the patients who are affected by this virus in the hospitals and in remotely monitoring patients. Figure 11.1 shows the number of ways that emerging technologies tackle coronavirus.

11.2.1 Preventive Measures

Coronavirus nature is transmittable means it can spread from the contacts of a healthy person with an infected person and it spreads very fast. Till now no vaccine is found for this kind of virus. The only solution is prevention. Main prevention is required in the hospitals, where health workers are performing the treatment to save lives and they come directly in contact with the infected patients. Face masks are the essential equipment used by medical examiners to diminish the threat of contact with the virus while performing their jobs. Also, great pressure on the manufacturing units of antiviral soap and sanitizers to fullfill the needs to keep the price in control. Autonomous sanitizing machines are required to deploy at affected clusters to bring the spread of the virus to an end. The most relevant solutions applied with the usage of emerging technologies that enable the faster and efficient way to battle with COVID-19 pandemic are as follows [7]:

- Disease Surveillance
- Air Filtration Systems
- Disinfectants
- Spit Disposal
- Antiviral Masks

11.2.2 Diagnostic Solutions

The WHO advised all health authorities throughout the world to test, detect, trace, and isolated coronavirus infected patients. Only social distancing is the one and only solution to diminish the spread of the virus and used home testing and diagnostic kits. Due to an increase in the number of infected patients and for the security measures, virtual medical visits and remotely diagnosis of patients are doing by the doctors. Chatbots and a number of mobile apps are used in the battle of COVID-19.

The most relevant solutions for the diagnosis of infections are applied with the usage of emerging technologies that enable a faster and efficient way to battle with COVID-19 pandemic are as follows [7]:

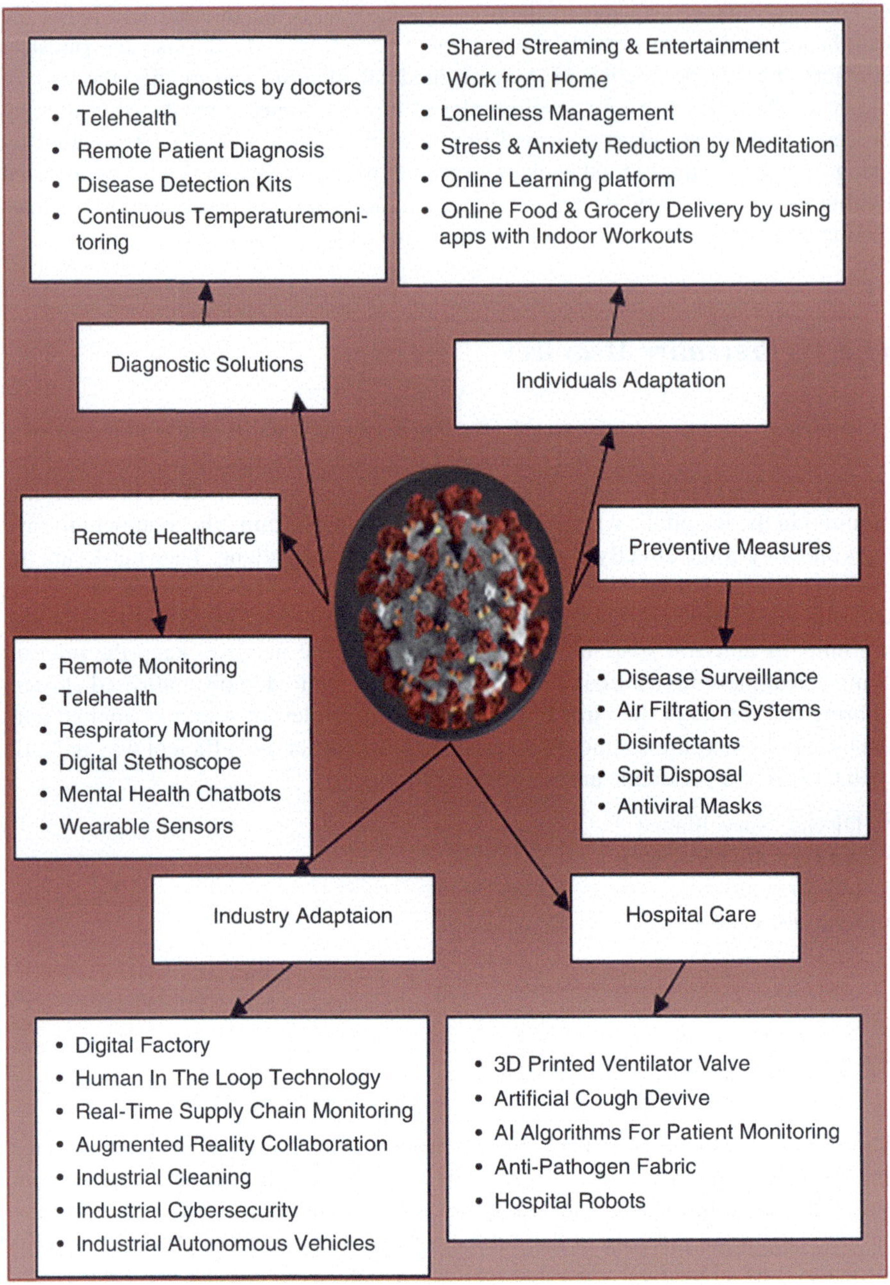

Fig. 11.1 Role of modern technology to quash COVID-19

- Mobile Diagnostics by doctors
- Telehealth
- Remote Patient Diagnosis
- Disease Detection Kits

11.2.3 Hospital Care

Hospitals are the main battlefield where health workers directly contact infected patients and provide treatment. To avoid physical contact, Robots are employed to supply food packets and pills to infected persons and help out to reduce the burden from health workers. Artificial ventilators are used to improve the patient's management. Health workers are the front line warriors who require safety goggles, PPE Kits, gloves, and surgical-grade essentials.

To battle with COVID-19 pandemic in a faster and efficient way in the hospital areas, the emerging technologies are providing the following solutions [7]:

- Hospital Robots
- 3D Printed Ventilator Valve
- Artificial Cough Device
- AI Algorithms For Patient Monitoring
- Antipathogen Fabric

11.2.4 Industry Adaptation

During this epidemic time, all the factories, industries, and businesses are locked due to the lockdown situation and result in heavy losses. To prevent the loss, many industries and businesses are circulating from bodily to virtual platforms by using the rising technologies. Robots and drones are employed to moving items from one place to another in industries and stop the stretch of the virus by minimizing social distancing. Machines and components in a factory are controlled by augmented reality to diminish the workers inside the factory. The most relevant solutions for industries adopted during this epidemic are the usage of emerging technologies that enable faster and efficient way are as follows [7]:

- Digital Factory
- Human In The Loop Technology
- Real-Time Supply Chain Monitoring
- Augmented Reality Collaboration
- Industrial Cleaning
- Industrial Cybersecurity
- Industrial Autonomous Vehicles

11.2.5 Remote Healthcare

In this pandemic time, hospitals are not able to give attention to normal patients and also it is not secure to visit the hospitals in that situation. But for their treatments, health workers are using lots of applications to provide assistance and treatment to them. The digital platform allows doctors and infected persons to remotely communicate with video conferencing and provides digital medical assistance by maintaining social distancing.

The most relevant solutions for remote healthcare are applied with the usage of emerging technologies that enable a faster and efficient way to battle with COVID-19 pandemic are as follows [7]:

- Remote Monitoring
- Telehealth
- Respiratory Monitoring
- Digital Stethoscope
- Mental Health Chatbots
- Wearable Sensors

11.2.6 Individuals Adaptation

During the lockdown and also to maintain the social distancing to prevent the spread of infection, smartphones-based applications are used to connect with each other. Due to coronavirus, schools, colleges, and universities are using the E-learning platforms to complete their syllabus and continue the teaching-learning process between the teachers and students. Offices are temporarily closed in this situation and finding innovative online tools to connect the employees remotely and provide the solution work from home to stop the spread of the virus. For entertainment, streaming and apps are used for passing time, because in this outbreak all the sources of entertainment like Malls, Cinema Halls, Gyms, Fun clubs, and many more are shutdown. Technology enables people to normally live their life by maintaining social distancing and self-isolation during this pandemic time.

The most relevant solutions for individuals adopted during the battle with the COVID-19 pandemic with the usage of emerging technologies that enable faster and efficient way are as follows [7]:

- Shared Streaming & Entertainment
- Work from Home
- Loneliness Management
- Stress & Anxiety Reduction by Meditation
- Online Learning platform
- Online Food & Grocery Delivery by using apps
- Indoor Workouts

11.3 Literature Review

The COVID-19 pandemic is dispersing all over the world and countries suffering from this infection are failed to predict the magnitude of the situation due to the heavy demand for medical care facilities broken down the top healthcare models in the world. Now activities of the person have moved to the binary platform by using emerging technologies like AI, Cloud Computing, IoT, Blockchain, 5G Network, Robotics, and Drones to prevent, diagnose, tracing of the virus, social distancing, workplace safety, and many more. These technologies get better consistency of treatment and also the power of decision making. The infected patients are increasing daily globally and at that time its need to utilize the emerging technologies in a robust, organized manner, and in an efficient way to enhance the battle against the COVID-19 pandemic. Figure 11.2 demonstrates the accomplishment of CI technologies to handle the COVID-19 pandemic situation.

Technology refers to techniques, frameworks, and devices which are the aftereffect of scientific information being utilized for practical purposes. Emerging technologies like AI, Cloud Computing, IoT, Big data, neural network are used to handle this pandemic situation. Table 11.1 summarized the literature review of AI technology-based research papers. Table 11.2 contains the literature review of IoT technology-based research papers written on this pandemic time to handle this situation. Big data, cloud computing, fuzzy logic, blockchain, neural network-based research papers written on the COVID-19 epidemic situation are reviewed in Table 11.3.

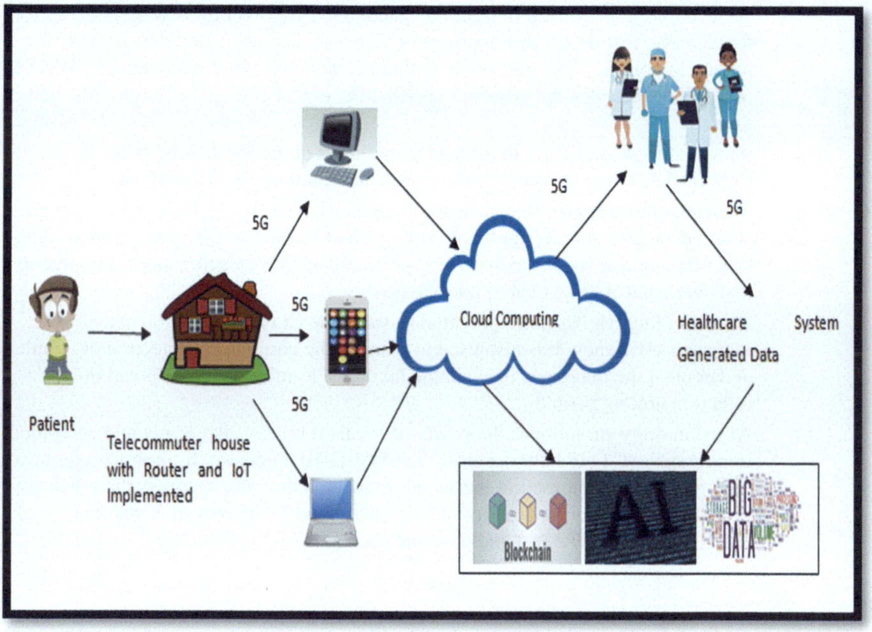

Fig. 11.2 Application of CI technologies for tackling COVID-19 pandemic

Table 11.1 Literature review on application of artificial intelligence (AI)

S. no.	Author	Study
1	[8]	AI-based mobile applications like ArogyaSetu are launched by the government of India for creating awareness among the citizens, self-assessment, and contact tracing for COVID-19 infection
2	[9]	AI-based applications play a vital role in this epidemic time. AI applications are used in the diagnosis of disease, contact tracing, and maintain social distancing for the safety of the people in the workplace
3	[10]	Many COVID-19 patients infected by coronavirus develop pneumonia which is called novel coronavirus pneumonia (NCP) and rapidly fails the respiratory system. The AI-based system is developed to identify NCP and also distinguish it from other common pneumonia by using computed tomography (CT). AI system performs quick diagnosis and helps the radiologists and physicians when the health system is overloaded
4	[11]	The collaboration of AI with pharmacology can improve the efficiency of drug repurposing. Implementation of AI technology can generate the learning prediction model and perform a quick virtual screening to accurately display output. AI technology can identify the drugs that fight against the disease like COVID-19
5	[12]	AI techniques are used in the discovery and recognition of COVID-19 medical images
6	[1]	AI technology improves the screening, prediction, tracking of contacts, forecasting, and development of drugs of COVID-19
7	[13]	AI technology plays an essential function in the processing of an enormous amount of medical data and is also used to extract the key points for several applications. For the repurposing drug, the existing datasets and mined
8	[14]	AI technology is utilized to fight this pandemic by extracting new approaches for the discovery of drugs, development of vaccines, and also spread awareness among the public. This also helps to find the new possible treatment of COVID-19 and also accelerates the process to predict the existing drugs or develop the new drug
9	[15]	AI technology is utilized to recognize marketed drugs for dealing with COVID-19. The potential of old drugs is identified by the AI platform
10	[16]	Presented the AI bases diagnosis tool named AI4COVID-19 by using the cough sound through a mobile application. By virtual testing for everyone through this tool offer unique functionality like timely, cost-effective, self-monitoring, tracing, and also control the widen of coronavirus
11	[17]	AI technology shows more potential to solve the COVID-19 problem and also increases efficiency. It is also used to manage the equipment, detection of a fault, and control the diagnosis in available facilities, to minimize the spread of infection among people
12	[18]	AI technology strengthens the power of medical images like X-ray and computed tomography (CT) to battle against the COVID-19 epidemic. It minimizes contact with patients by automating the scanning method and also recovers the efficiency of work by an accurate description of infection in the images of X-ray and CT. Radiologists take fast and accurate decisions

(continued)

Table 11.1 (continued)

S. no.	Author	Study
13	[19]	The process of diagnosis and treatment of COVID-19 disease are accelerating by the use of AI technology. A number of techniques have been developed to fight COVID-19
14	[20]	With AI technology, COVID-19 infection is identified in the early stage. AI model is designed to recognize COVID-19 infection on initial chest CT scans
15	[21]	For the recognition of COVID-19 images of the X-rays are used. Construct a model for detecting COVID-19 with high-resolution X-rays. Reduce the work pressure of radiologists and also help to stop the spread of COVID-19
16	[22]	AI is the upcoming and valuable technology to recognize the infection in an early-stage and also helpful in monitoring the infected person. It improves the treatment and decision-making process and is used to develop the proper treatment, prevention of the COVID-19, and also helps in the drug and vaccine development of COVID-19
17	[23]	Proposed a new framework that can be used by doctors and radiologists based on using only smartphone sensors at any time and anywhere. Does not require any external sensors to provide an accurate result by this framework
18	[24]	AI technology is used to design effective robots and autonomous machines for working, disinfection, and deliver food and medicines to the patients in the hospitals. AI and natural language processing (NLP) technologies are utilized to design the chatbot which helps in remotely communicate and provide consultations to the people about the COVID-19
19	[25, 26]	AI is the most used technology and if it is used properly, it should be highly effective technology against the COVID-19 pandemic time. This technology is used in disease surveillance, prediction of risk, host identification, medical diagnosis, busting fake news, and also used in the implementation of lockdown properly
20	[27]	The spread of coronavirus in real-time and plan to improve the health of people by monitoring their effectiveness. Also, help to discover new drugs and also identify the potential vaccine from the existing vaccines
21	[28]	AI is a very useful technology for helping in the outbreak prediction and detection of coronavirus. It also an attractive tool for the discovery of vaccines and drugs by using the datasets provided by healthcare organizations, governments, and also from patients
22	[29]	DL domain changes the traditional paradigm of the medical field. With this technology, doctors have more time to provide more care to patients. It increases the assessing level of satisfaction of both doctors and patients by the integration of real and binary data
23	[30]	In the machine learning domain, DL is the new branch that motivates the doctors to establish and simulate a NN for the analysis of the brain of the human being. In the medical domain, analysis of medical images for the diagnosis of the disease is a crucial part but it can be sort-out by the implementation of DL
24	[31]	Computer science branches like biomedical big data and AI play an essential role in the crucial time of the COVID-19 pandemic. Images of CT and X-rays are used for monitoring and detection of disease

Table 11.2 Literature review on application of internet of things (IoT)

S. no.	Author	Study
1	[32, 33]	With IoT technology, all the medical types of equipment are connected with the internet and make available information timely to healthcare workers. With well-connected devices, infected cases are easily handled remotely
2	[34, 35]	IoT technology assists the patients, physicians, healthcare workers, and hospital management to recognize the symptoms of the COVID-19 and also managed the infected cases globally. This technology also helps to minimize the complexity and time taken for effective management during this pandemic time IoT technology provides a variety of applications like telehealth, digital scanning, digital staff, and many more. IoT-based telemedicine is a way for health workers during this pandemic time to provide treatment to infected patients
3	[36]	In the current situation, the performance of IoT in the medical field helps the patients to receive proper healthcare at home and also creates a comprehensive management database for governments and healthcare workers
4	[37]	IoT-enabled applications to monitor health in real-time and improve global health. This technology develops the smart disease surveillance system to control the situation during this pandemic time
5	[38]	Cognitive internet of medical things (CIoMT) technology is used for smart health care and also helps to handle the pandemic situation. It helps in rapid diagnosis, dynamic monitoring, provides better treatment, and also controls the spread of coronavirus to others
6	[39]	IoMT develops a quality environment for smart healthcare. It helps in the monitoring and tracking of infected persons remotely and provides quality services
7	[40]	Internet of health things (IoHT) is an extension of IoT, whose main motive is to connect the infected patient to healthcare facilities to monitor and control the patient's body by using the sensors
8	[41]	With the help of IoMT, healthcare workers get relief and also ensure quarantine, implementation, and origin of pandemic. By using sensors, data can be collected and sent to a central server for analysis. It is the better method for the medical helpers and government agencies for the updated information on the COVID-19 crisis
9	[42]	Proposed the smart helmet with a mounted thermal imaging system capable to detect the COVID-19 infected person with minimum human interactions
10	[43]	IoT technology helps in the identification of risk and infection of COVID-19 and also minimizes the load of health workers and manufacturing units
11	[44]	Proposed the IoT-based framework to minimize the impact of a communicable disease like COVID-19. The records of confirmed cases of COVID-19 are used to develop an ML-based predictive model infection as well as provide the treatment responses
12	[45, 46]	IoT technology helps to monitor, tracking, delivering, and collecting of data from the users and assists the healthcare by using IoT-enabled technologies like wearables, drones, robots, IoT buttons, and smartphone application

Table 11.3 Literature review on application of other technologies like big data, blockchain, drones, cloud computing, robotics

S. no.	Author	Study	Technology used
1	[27]	Big data technology is used to handle the large amount of data produced from public health observation, monitoring of real-time epidemic, and also used in the forecasting of the situation	Big data
2	[28]	Integration of big data and AI technology helps to understand the COVID-19 in terms of tracking, the structure of the virus, its treatment, and also search and manufacturing of vaccine	
3	[47]	Big data technology is used to handle the huge amount of infected person data and helps to understand the structure and nature of coronavirus. This technology helps scientists, health workers, and epidemiologists in the decision-making process to fight COVID-19	
4	[25]	Drone technology minimizes human interaction and also reaches inaccessible areas by the people. Drone technology is adopted for crowd surveillance to maintain social distancing, to broadcast important information particularly in those areas where communication channels are lack during the lockdown period. Also used to spray disinfectants in the contaminated zones	Drone
5	[48]	With the help of blockchain technology, the public and organizations become part of interconnected networks to share secure data globally. Blockchain-based applications are used to monitor the COVID-19 patients and minimize some burden from the health workers. Algorithms help to provide real-time information and also help in the effective management of the supply chain	Blockchain
6	[49]	With blockchain technology, data of infected patients are automatically reported to the health workers at the same time when it is stored in the blockchain and data are transparent with completely open for the public without any manipulation. With the use of blockchain monetary donations become transparent and also prevent the spread of false information related to COVID-19	
7	[50]	Blockchain technology plays an essential l role in the field of medicine with the management of digital medical data, biomedical research, remotely monitoring the patients, control the drugs, and pharmaceuticals supply chain management	
8	[51]	In the pandemic time, the diagnosis of infected patients is difficult because of the shortage of testing kits. Combination of blockchain with other technology helps to collect the digital data from the various sources without leakage of data and also maintains the confidentiality of data	

(continued)

Table 11.3 (continued)

S. no.	Author	Study	Technology used
9	[52]	The blockchain system generates an account for every person and contact tracing becomes easier when mobile devices of persons are connected with blockchain account. When the person comes in contact with another person, then blockchain adds the transaction with geo-location and time stamp and the healthcare official able to verify that the person makes contact with the COVID-19 infected person or not	
10	[53]	Blockchain technology is used to control the pandemic of COVID-19 with solutions like tracking, protection of user privacy, safely daily operations, medical supply chain, and also tracking the donations	
11	[54]	Designed the tracing and notification system based on blockchain with three types of tracing services based on Bluetooth, location, and health. The system will provide the remainder to the user about their previous contacts that may cause infection based on user travel and contact history	
12	[55]	Blockchain technology plays an essential role in the management of the post COVID-19 world. It is used to implement various key functions like contact tracing, sharing of patient information, E-government, online learning, management of immigration, contact-free delivery, and automated surveillance	
13	[56]	Blockchain technology has the potential to change healthcare systems. This technology provides the secure transfer of health information of patients between the healthcare workers	
14	[57]	Blockchain technology provides five perspectives as tracing the origin of the pandemic, social distancing, quarantining, smart hospitals, remote healthcare, and telemedicine	
15	[58]	A blockchain-enabled system named BeepTrace is proposed to resolve the privacy issues during the binary contact tracing for coronavirus pandemic	
16	[59]	Cloud computing technology provides the resources of the computer system over the internet like servers for the storage, database, etc. by using this technology, all the resources are faster available and flexible which minimized the processing coat and also increased efficiency	Cloud computing
17	[60, 61]	Cloud-based tools are used for the screening and also alert the authorities if quarantine is breached. Cloud-based AI-assisted services are used to identify the cases of COVID-19. The cloud application can transform the healthcare system from capital intensive to pay per usage model	
18	[62]	During the COVID-19 pandemic, patient-generated health data (PGHD) play a very important role. Coronavirus tracking apps are used in smartphones to collect and share PGHD and store them on the cloud. Users are easily checked by entering personal information on apps by comparing their data with cloud data whether the user has contact with an infected person or not	

(continued)

Table 11.3 (continued)

S. no.	Author	Study	Technology used
19	[63]	Doctors are the first line of defense to slow the spread of the virus by maintaining social distancing and provide the services by call or video conferencing with patients. 5G technology is the main source of telemedicine. 5G provides the high bandwidth required for video conferencing	5G network technology
20	[25]	Hospitals with 5G enabled medical imaging platforms are used to real-time diagnosis of COVID-19 patients and also reduce the load of healthcare warriors	
21	[64]	5G smartphones are used as the virtual communication device between the patients and doctors by reducing healthcare costs and also maintaining the social distancing in this pandemic tie	
22	[65]	By the integration of the fractal dimension and fuzzy logic system, the proposed hybrid intelligent approach for accomplishing the efficient and accurate forecasting of the COVID-19 time series	Fuzzy logic
23	[66]	The fuzzy logic-based model is used to find the appropriate conditions for the growth of COVID-19 infection. The spread of COVID-19 disease decreases with higher temperature and low RH and on the other hand, lower temperature with high RH provides an enviable atmosphere for coronavirus	
24	[67]	Introduced the COVID-net named system based on a neural network for the detection of coronavirus cases from the CXR images. It is open-source and easily available to the public	Neural network
25	[68]	Proposed a deep learning approach to identify COVID-19 infected cases by the usage of radiography images named CoroNet based on a neural network	

11.3.1 Applications of Artificial Intelligence

- Used to identify the COVID-19 infection through chest CT images.
- COVID-19 suspected patients are detected with signs and symptoms.
- Mobile applications based on AI are used to spread awareness and tracing for COVID-19 infection.
- Improve the discovery of COVID-19 drugs.
- Reducing the workload of health workers.

AI technology is playing an essential role in the fight with COVID-19 and also provides quick solutions to prevent this virus. Many applications are designed on AI technology like ArogyaSetu App in India which is used to create awareness, self-assessment, and also help to trace the contacts for COVID-19 infection. During this pandemic time, front line worriers are facing overload problems due to the huge increase of infected patients and have limited health workers. AI technology-based systems help to minimize the burden by performing quick diagnosis. It also helps in prediction and detection of coronavirus. AI technology is used to design and develop robotics and drones. Robotics is used for the supply of food packets and medicines to the infected patients in the hospitals and help to maintain social distancing. Drones are used to spry the disinfectant in the quarantine zones and help to stop the spread of coronavirus.

11.3.2 Applications of IoT

- IOT technology helps in remote monitoring of self-quarantine and self-assessment and sends the data to health workers for the assessment.
- IOT technology helps in the rapid diagnosis of a human being with a history of traveling in COVID-19-affected countries.
- Support remote consultations between healthcare workers and patients with smart video conferencing and telemedicine.
- Smart thermometers are used to check the temperature of the person.

In the pandemic time, IoT technology has been used in the medical domain and also gives a positive result to handle this disease. IoT technologies are used in three phases including early identification, quarantine time, and after recovery. IoT-enabled devices like wearable, drones, robots, IoT buttons, and smartphone applications are used in fighting with COVID-19 [45].

IoMT is the extended version of IoT in the field of medicine. IoMT technology helps to provide an integrated network of medical equipment to healthcare workers to battle this pandemic situation and automatically convey a message to the medical staff. With this technology, infected cases are easily handled in a remote location with well-connected teleservices. IoMT technology excellently screens the infected patients and also handles all the cases smartly. A better environment can be created with the proper accomplishment of this technology which helps to fight this invisible enemy.

11.3.3 Applications of Other Technologies

- Big data is used to track COVID-19 cases and provides a large amount of space to store data.
- Drones are used for disinfecting and sterilizing COVID-19 contaminated areas.
- Autonomous robots are used to provide medicines and food to COVID-19 patients and reduce health worker's risks of infection.
- With the help of blockchain, verification and validation of COVID-19 data are done in an easy way.
- Facilitates the secure sharing of data.
- 5G technology supports real-time sharing of health data and high-quality video conferencing.

- Home quarantine patients are tracked using GPS and mobile phones.
- Reduce the load of healthcare warriors.
- Help in the recognition of coronavirus cases with radiography images.

Other technologies like Cloud computing, Blockchain, 5G network technology, Big data, and many more are playing a vital role during this epidemic time. In the current situation, a large amount of data are collected from various sources like applications used on smartphones, patient's records from hospitals, and Government released data are stored on the cloud which helps to provide the updated information. To maintain social distancing, a number of activities are moved from physical to virtual platforms with the help of 5G network technology. 5G network technology provides the high bandwidth of the internet which helps to video conferencing, teleconferencing, and sharing of videos and images of huge size at very fast speed.

11.4 Challenges During Implementation of CI Technologies

CI technologies provide new inventions in the binary world. By using CI technologies, simulated expertize is to develop and design which is to some extent similar to the real-time situation. These technologies are given a number of applications in various domains that are used in daily work. But as usual, every coin has two sides, one side of CI technologies is very useful in every domain but on the other side, these technologies face several challenges during the implementation which highlight in Fig. 11.3. Some of them are listed as:

1. **Lack of Awareness**: Generally users are not aware of the applications of CI technologies. The value of CI technologies is best understood when mass users adopted these technologies.
2. **Network Load**: In some applications of CI technologies environment, data are streaming live over the internet with minimum local caching of frequently used data.
3. **Congestion in Communication**: In CI technologies, communication can be occurring in between servers and the asset cluster and which causes congestion problems in communications.
4. **Cost:** The initial cost to develop the CI technologies-based environment is so high. A large scale of people is not able to afford these technologies in their daily routine.
5. **Internet:** The Internet is the main source to implement the CI technologies-based environment. So 5G internet bandwidth is required but still, 5G internet service is not fully implemented in most areas.
6. **Experience issue**: Users are not skilled in how to use the applications based on CI technologies and sometimes users do not easily adopt the new technologies because of less experience.

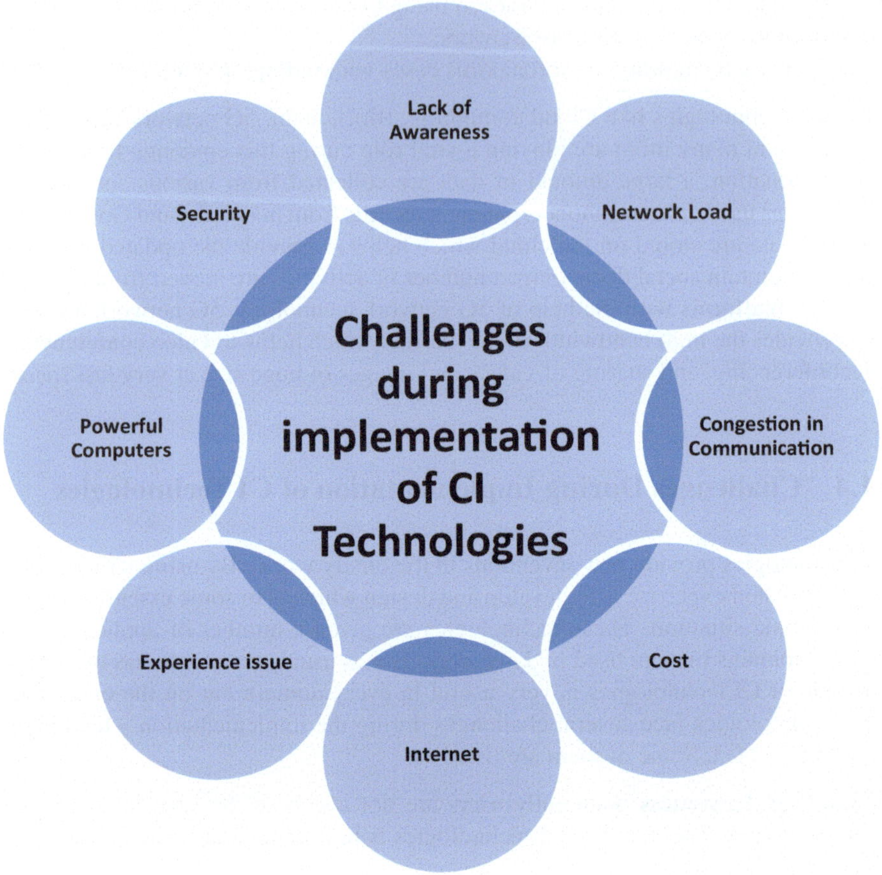

Fig. 11.3 Challenges during the implementation of CI technologies

7. **Security:** Cybersecurity and data privacy are sensitive issues in the digital platform. Due to these reasons, some users are not using these technologies even do not try to adopt them.
8. **Powerful Computers**: To use the CI technologies, the main necessity is powerful computer systems with a high power processor with high configuration and resolution.

11.5 Conclusion

COVID-19 pandemic is a public health emergency globally and has become the most challenging area for global researchers. Academic research helps to a proper understanding of COVID-19. Researchers are investigating each and every possible option to battle the COVID-19 pandemic and a new way is opened by the emerging technologies. Now technologies have become an important part of the life of people to execute their day-to-day activities and help to save a life. This chapter talks about the symptoms and preventions against the COVID-19. It also highlighted the emerging technologies used to fight COVID-19. IoT technology is used to integrate the medical equipment with the internet and provide remote treatment to the infected patients and many more technologies are highlighted. Emerging technologies like IoT, AI, Blockchain, 5G, and many more give complementary efforts to the world to fight against the COVID-19 and future pandemics.

References

1. Lalmuanawma, S., Hussain, J., & Chhakchhuak, L. (2020). Applications of machine learning and artificial intelligence for Covid-19 (SARS-CoV-2) pandemic: A review. *Chaos, Solitons and Fractals, 139*. https://doi.org/10.1016/j.chaos.2020.110059.
2. Montemurro, N. (2020). The emotional impact of COVID-19: From medical staff to common people. *Brain, Behavior, and Immunity, 1591*, 1–2. https://doi.org/10.1016/j.bbi.2020.03.032
3. Haleem, A., Javaid, M., Vaishya, R., & Deshmukh, S. G. (2020). Areas of academic research with the impact of COVID-19. *The American Journal of Emergency Medicine, 38*, 1524–1526. https://doi.org/10.1016/j.ajem.2020.04.022
4. Shaw, R., Kim, Y., & Hua, J. (2020). Governance, technology and citizen behavior in pandemic: Lessons from COVID-19 in East Asia. *Progress in Disaster Science, 6*, 100090. https://doi.org/10.1016/j.pdisas.2020.100090
5. Manjunath, B. S. (2020, April). Covid-19: 8 ways in which technology helps pandemic management. IT News, ET CIO.
6. Kumar, A., Gupta, P. K., & Srivastava, A. (2020). A review of modern technologies for tackling COVID-19 pandemic. *Diabetes and Metabolic Syndrome: Clinical Research & Reviews, 14*(4), 569–573. https://doi.org/10.1016/j.dsx.2020.05.008
7. Startus Insight. (2020). 8 ways emerging technologies tackle the global coronavirus pandemic.
8. Ransing, R., Nagendrappa, S., Patil, A., Shoib, S., & Sarkar, D. (2020). Potential role of artificial intelligence to address the COVID-19 outbreak-related mental health issues in India. *Psychiatry Research, 290*, 113176. https://doi.org/10.1016/j.psychres.2020.113176
9. Sipior, J. C. (2020). Considerations for development and use of AI in response to COVID-19. *International Journal of Information Management, 55*, 102170. https://doi.org/10.1016/j.ijinfomgt.2020.102170
10. Zhang, K., et al. (2020). Clinically applicable AI system for accurate diagnosis, quantitative measurements, and prognosis of COVID-19 pneumonia using computed tomography. *Cell, 181*(6), 1423–1433.e11. https://doi.org/10.1016/j.cell.2020.04.045
11. Mohanty, S., Harun, M., Rashid, A. I., Mridul, M., Mohanty, C., & Swayamsiddha, S. (2020). Application of artificial intelligence in COVID-19 drug repurposing. *Diabetes and Metabolic Syndrome: Clinical Research & Reviews, 14*(5), 1027–1031. https://doi.org/10.1016/j.dsx.2020.06.068
12. Albahri, O. S., et al. (2020). Systematic review of artificial intelligence techniques in the detection and classification of COVID-19 medical images in terms of evaluation and benchmarking: Taxonomy analysis, challenges, future solutions and methodological aspects. *Journal of Infection and Public Health, 13*, 1381–1396. https://doi.org/10.1016/j.jiph.2020.06.028

13. Park, Y., Casey, D., Joshi, I., Zhu, J., & Cheng, F. (2020). Emergence of new disease: How can artificial intelligence help? *Trends in Molecular Medicine, 26*(7), 6–8. https://doi.org/10.1016/j.molmed.2020.04.007
14. Ahuja, A. S., Reddy, V. P., & Marques, O. (2020). Artificial intelligence and COVID-19: A multidisciplinary approach. *Integrative Medicine Research, 9*(3), 100434. https://doi.org/10.1016/j.imr.2020.100434
15. Ke, Y. Y., et al. (2020). Artificial intelligence approach fighting COVID-19 with repurposing drugs. *Biomedical Journal, 43*(4), 355–362. https://doi.org/10.1016/j.bj.2020.05.001
16. Imran, A., et al. (2020). AI4COVID-19: AI enabled preliminary diagnosis for COVID-19 from cough samples via an app. *Informatics in Medicine Unlocked, 20*, 100378. https://doi.org/10.1016/j.imu.2020.100378
17. Wang, B., Yang, Z., Xuan, J., & Jiao, K. (2020). Crises and opportunities in terms of energy and AI technologies during the COVID-19 pandemic. *Energy AI, 1*, 100013. https://doi.org/10.1016/j.egyai.2020.100013
18. Shi, F., et al. (2020). Review of artificial intelligence techniques in imaging data acquisition, segmentation and diagnosis for COVID-19. *IEEE Reviews in Biomedical Engineering*, 1–13. https://doi.org/10.1109/RBME.2020.2987975
19. Jamshidi, M., et al. (2020). Artificial Intelligence and COVID-19: Deep Learning Approaches for Diagnosis and Treatment. *IEEE Access, 8*, 109581–109595. https://doi.org/10.1109/ACCESS.2020.3001973
20. Mei, X., et al. (2020). Artificial intelligence–enabled rapid diagnosis of patients with COVID-19. *Nature Medicine, 26*(8), 1224–1228. https://doi.org/10.1038/s41591-020-0931-3
21. Salman, F. M., Abu-Naser, S. S., Alajrami, E., Abu-Nasser, B. S., & Ashqar, B. A. M. (2020). COVID-19 detection using artificial intelligence. *International Journal of Computer Engineering Research, 4*(3), 18–25.
22. Vaishya, R., Javaid, M., Khan, I. H., & Haleem, A. (2020). Artificial intelligence (AI) applications for COVID-19 pandemic. *Diabetes and Metabolic Syndrome: Clinical Research & Reviews, 14*(4), 337–339. https://doi.org/10.1016/j.dsx.2020.04.012
23. Maghdid, H. S., Ghafoor, K. Z., Sadiq, A. S., Curran, K., & Rabie, K. (2020). A novel AI-enabled framework to diagnose coronavirus COVID 19 using smartphone embedded sensors: Design study (pp. 1–7).
24. Nguyen, T. T., Waurn, G., & Campus, P. (2020). Artificial intelligence in the battle against coronavirus (COVID-19): A survey and future research directions. Researchgate.Net (pp. 1–13). https://doi.org/10.13140/RG.2.2.36491.23846.Artificial
25. Chamola, V., Hassija, V., Gupta, V., & Guizani, M. (2020). A comprehensive review of the COVID-19 pandemic and the role of IoT, drones, AI, blockchain, and 5G in managing its impact. *IEEE Access, 8*, 90225–90265. https://doi.org/10.1109/ACCESS.2020.2992341
26. Sohrabi, C., Alsafi, Z., Neill, N. O., Khan, M., & Kerwan, A. (2020, January). Since January 2020 Elsevier has created a COVID-19 resource centre with free information in English and Mandarin on the novel coronavirus COVID- 19. The COVID-19 resource centre is hosted on Elsevier Connect, the company's public news and information.
27. Barragán, D., & Manero, J. (2020). *How big data and artificial intelligence can help against COVID-19* (pp. 4–11). IE Business School.
28. Pham, Q. V., Nguyen, D. C., Huynh-The, T., Hwang, W. J., & Pathirana, P. N. (2020). Artificial intelligence (AI) and big data for coronavirus (COVID-19) pandemic: A survey on the state-of-the-arts. *IEEE Access, 8*, 130820–130839. https://doi.org/10.1109/ACCESS.2020.3009328
29. Piccialli, F., Di, V., Giampaolo, F., & Cuomo, S. (2021). A survey on deep learning in medicine: Why, how and when? *Information Fusion, 66*, 111–137.
30. Wong, K. K. L., Fortino, G., & Abbott, D. (2020). Deep learning-based cardiovascular image diagnosis: A promising challenge. *Future Generation Computer Systems, 110*, 802–811. https://doi.org/10.1016/j.future.2019.09.047
31. Amini, A., Chen, W., Fortino, G., Li, Y., Pan, Y., & Wang, M. D. (2020). Editorial: Special issue on 'AI-driven informatics, sensing, imaging and big data analytics for fighting the COVID-19 pandemic. *IEEE Journal of Biomedical and Health Informatics, 24*(10), 2731–2732. https://doi.org/10.1109/JBHI.2020.3025594

32. Singh, R. P., Javaid, M., Haleem, A., & Suman, R. (2020). Internet of things (IoT) applications to fight against COVID-19 pandemic. *Diabetes and Metabolic Syndrome: Clinical Research & Reviews, 14*(4), 521–524. https://doi.org/10.1016/j.dsx.2020.04.041
33. Rahman, A., Hossain, M. S., Alrajeh, N. A., & Alsolami, F. (2020). Adversarial examples – Security threats to COVID-19 deep learning Systems in Medical IoT devices. *IEEE Internet of Things Journal*, 1–1. https://doi.org/10.1109/jiot.2020.3013710
34. Oyeniyi, J., Ogundoyin, I., & Oyeniran, O. (2020, June). Application of internet of things (IoT) to enhance the fight against covid-19 application of internet of things (IoT) to enhance the fight against covid-19 pandemic. *Diabetes & Metabolic Syndrome: Clinical Research & Reviews, 14*, 521–524.
35. Alam, T. (2020). Coronavirus disease (Covid-19): Reviews, applications, and current status. SSRN Coronavirus & Infectious Disease Research eJournal. https://doi.org/10.2139/ssrn.3660497.
36. Yang, T., Gentile, M., Shen, C. F., & Cheng, C. M. (2020). Combining point-of-care diagnostics and internet of medical things (IOMT) to combat the Covid-19 pandemic. *Diagnostics, 10*(4), 4–6. https://doi.org/10.3390/diagnostics10040224
37. Rahman, M. S., Peeri, N. C., Shrestha, N., Zaki, R., Haque, U., & Hamid, S. H. A. (2020). Defending against the novel coronavirus (COVID-19) outbreak: How can the internet of things (IoT) help to save the world? *Health Policy Technology, 9*, 136–138. https://doi.org/10.1016/j.hlpt.2020.04.005
38. Swayamsiddha, S., & Mohanty, C. (2020). Application of cognitive internet of medical things for COVID-19 pandemic. *Diabetes and Metabolic Syndrome: Clinical Research & Reviews, 14*(5), 911–915. https://doi.org/10.1016/j.dsx.2020.06.014
39. Pratap, R., Javaid, M., Haleem, A., Vaishya, R., & Ali, S. (2020). Internet of medical things (IoMT) for orthopaedic in COVID-19 pandemic: Roles , challenges , and applications. *Journal of Clinical Orthopaedics and Trauma, 11*(4), 713–717. https://doi.org/10.1016/j.jcot.2020.05.011
40. Kamal, M., Aljohani, A., & Alanazi, E. (2020). IoT meets COVID-19: Status, challenges, and opportunities.
41. Tsikala Vafea, M., et al. (2020). Emerging technologies for use in the study, diagnosis, and treatment of patients with COVID-19. *Cellular and Molecular Bioengineering, 13*, 249–257. https://doi.org/10.1007/s12195-020-00629-w
42. Mohammed, M. N., Syamsudin, H., Al-Zubaidi, S., Sairah, A. K., Ramli, R., & Yusuf, E. (2020). Novel covid-19 detection and diagnosis system using iot-based smart helmet. *International Journal of Psychosocial Rehabilitation, 24*(7), 2296–2303. https://doi.org/10.37200/IJPR/V24I7/PR270221
43. Kumar, M. S., Raut, D. R. D., Narwane, D. V. S., & Narkhede, D. B. E. (2020). Applications of industry 4.0 to overcome the COVID-19 operational challenges. *Diabetes and Metabolic Syndrome: Clinical Research & Reviews, 14*(5), 1283–1289. https://doi.org/10.1016/j.dsx.2020.07.010
44. Otoom, M., Otoum, N., Alzubaidi, M. A., Etoom, Y., & Banihani, R. (2020). An IoT-based framework for early identification and monitoring of COVID-19 cases. *Biomedical Signal Processing and Control, 62*, 102149. https://doi.org/10.1016/j.bspc.2020.102149
45. Nasajpour, M., Pouriyeh, S., Parizi, R. M., Dorodchi, M., Valero, M., & Arabnia, H. R. (2020). Internet of things for current COVID-19 and future pandemics: An exploratory study. *Journal of Healthcare Informatics Research, 4*, 325–364.
46. Prabhu, J., et al. (2020). IoT role in prevention of COVID-19 and health care workforces behavioural intention in India - an empirical examination. *International Journal of Pervasive Computing and Communications, 16*(4), 331–340. https://doi.org/10.1108/IJPCC-06-2020-0056
47. Haleem, A., Javaid, M., Khan, I. H., & Vaishya, R. (2020). Significant applications of big data in COVID-19 pandemic. *The Indian Journal of Orthopaedics, 54*(4), 526–528. https://doi.org/10.1007/s43465-020-00129-z
48. Vaishya, R., Haleem, A., Vaish, A., & Javaid, M. (2020). Emerging technologies to combat the COVID-19 pandemic. *Journal of Clinical and Experimental Hepatology, 10*(4), 409–411. https://doi.org/10.1016/j.jceh.2020.04.019

49. Chang, M. C., & Park, D. (2020). How can blockchain help people in the event of pandemics such as the COVID-19? *Journal of Medical Systems, 44*(5), 102. https://doi.org/10.1007/s10916-020-01577-8
50. Mashamba-Thompson, T. P., & Crayton, E. D. (2020). Blockchain and artificial intelligence technology for novel coronavirus disease-19 self-testing. *Diagnostics, 10*(4), 8–11. https://doi.org/10.3390/diagnostics10040198
51. Kumar, R., et al. (2020). Blockchain-federated-learning and deep learning models for COVID-19 detection using CT imaging. 14(8), 1–12.
52. Bansal, A., Garg, C., & Padappayil, R. P. (2020). Optimizing the implementation of COVID-19 'immunity certificates' using Blockchain. *Journal of Medical Systems, 44*(9), 19–20. https://doi.org/10.1007/s10916-020-01616-4
53. Nguyen, D. C., Ding, M., Pathirana, P. N., & Seneviratne, A.. (2020). Blockchain and AI-based solutions to combat coronavirus (COVID-19)-like epidemics: A survey (pp. 1–15).
54. Song, J., Gu, T., Feng, X., Ge, Y., & Mohapatra, P. (2020). Blockchain meets COVID-19: A framework for contact information sharing and risk notification system.
55. Kalla, A., Hewa, T., Mishra, R. A., Ylianttila, M., & Liyanage, M. (2020). The role of blockchain to fight against COVID-19. *IEEE Engineering Management Review, 48*, 85–96. https://doi.org/10.1109/EMR.2020.3014052
56. Alam, T. (2020). Internet of things and blockchain-based framework for coronavirus (COVID-19) disease. SSRN Electronic Journal. https://doi.org/10.2139/ssrn.3660503.
57. Dai, H.-N., Imran, M., & Haider, N. (2020). Blockchain-enabled internet of medical things to combat COVID-19. *IEEE Internet of Things Magazine, 3*, 52–57.
58. Xu, H., Zhang, L., Onireti, O., Fang. Y., Buchanan, W. B., & Imran, M. A. (2020). BeepTrace: Blockchain-enabled privacy-preserving contact tracing for COVID-19 pandemic and beyond (pp. 1–13). https://doi.org/10.13140/RG.2.2.25101.15849/1.
59. Javaid, M., Haleem, A., Vaishya, R., Bahl, S., Suman, R., & Vaish, A. (2020). Industry 4.0 technologies and their applications in fighting COVID-19 pandemic. *Diabetes and Metabolic Syndrome: Clinical Research & Reviews, 14*(4), 419–422. https://doi.org/10.1016/j.dsx.2020.04.032
60. Whitelaw, S., Mamas, M. A., Topol, E., & Van Spall, H. G. C. (2020). Applications of digital technology in COVID-19 pandemic planning and response. *Lancet Digital Health, 2*(8), e435–e440. https://doi.org/10.1016/S2589-7500(20)30142-4
61. Kumar, P. (2020, June). Literature based study on cloud computing for health and sustainability in view of covid19. *Core.Ac.Uk.*
62. Ye, J. (2020). The role of health technology and informatics in global public health emergency: Practices and implications from the COVID-19 pandemic (preprint). *JMIR Medical Informatics, 8*, e19866. https://doi.org/10.2196/19866
63. Vidal-Alaball, J., et al. (2020). Telemedicine in the face of the COVID-19 pandemic. *Atencion Primaria, 52*(6), 418–422. https://doi.org/10.1016/j.aprim.2020.04.003
64. Iyengar, K., Upadhyaya, G. K., Vaishya, R., & Jain, V. (2020). COVID-19 and applications of smartphone technology in the current pandemic. *Diabetes and Metabolic Syndrome: Clinical Research & Reviews, 14*(5), 733–737. https://doi.org/10.1016/j.dsx.2020.05.033
65. Lalmuanawma, S., Hussain, J., & Chhakchhuak, L. (2020). Applications of Machine Learning and Artificial Intelligence for Covid-19 (SARS-CoV-2) pandemic: A review. *Chaos, Solitons Fractals, 139*, 110059. https://doi.org/10.1016/j.chaos.2020.110059
66. Chowdhury, M. A., Shah, Q. Z., Kashem, M. A., Shahid, A., & Akhtar, N. (2020). Evaluation of the effect of environmental parameters on the spread of COVID-19: A fuzzy logic approach. *Advances in Fuzzy Systems, 2020.*
67. Wang, L., Lin, Z. Q., & Wong, A. (2020). COVID-Net: A tailored deep convolutional neural network design for detection of COVID-19 cases from chest x-ray images. *Scientific Reports*, 1–12.
68. Khan, A. I., Shah, J. L., & Bhat, M. M. (2020). CoroNet: A deep neural network for detection and diagnosis of COVID-19 from chest x-ray images. *Computer Methods and Programs in Biomedicine, 196*, 105581. https://doi.org/10.1016/j.cmpb.2020.105581

Chapter 12
Exploring the Role of Artificial Intelligence in Healthcare Management and the Challenge of Coronavirus Pandemic

Maryam Mohamed Zainal, Allam Hamdan, and Muneer Al Mubarak

12.1 Introduction

Artificial intelligence (AI) is a technology that enables database system and software to be used in healthcare management decisions. It is a simulation of human intelligent behavior in Healthcare facilities. It is about sing this modern technology in our lives and healthcare sector. AI is being used in many sectors but in the medical section is still not clear and whether it has major contribution currently and, in the future [1]. The database and information gathered using AI in healthcare could be applied successfully on pathology, dermatology, and image analysis (medical imaging) of radiology. All these areas are affected by AI with a diagnostic speed exceeding medical experts to reach the 100% perfection system performance besides the physician knowledge and the knowledge management system that is applying in the healthcare sector.

This research focuses mainly on medical imaging and the effect of artificial intelligence on radiology services improvement in the healthcare sector and how it can help the doctors and the patients to discover and define the early stage of any type of diseases that could be missed during the human practice and human errors. AI and machines will not replace the physicians, but will help them make better medical decision and replace the human error judgments in certain functional areas in healthcare by unlocking the clinical information database which will help in decision making in the medical practice. In this research, it discusses present and future use of AI in healthcare.

M. M. Zainal
Al Hilal Healthcare Group, Manama, Bahrain

A. Hamdan (✉) · M. Al Mubarak
Ahlia University, Manama, Bahrain

P. Siarry et al. (eds.), *The Fusion of Internet of Things, Artificial Intelligence, and Cloud Computing in Health Care*, Internet of Things,
https://doi.org/10.1007/978-3-030-75220-0_12

We will first briefly review the main four relevant aspects for the medical investigation and the AI usage [2]:

1. The impact of AI in healthcare motivation by providing the physician with up-to-date information and feedback from a big base of population and from all over aspects that can encourage and motivate them in taking a better decision for them and for the patients.
2. Healthcare data can be available all over for all medical practitioner especially for the diagnostic procedures that are being used by the radiology department in different kinds of modalities and machines.
3. AI devices according to a previous study can be divided into two main categories (ML and NLP) that will be discussed more about it later.
4. Diseases types that the AI can help in defining and discover like cancer, nervous system diseases, and cardiovascular system disease (all will be discussed later in more details).
   Still, the raised question is what is the difference between artificial intelligence in healthcare practice and the normal technology?
   We can briefly say that artificial intelligence is all about gaining the information, re-process it, and give back to the end-user to be used in decision making. Moreover, during the global situation of Coronavirus pandemic that more than 130 countries including the Kingdom of Bahrain, have been facing rapid spread of this disease all over the cities and between people. Therefore, this research also looks for the role of AI in fighting against the COVID-19 virus and the impact of using the medical imaging technology in promptly discovering the virus by using the most familiar imaging technique between people (the Chest X-ray) as well as other techniques [3].

12.2 Literature Review

As part of the global crisis we are facing, the Kingdom of Bahrain is trying to be up to date with the new technologies and Artificial intelligence tools that are being used in the war against the Coronavirus. The most shown Implementations in Bahrain are the websites and mobile applications that have been created by the government to keep all the society aware of whatever we are facing [4, 5].

In this chapter we are going to focus on Artificial intelligence in Healthcare in the first part then will go through the Medical imaging in specific in the second part, ending the research with the role of AI in fighting the Coronavirus [6].

Artificial intelligence includes intelligent aspects and agents that are taking the surrounding situations to take actions and decisions to maximize the advantages and increasing the efficiency in reaching the goals and objectives. As a basic science, artificial intelligence is used to enhance the use of modern technology and computer systems and science in order to utilize the knowledge for best use. Artificial intelligent with its capability and advantages to analyzing the big amount of data to small information and easy to access is one of the important processes that are being used in medicine in general and healthcare sector in particular especially when there are scenarios and situation that the medical practitioner cannot take a discussion in it without the reference to the big database of information. Putting in mind that the pressure and timeless in the work lives of the medical practitioner especially during the catastrophes happening in the world just like what the essay is going to talk about it (COVID-19) [4, 7, 8].

Important figures can be used in healthcare to switch the artificial intelligent key to a useful tool in the health sector, some of the new systems and programs are offering a question-answer tool for all public based on hypothesis generations and evidences that are taking from medical professionals and decision making in the health sector [9]. The two main goals to be reached while converting AI to HC tool are to reduce the pressure on medical practitioners and to increase the people awareness and knowledge about different types of diseases and keep them up to date, in the situation of Coronavirus we are facing now. The advance technology and AI use in the health sector reduce the healthcare facilities visits to more than half of the numbers, which will automatically reduce the number of infected people by lowering the admixture between the public [10]. As a base of professional information that can be allowed for doctors and patients, this will help both parts of people by using the telemedicine and trustable applications [11].

According to [12], AI usage and the new technology will be part of the routine of each healthcare facility in the near future, starting from answering the medical questions for patients going through suggestions and ending with giving treatments based on the explanation and negotiations will be taking place between the system and the patient. As part of global development according to [13], companies are facing the problem of diversity of the base of the artificial intelligence that is being used in the companies, which cannot fit the traditional and culture of people in the companies. Another problem facing the AI in this time especially for the large companies with a large number of accesses and servers is that a large number of databases and information and the way to store it in safe storage from any changes and reachable at the same time. As part of this procedure, a website has been distributed among the public since the start of Coronavirus crisis in the world, the website is based on some questions for the people and according to it, they give suggestion to take advance concern and contact the responsible governmental side in the country, or consider it as the normal flu or any other disease that can be treated by normal medications at home, still, the raised question is it affected and accurate to trust? [14].

As a new technology being used by people, defiantly there will be some problems and a reduction of people responded. As the main problem facing the global development (AI dangerous) word still in mind especially for non-IT and techniques people, this problem has been suggested to be solved by raising public awareness and targeting the development and learning for the governments to help in aware and train the public later. Another problem facing the development of AI in the modern countries is the privacy and safety of informations which are being shared in the servers and networks and the limitation of the access to these details. As a healthcare user, saving the documents related to the history of diseases is a very sensitive goal, saving these data from any misusing or any changes to make sure that all information related to treating the new cases will get to the right person with every single letter as per original basis. AI in healthcare is directly related to the lives and health of the public that cannot play in it in any way, therefore devices must be protected from external reliable. Still, the raised question is how AI can be helpful in the healthcare sector? To answer this question, AI is being used by the doctors and patients to help them in reaching the related case data and information. On the second hand, some are expecting to replace doctors with technology soon. Still replacing the human with technology is way complicated to be a concern, the human body and the sense of feeling between the doctor and the patient are too complicated to be known and practice by a machine [15].

The difference between the AI technology from the traditional technology in the healthcare sector, that AI has the ability to gain, process, and give the final discussion to the user according to the information stored in it by doctors and professional people, still the problem here is that the AI and the modern systems cannot take any urgent situation from outside the database stored in it, this will put the users in a position to switch off the technology and get back to use the human mind to deal with the urgent threatening of the human lives. Here we will discuss some of the useful uses for AI in the healthcare sector [5].

Radiology	A study in [16] developed a system of an algorithm that could find pneumonia in the Chest X-ray at any specific site of it in the chest. This new technology in detecting the simple diseases in one of the medical imaging modality can reduce the timing being used in checking each image, reduce the missing errors made by the specialist Radiologist between the large number of images being seen every day, increasing the accuracy and efficiency, and all these will guide to the most important goal to reduce the recall cases in the hospitals and clinics which in accompanied will reduce the radiation exposure to the patients and medical staff. Still, some of the specialists according to the annual meeting held in North America have a concern about replacing them with uncompleted technology
Imaging	In a paper published by [17] in the journal "annals of oncology" consists that determine the skin cancer can be 95% more accurate than the dermatologists with 86.6% accuracy. This can approve that some of the scanning and imaging are more accurate with the help of artificial intelligent technology, using these technologies cannot replace the human being in the health sector, but can help them to reach the perfection in determining the diseases and taking care of human health and lives
Diseases diagnosis	Being accurate in diagnosis diabetes and cardiovascular disease has taken a place in many recent kinds of research and modern technologies are being developed to help in finding the causes of these diseases as they are categorized as two of the ten top diseases that lead to death in the world An article has been published by [18] about the multiple types of AI being used in the healthcare sector. Over the years between 2008 and 2017, several types of research and studies took a place to determine the best technology in AI to define and used in diseases diagnosis, still, the field is too big to end it and all studies are being re-concern every day to conclude it and find the solution

Telehealth	Telehealth or telemedicine started taking place all over the world. In the kingdom of Bahrain and as a small country, the only one radiology Centre in the Kingdom, its working is based on the telemedicine used by, first outsourcing the radiology departments in the small clinics and hospital to reduce the expenses and cutting the cost of the operations cost and the salaries of radiology staff. Secondly, they are putting their telemedicine devices instead of doctors all over the branches and start reading all types of medical imaging examinations are being done from the main branch, so the idea is instead of putting one doctor in each branch, a bulk of doctors are setting in the reporting center, reporting for more than 20 centers and hospitals in the same time. This idea is a very modern application of artificial intelligence in Bahrain and in medical imaging in specific that has been agreed and approved by the governmental sides
Drugs interactions	As a chronic disease patient, a variety of people aged more than 50 years are talking more than one type of medication, to avoid to interactions of medication with each other, they created an artificial intelligence system that can collect the information about the drugs and warn any medication's user to not fall in the error of interaction of drugs. This can be more accurate and efficient than depending on the human mind in memorizing the consequences of each medication [19]
Creation of new drugs	In Jan 2020, BBC News talked about a medication for (obsessive-compulsive disorder) that has been developed by artificial intelligence machines within 1 year and it is ready to be used by humans. Normally the companies and pharmaceuticals are taking around 5 years to produce such the same drug before publishing it and start the human trail
Others	As part of the COVID-19 war in the Kingdom of Bahrain, some of the physicians switched their actual clinics to digital consultations. This is an ideal application of artificial intelligence that has been used and talk about it by [7]. The idea of this to reduce the number of visitors in the clinics and priorities the appointments to urgent and chronic cases. The application is based on entering the patient medical history and syndromes, using the database and online consulting for the doctor's treatment is being given and rescheduling an actual appointment for the severe cases

The developing nations are the countries will behind technology and fewer opportunities in different aspects of life. Focusing on the healthcare and medical sector in these countries can lead us to the fact of using AI in the world can help them improved and learn remotely. By treating and teaching them, the doctors can diagnose the diseases faster and in wider ranges besides improving the patient care [20]. The rapid development in Artificial intelligence technology is a reflection of the need for urgent techniques that can help in the diagnostic of different types of chronic and dangerous diseases. A variety of essays and research papers took place in this area to give accurate and early diagnostic of the different types of diseases [21].

AI can help in preventing and discover a different type of diseases such as

- (Gene Expression) – in this century and with the technology and developed tools are being used in the healthcare, AI plays a very important role in interrupting the microarray of the Genes to detect any abnormalities any example that can be found in most of the modern countries is the IVF, where doctors are interfering

in Industrial insemination to change the abnormalities in the genes like the sickle cell disease or just to change the color of the fetus eyes [8, 22, 23].
- (Cancer Diagnosis) – the cancer cells are about a tortuous cell with extra pulps and nodulous that can be seen and defined by different types of medical imaging. With the modern techniques of Artificial intelligence, these cells can be determined by the advance technology which can be missed by the human due to human errors [24].
- (Cardiovascular diseases) – again the artificial technology can help in preventing and reducing the heart attacks be defining the places and sites of the thrombus in the blood before reaching blocked veins in the human body [25].
- (Medical Imaging) – instead of wasting half an hour of the doctor's time, the artificial intelligence applications can do the (ECG) and determine the sites and any abnormalities in the reports [26].

Overall, artificial intelligence has been recently involved in the management and development of a different type of the ten top causes disease and classified as the basic element in helping the physician and patients in a different type of applications (like the mobile phone application being used now in the Kingdom of Bahrain during the COVID-19 pandemic) [1].

As one of the most important technologies has been developed and used in the healthcare sector and concerning human health and lives, investors are competing for each other to invest in the development of diverse applications in healthcare. In association with encouraging the use of artificial intelligence in medical practice, [27] published a white paper to explain the impact, usage, policies, and the application can be used to improve the impact of AI in medical imaging. As per [6], number of AI applications have been discussed, including the nursing assistance inpatient care and surgeries, helping in the administrative work, medical records, improving the diagnostic accuracy, and dosage error reduction by reducing the recall of medical imaging. Much more applications can be applied in healthcare and depend on the speed of developing these technologies and medical staff training.

This new field in medical sector created a market and competition between the investors from entrepreneurial and corporate institutions, "recent research estimated that over 50$ billion USD has been invested in AI start-ups since 2011 till the first half of 2018, in a percent of 12% attacking the worldwide investments" [28].

Emphasizing diversity in public all over the world should take in mind while developing artificial intelligence systems in healthcare. The nature of the human being and the environment in Asia from example is different than the one in South Africa, about the type of disease, treatment types, education, investments, and the availability of the technology will be diverting from side to side. In another hand according to a study has been adopted in 2019, Medical innovation and developing of heart attacks diseases discovery have been focused on male patients only, in fact recently has been approved that female are getting the same heart attack but with different symptoms. All these should be taken in mind while developing the techniques of artificial intelligence [29].

12.2.1 The Physician–Patient Relationship

The physician-patient relationship based on ethics and trust is the major decision in choosing the right doctor or the specific hospital/Medical center. How could we save this trust and relationship between humans and machines developed by Artificial intelligence? To answer this, the patient is searching first for the Serenity from the doctor before starting the physical treatment and diagnosis. Replacing the medical workers with machines will destroy this relationship. Doctors usually and by the social life refereeing the patients from one specialty to another in the process of diagnosis, with the use of applications and machines this advantage will be deleted from the process where the patient should ask and try by themselves.

12.2.2 Artificial Intelligent in Medical Imaging

As a very fast developing path in the medical care, Radiology has been taking a very advanced stage in rapidly developing and increasing the data basis, with the fast developed. Artificial intelligence took a place in the medical imaging to catch the growth during the lack of the number of readers, radiologists, and medical staff who are specialists in radiology and imaging reading. With the force to increase the productivity in the healthcare, the pressure on Radiologist has been increased, the average has been reduced to 3–4 s per image to interpret in it, with 8 hours duty for the radiologist and in compensating with visual perception and decision making discussions and under this uncertain pressure, the human errors percent is increased in a very notable way [30]. By compensating the Artificial intelligence with the human effort, it is obvious that we can note the efficiency increment, errors reduction, and achieve objectives with minimal interrupt by the human, to give the chance for the radiologist for more focus and interfere in the image reading in a way that will help the patients and the human health [31, 32].

Two methods are being used in radiology to utilize the use of Artificial intelligence in medical imaging, first one is the term of mathematical equations usage (e.g., determine the tumor texture and feature being shown in the images) [33], this can be automatically used by the computers with the bulk of images to give the reader or the radiologist more chance for more accrue diagnosis and decision making. The second method has been focused more on it in recent years. The deep learning method is a way that is used by an automatic configuration of the algorithm that is being done without any human interruption and experts. By directly noticing the changes of the human tissue, the errors percent of mass diagnosis or any unclear features for the radiologists will be reduced [34]. Putting in mind with the rapid increase of the methods and the usage of Artificial intelligence in medical imaging, we can see that the radiologist and specialist technologist can be equalized in some of the modalities images reading, costing a reduction in time-consuming, and giving more chance to avoid errors and to see more patients [35–38].

12.2.3 Impact on Oncology Imaging

To be able to fill the gap of determining the oncology diseases (especially the most common between people, the Cancer), you have to be familiar with three main topics Abnormality detection, characterization, and subsequence monitoring of change or to bring a team of people with all knowledge related to it, to accurately determine the diseases [39].

1. Abnormality detection: in the normal steps of detecting the abnormalities and findings, the radiologist is using the normal steps they learned and dictionaries to start finding and either confirming or rejecting according to their skills that are relying on education, experience, and understanding of the patients' health and the environment and society with lifestyle coming from it and then make the decisions that are usually made by the specialist or consultants based on the appearance of any abnormalities and unusual patterns [40].
2. Characterization: It is categorizing the stage and age of the diseases and tumors by determining the segmentation and diagnosis (such as size, extent, and internal texture). Humans are not able to count or find some of the characteristics and changes in the tissue due to the limitation of brain work and the number of cases that are being seen by each reader every day. For example, it is different for the human being to define the difference between malignant and benign tumor seen by CT scan, and preferably to take a biopsy for more accurate results, this can cost more money, time, and consume the patient power, all this can be solved with modern technologies and usage of Artificial intelligence [41].
3. Monitoring: As a tumor monitoring to define the stages and development of diseases like Cancer, any small error can cost the human life and public health. The Artificial intelligence usage in these cases can put a comparable image between each period and gives a specific diagnosis and measuring in a way that will save the patient health, and to be ready in case of any urgent response needed.

12.2.4 AI Challenges in Medical Imaging

Due to the fast development in public health in general and Radiology imaging in specific and in the types of a new disease that are being introduced every period (e.g., the Coronavirus), it is difficult to catch up with the updates and keep the artificial intelligence technology up to date. Now the world is facing the Coronavirus with no ability to find any medication or solution to kill this disease, still, the studies are slower than the virus development [16, 42, 43].

Another problem is facing the artificial intelligence in the healthcare, that some of the techniques require the interfere of human expertize, which will not be available full time to attend the start of technology practice [4]. In the case of multiple tumors or mass, the technology cannot mark all the up normal findings in one time, which will cause a technology error that will affect the disease's discovery percent. Using the Picture Achieving and Communications system (PACS), ensured that medical imaging is electronically organized in a system that can be destroyed by the loss of internet connection and internet hackers, and results in losing all the images if no proper storage has been done [44].

12.2.5 Future Perspectives

From the early days of discovering the X-rays imaging in the 1890s to the more recent modalities are used in healthcare such as CT, MRI, and PET/CT, medical imaging is developing to keep as a pillar for the medical treatment. As a basic advantage, enabling the differentiating between the densities in the soft tissue and discovering the up normality that the trained eye cannot recognize it. With the new algorithm scales and recent development, the use of artificial intelligence promised to be more accurate and see a relative improvement in performance that will help to increase in the health services given to the patients.

12.2.6 Role of Medical Imaging in Fighting the CoronaVirus

COVID-19 or as it is known Coronavirus disease is infectious that attacks the lungs or the respiratory system directly, where it causes a severe acute respiratory syndrome. It has been announced as a global pandemic in 11th March 2020, after reporting the first case on late December 2019.

Since the first report of the COVID-19 case in Wuhan, China, the competition has been started between the technology companies to build teams with the clinicians, academics, and government entities to fight together in the war against this new virus, and to stop it from spreading after reaching more than 100 countries with millions of cases all around the world [45–47].

In the last part of this research, we are going to talk about the use of artificial intelligence in this war and some of the ways they are using in managing.

- AI is used to identifying, track, and forecast outbreaks, by using a new application that has been built by Kingdom of Bahrain government, they are tracking the suspected cases by allowing a full location share from each citizen, and give a warning for any of the public who has been in contact with the positive cases in the last 14 days.
- AI can help in diagnosis of the virus. Back to the same topic has discussed in the second part of the lecture review in this research, artificial intelligence is being used in diagnosis of the COVID-19 symptoms in medical imaging due to the

overload on the Radiology departments in this crisis. Still, this has not been applied in Bahrain and a study is going on it at Gulf Medical University, to start using the portable CT scan to scan the patients faster than waiting for the Lab results.

- Processing healthcare claims, the new technologies can be offered to the administrative parts of the hospitals and healthcare facilities as well as the medical staff. New insurance companies in Bahrain start using the E-cards and E-claims to reduce the direct contact between the public or the patients and the staff in the back offices. As part of reducing direct contact also, some of the healthcare facilities and business centers, in general, offered the nonwallet payment method which can give the chance for the customer to pay directly from their mobile phones without using the cards or tangible money.
- Using Drone in delivering the medical supplies and to keep an eye on the streets and gatherings more than five as per the Bahraini's government put the new rules. Drones can be the fastest and easiest way to deliver the medical supplies without the need for direct contact between the sender and receiver and can be a good option in countries that are applying the quarantine to the public during the day hours yet this technique has not been applied in Bahrain [48].
- Using robots in cleaning and sterilizing the streets and suspected places with spreading of the virus as a precaution from more spreading to the virus, as the robots are not containing soft tissue that can be the perfect place for the virus to grow.
- Developing the drugs can be done by the new technology with the algorithm scales to discover the protein type and whatever is best to destroy it without the risky part of dealing with the virus directly by the lab technologist and the scientists.
- Temperature detection technology is used to detect the human temperature by capturing it in seconds with the need for direct contact or the reduction in distance to measure it. Bahrain's government applied this technique months ago in the entrance of the kingdom on King Fahad causeway and Bahrain international airport as the first precaution system for the new coming travelers who are entering the kingdom.
- Online consultations have been approved in Bahrain by the national health regulatory authority, to reduce the working hours in the private medical centers and decrease face- to-face contact especially for the front-line medical staff; that is the government in need to their effort in this war.

Yet the CT scan medical imaging is not approved as a way of COVID-19 diagnosis, as the findings on the images can be related to another respiratory system disease. In general, during this crisis, the governments and public noticed the importance of using the new technology rather than depending on healthcare technology only to fight against it and to protect the public health [49, 50].

Still, the question is being raised, could the artificial intelligence technology fight against the spread of COVID-19 and win the war?

12.3 Method

This section will analyze demographic data that are collected via a questionnaire survey (which is the primary information and the main tool in the study), to collect bulk of information such as age, gender, education, etc. The survey is consisting of multiple-choice questions to random group of people who have received the survey by social media channels like (WhatsApp and Instagram).

To address the key research objectives, multiple choice has been divided into mandatory questions for all participants talking generally about the population knowledge and awareness about the COVID-19 in Kingdom of Bahrain, and a specific questions targeting the medical students and staff only with medical backgrounds. The study population consisted of random people from Bahrain's society with different backgrounds and education levels as the questioner was targeting the COVID-19 updates in Bahraini's society which all type of people are leaving it in the current pandemic, some of the sample were not Bahraini, but according to the research needs, the study was targeting the Bahrain's citizens in general regardless the nationality or the gender. A total of 60 samples have been collected with random size of each industry. Mostly the targeted sample was between medical and staff and students but the sample was containing only 25% from them.

12.4 Descriptive Analysis

According to Table 12.1, the results of the first question which is asking about participants' age, show that most of the survey participants are aged between 30 and 40 years old (33.9%) of the total sample population, the second majority are participants aged between 25 and 29 years old (32.1%), then above 40 years old (19.6%), between 20 and 24 (8.9%), and finally between 15 and 19 (5.4%). The majority of participants' genders were females (66.1%) who were higher than males (33.9%). This will provide the chance unequally between both genders to express their perceptions toward the role of Artificial Intelligence in fighting during the crisis of COVID-19, this unequally between the genders is due to the fact that most interested and workers in the medical field are females.

The findings showed the majority of participants were Bachelor's Degree holders (66.1%), then High school Diploma degree with (14.3%), after that Master degree with (10.7%), Ph.D. degree with (5.4%), and others (Undergraduates) with (3.6%). The findings show that High School degree holders are close to Master Degree holders. Therefore, different perceptions and background may not affect that much because such topic is being discussed according to the global sorting as an international crisis and being talked about it more in details in all the social media and the news channels (i.e., Instagram, Google, Social Groups) rather than the educational institutions.

Table 12.1 Participants' responses to demographic questions

Demographic	Answer	Frequency	Percent %
Age	15–19	3	5.4
	20–24	5	8.9
	25–29	18	32.1
	30–40	19	33.9
	Above >40	11	19.6
	Total	56	100
Gender	Male	19	33.9
	Female	37	66.1
	Total	56	100
Education	Under graduate	2	3.6
	High school diploma	8	14.3
	Bachelor degree	37	66.1
	Master degree	6	10.7
	PhD	3	5.4
	Total	56	100
Are you medical staff/student	Yes	14	25
	No	42	75
	Total	56	100

The survey showed that most participants are Medical Staff / Students with (75%); however, nonmedical Staff / Students participants came in the second and last place with (25%). We can notice that the majority of participants have Medical Background and can see clearly from their working places, the effect of using the Artificial Intelligence in Healthcare sector in General and in fighting the COVID-19 during this crisis in specific.

Based on Table 12.2, we will discuss and explain different factors that impact using Artificial intelligence in the Healthcare sector in Bahrain and how it can be helpful in quickly discover and reduce the dangers of the virus. There are three main factors that need to be addressed in this study, awareness and Knowledge, Using the technology and the expectations for the crisis future. There are other factors that may impact participants' intention to be involved in using Artificial intelligence channels. The above-mentioned factors are considered as a major factor that impacts consumers' decision to purchase any kind of product. People's perception is built based on their knowledge and background of any new technology pop-up in the social media and between the populations in Bahrain. Therefore, a source of knowledge and communication channels of certain awareness is very important as it is going to impact people's perception.

From the above table, we can see that most of the participants are following the updated of COVID-19 news and Bahrain and the new ways that are being used to speed up the discovery of the virus with the location used to alert anyone are going near an active case in the last 14 days. Of course, with multi Social media, applications, and news channels in Bahrain that already launched and developed by using

Table 12.2 Awareness and knowledge, using the technology and the expectations for the crisis future

Questions	Answer	Frequency %	Mean
Due to artificial intelligence awareness in Bahrain, the number of COVID-19 cases in Bahrain is under control	Strongly agree	16 28.6%	0.29
	Agree	23 41.1%	0.41
	Natural	15 26.8%	0.27
	Disagree	1 1.8%	0.02
	Strongly disagree	1 1.8%	0.02
Using artificial intelligence in healthcare can reduce the diagnosis errors in finding the COVID-19 and spread of the virus	Agree	28 50%	0.61
	Natural	16 28.6%	0.35
	Disagree	2 3.6%	0.04
Have you been following the updates of COVID-19 in Bahrain	No	1 1.8%	0.02
	Yes	55 98.2%	0.98
How do you assess your knowledge you gained from artificial intelligence channels about the coronavirus	Good	39 30.4%	0.7
	Average	17 69.6%	0.3
Do you spread any instructions and directions you are getting through artificial intelligence channels	Yes	22 39.3%	0.39
	Sometimes	25 44.6%	0.45
	No	9 16.1%	0.16
Can we use other modalities to diagnose the COVID-19 (e.g., X-ray chest? CT chest?)	Yes	16 28.6%	0.41
	Maybe	19 33.9%	0.49
	No	4 7.1%	0.10

the new technology and artificial intelligence, it was expected that the majority had heard about the virus and being updated. In spite that the second-highest percentage of participants' education level is high school Diploma, the majority have been part of the social media life. This is an indicator that awareness is not related to educational level especially (69.6%) of people's assess. Their knowledge about the topic is average and 30.4% as good. Social media, applications, news channels, and other sources of knowledge may have an impact more than educational entities. The findings showed that the majority of participants with (25%) yes answers and (22%) are involved in Bahrain Team goals are participating in the campaign against COVID-19 by helping in spreading the updated news and instructions to their contacts, friends, and families.

In related to multichoice questions, people went for Mobile applications mostly, google search and online consultation with some physicians as a basic knowledge to know more about whatever is related to the virus symptoms and the global news related to any reductions or increased in the number of cases, any vaccination or medications are being developed and tried (Table 12.2).

12.5 Conclusion

The research was made according to the current situation of the new technology in general and COVID-19 in specific and based on the research and articles have been found from different backgrounds and dates of an issue without taking in mind any other financial or country developments and backgrounds.

In the research we started talking about the Artificial intelligence in general in the healthcare facilities, how the definition has been started to be used and catch up the development up to date, use of AI with some applications from different countries, going through the limitations, and the question of replacing the human with robots. In the second part of the lecture review, we went through the use of Artificial intelligence in the medical imaging and the future expectations, advantages and disadvantages of using it. In the last part of the research, we talked about the applications of using Artificial intelligence in the current situation during the COVID-19 spread in the world. A questioner has been distributed to a different type of people in Bahraini society and has discussed and analyzed according to questions has been raised about the impact of using the Artificial intelligence in fighting the spread of Coronavirus.

After more than 60 years of research, we can say that the artificial intelligence tools are being considered and used in best practice these days, after noticing the importance of it in our lives, especially with the last update of the world crisis of COVID-19 *(Heller N 2018)*. The crisis showed how AI has been utilized to cover most of lives needs, starting from working at home for almost 70% of Bahraini's governmental employees, passing through the online school and university's class, going to online consultations in the healthcare facilities, and ending with the online shopping for all public needs. Ultimately, there has never been a better time to start practicing this type of technology in our lives. As to the main question raised at the beginning of this research, could the robots take a place in the hospitals and physician's lives to take the responsibility of operating and managing the medical practice? In the conclusion, we can say that the artificial intelligence can play an important role in fighting the diseases and a very important tool in the diagnosis and reducing the human errors, yet the human cannot be replaced or compared with the technology and machines. Human physicians and medical staff are not a tool to be replaced or changed; choosing the right person at the right time for the right job beside the artificial intelligence tools can generate a powerful team with almost the perfection percent of reducing the errors.

Artificial intelligence tools as per *(Chander Mohan 2018)* can be an assist for the radiologists or readers in the medical imaging reading and cannot defiantly replacing them, be highlighting the findings of the advanced cases, to be seen by the human team and mark the other normal images as normal and pass it, another advantage can be the memorization and linking between the patients' history and the diagnosis and complains to achieve a better understanding of the patient condition. This will help them reduce the time of reading and increase the quality and efficiency of the radiology departments all over the healthcare facilities. Artificial intelligence will play a more important role in the coming years, and all medical practitioners should be aware and well trained to use this technology, in fact, they are saying that the technology will affect mostly the radiology department before any other facility *(Ravi D, Wong C, Deligianni F 2017).* In fact, the most advanced and technological airplanes with the developed system and all artificial intelligence technology still need at least two human pilots on board. Simply anything deals with human lives should be trusted to be handled for human only.

References

1. Amini, A., Chen, W., Fortino, G., Li, Y., Pan, Y., & Wang, M. D. (2020). Editorial: Special issue on 'AI-driven informatics, sensing, imaging and big data analytics for fighting the COVID-19 Pandemic'. *IEEE Journal of Biomedical and Health Informatics, 24*(10). https://doi.org/10.1109/JBHI.2020.3025594
2. Salman, M., & Battour, M. (2020). Career excellence between leadership roles and achievement motivation for employees in the Ministry of Education in the United Arab Emirates. *International Journal of Business Ethics and Governance, 3*(1), 46–96. https://doi.org/10.51325/ijbeg.v3i1.33
3. Piccialli, F., Di Somma, V., Giampaolo, F., Cuomo, S., & Fortino, G. (2021). A survey on deep learning in medicine: Why, how and when? *Information Fusion, 66*, 111–137.
4. Wong, K., Fortino, G., and Abbott, D. (2019). Deep learning-based cardiovascular image diagnosis: A promising challenge. *Future Generation Computer Systems, 110*. https://doi.org/10.1016/j.future.2019.09.047.
5. Racine, E., Boehlen, W., & Sample, M. (2019). Healthcare uses of artificial intelligence: Challenges and opportunities for growth. *Healthcare Management Forum, 32*(5), 272–275. https://doi.org/10.1177/0840470419843831
6. Jiang, F., Jiang, Y., Zhi, H., Dong, Y., Li, H., Ma, S., Wang, Y., Dong, Q., Shen, H., & Wang, Y. (2017). Artificial intelligence in healthcare: Past, present and future. *Stroke and Vascular Neurology, 2*(4), 230–243. https://doi.org/10.1136/svn-2017-000101
7. Dilsizian, M. E., & Siegel, E. L. (2018). Machine meets biology: A primer on artificial intelligence in cardiology and cardiac imaging. *Current Cardiology Reports, 20*(12), 1–7. https://doi.org/10.1007/s11886-018-1074-8
8. Gupta, I., Mishra, N., & Tandon, D. (2020). Triple bottom line: Evidence from aviation sector. *International Journal of Business Ethics and Governance, 3*(1), 97–104. https://doi.org/10.51325/ijbeg.v3i1.32

9. Shinners, L., Aggar, C., Grace, S., & Smith, S. (2019). Exploring healthcare professionals' understanding and experiences of artificial intelligence technology use in the delivery of healthcare: An integrative review. *Health Informatics Journal, 26*(2), 1225–1236. https://doi.org/10.1177/1460458219874641
10. Ellis, L. (2019). Artificial intelligence for precision education in radiology – Experiences in radiology teaching from a UK foundation doctor. *The British Journal of Radiology, 92*(1104), 20190779. https://doi.org/10.1259/bjr.20190779
11. Emanuel, E. J., & Wachter, R. M. (2019). Artificial intelligence in health care. *JAMA, 321*(23), 2281. https://doi.org/10.1001/jama.2019.4914
12. Salman, M., & Laouisset, J. (2020). The governance in the corporate excellence model – The 4th generation model. *International Journal of Business Ethics and Governance, 3*(2), 73–95. https://doi.org/10.51325/ijbeg.v3i2.34
13. Tekkeşin, A. I. (2019). Artificial intelligence in healthcare: Past, present and future. *The Anatolian Journal of Cardiology*. https://doi.org/10.14744/anatoljcardiol.2019.28661.
14. Racine, E., Boehlen, W., & Sample, M. (2019). Healthcare uses of artificial intelligence: Challenges and opportunities for growth. *Healthcare Management Forum, 32*(5), 272–275. https://doi.org/10.1177/0840470419843831
15. Meyer, A. (2020). Machine-learning based wind turbine operating state detection and diagnosis. https://doi.org/10.5194/egusphere-egu2020-6532.
16. Martinez-Vernon, A. S., Covington, J. A., Arasaradnam, R. P., Esfahani, S., O'Connell, N., Kyrou, I., & Savage, R. S. (2018). An improved machine learning pipeline for urinary volatiles disease detection: Diagnosing diabetes. *PLoS One, 13*(9). https://doi.org/10.1371/journal.pone.0204425.
17. Yu, K., Beam, A. L., & Kohane, I. S. (2018). Artificial intelligence in healthcare. *Nature Biomedical Engineering, 2*(10), 719.
18. Mokadem, W., & Muwafak, B. M. (2020). The difference of the theoretical approach of corporate social responsibility between the European Union and United States of America. *International Journal of Business Ethics and Governance, 3*(1), 1–14.
19. Greenspan, H., San José Estépar, R., Niessen, W. J., Siegel, E., & Nielsen, M. (2020). Position paper on COVID-19 imaging and AI: From the clinical needs and technological challenges to initial AI solutions at the lab and national level towards a new era for AI in healthcare. *Medical Image Analysis, 66*, 101800–101800. https://doi.org/10.1016/j.media.2020.101800
20. Aminova, M., Mareef, S., & Machado, C. (2020). Entrepreneurship ecosystem in Arab world: The status quo, impediments and the ways forward. *International Journal of Business Ethics and Governance, 3*(3), 1–13. https://doi.org/10.51325/ijbeg.v3i3.37
21. Martinez-Vernon, A. S., Covington, J. A., Arasaradnam, R. P., Esfahani, S., O'Connell, N., Kyrou, I., & Savage, R. S. (2018). An improved machine learning pipeline for urinary volatiles disease detection: Diagnosing diabetes. *PLos One, 13*(9), e0204425. https://doi.org/10.5281/zenodo.1419251
22. Alremaidhi, Y., Hasan Saleh, A. O., & Abdullah Othman, A. H. (2020). Assessing the relationship between the economic feasibility study and the guarantees provided by small and medium enterprises with the financing decisions in Kuwait. *International Journal of Business Ethics and Governance, 3*(2), 34–54.
23. Yang, H., Kundakcioglu, E., Li, J., Wu, T., Mitchell, J. R., Hara, A. K., … Tsui, K. (2014). Healthcare intelligence: Turning data into knowledge. *IEEE Intelligent Systems, 29*(3), 54–68. https://doi.org/10.1109/MIS.2014.45
24. Gandhi, S., Mosleh, W., Shen, J., & Chow, C. (2018). Automation, machine learning, and artificial intelligence in echocardiography: A brave new world. *Echocardiography (Mount Kisco, N.Y.), 35*(9), 1402–1418. https://doi.org/10.1111/echo.14086
25. Razzaque, A., & Hamdan, A. (2020). Artificial intelligence-based multinational corporate model for EHR interoperability on an e-health platform. Artificial intelligence for sustainable development: Theory, practice and future applications studies in computational intelligence (pp. 71–81). https://doi.org/10.1007/978-3-030-51920-9_5

26. Alareeni, B. (2019). A review of auditors' GCOs, statistical prediction models and artificial intelligence technology. *International Journal of Business Ethics and Governance, 2*(1), 19–31.
27. Unberath, M., Ghobadi, K., Levin, S., Hinson, J., & Hager, G. D. (2020). Artificial intelligence-based clinical decision support for COVID-19–where art thou? *Advanced Intelligent Systems, 2*(9), 2000104-n/a. https://doi.org/10.1002/aisy.202000104
28. Nassar, M., R. M, & Battour, M. (2020). The impact of marketing ethics on customer loyalty: A conceptual framework. *International Journal of Business Ethics and Governance, 3*(2), 1–12.
29. Alzaneen, R., & Mahmoud, A. (2019). The role of management information systems in strengthening the administrative governance in ministry of education and higher education in Gaza. *International Journal of Business Ethics and Governance, 2*(3), 1–43. https://doi.org/10.51325/ijbeg.v2i3.44
30. Dananjayan, S., & Raj, G. M. (2020). Artificial intelligence during a pandemic: The COVID-19 example. *The International Journal of Health Planning and Management, 35*(5), 1260–1262. https://doi.org/10.1002/hpm.2987
31. Jamile, Y., & Diab, S. (2021). Does quality of governance contribute to the heterogeneity in happiness levels across MENA countries? *Journal of Business and Socio-economic Development, 1*(1), 58–70. https://doi.org/10.1108/JBSED-03-2021-0027
32. Hasan, M., & Hassan, A. (2021). The impact of team management on the organizational performance in bahrain government sector. *TechManagement and Innovation Journal, 1*(1), 1–25.
33. Stebbing, J., Krishnan, V., Bono, S., Ottaviani, S., Casalini, G., Richardson, P. J., ... the Sacco Baricitinib Study Group. (2020). Mechanism of baricitinib supports artificial intelligence-predicted testing in COVID-19 patients. *EMBO Molecular Medicine, 12*(8), e12697-n/a. https://doi.org/10.15252/emmm.202012697
34. Kaushik, A., Patel, S., & Dubey, K. (2020). Digital cardiovascular care in COVID-19 pandemic: A potential alternative? *Journal of Cardiac Surgery, 35*(12), 3545–3550. https://doi.org/10.1111/jocs.15094
35. Emile, S. H., & Hamid, H. K. S. (2020). Fighting COVID-19, a place for artificial intelligence. *Transboundary and Emerging Diseases, 67*(5), 1754–1755. https://doi.org/10.1111/tbed.13648
36. Awad, I., Al-Jerashi, G., and Alabaddi, Z. (2021). Determinants of private investment in Palestine: Time series analysis. *Journal of Business and Socio-economic Development, 1*(1), 58–70. https://doi.org/10.1108/JBSED-04-2021-0038
37. Alnoaimi, F., & Mazzuchi, T. (2021). Risk management application in an oil and gas company for projects. *TechManagement and Innovation Journal, 1*(1), 26–45.
38. Derbali, A. (2021). Determinants of the performance of Moroccan banks. *Journal of Business and Socio-economic Development, 1*(1), 60–72. https://doi.org/10.1108/JBSED-01-2021-0003
39. Ali Saad, A. Z., Azman Bin, M. N., & Sharofiddin, A. (2020). Effect of applying total quality management in improving the performance of al-waqf of albr societies in Saudi Arabia: A theoretical framework for "Deming's model". *International Journal of Business Ethics and Governance, 3*(2), 13–33.
40. Tsiknakis, N., Trivizakis, E., Vassalou, E., Papadakis, G., Spandidos, D., Tsatsakis, A., ... Marias, K. (2020). Interpretable artificial intelligence framework for COVID-19 screening on chest X-rays. *Experimental and Therapeutic Medicine, 20*(2), 727–735. https://doi.org/10.3892/etm.2020.8797
41. Anjum, R., Mukhtar, A. H., Allam, M., Abdulmuttaleb, M., Ahlam, H., Esra, S., Bahaa, A., & Sameh, R. (2019). Learning readiness when sharing knowledge while e-learning, *Journal OPTION, Bolivarian, 34*(86), 3029–3044.
42. Ramaano, A. (2021). Potential of eco-tourism as a mechanism to buoy community livelihoods: The case of musina municipality, limpopo, South Africa. *Journal of Business and Socio-economic Development, 1*(1), 37–40. https://doi.org/10.1108/JBSED-02-2021-0020
43. Rahim, K. (2021). Assessment of implementation of key performance indicators (kpis) in driving the manufacturing industry in bahrain. *TechManagement and Innovation Journal, 1*(1), 46–62.

44. Zarzeczny, A., Babyn, P., Adams, S. J., & Longo, J. (2020). Artificial intelligence-based imaging analytics and lung cancer diagnostics: Considerations for health system leaders. *Healthcare Management Forum*. 084047042097506. https://doi.org/10.1177/0840470420975062.
45. Awad, A., & Awwad, B. (2019). Evaluating mergers as a tool to strengthen and modernize the palestinian banking system, an analytical study of palestinian banking system 2010-2017. *International Journal of Economics, Business and Management Research, Alicon Publications, India, 4*(3), 100–125.
46. Sisaye, S. (2021). The influence of Non-Governmental Organizations (NGOs) on the development of voluntary sustainability accounting reporting rules. *Journal of Business and Socio-economic Development, 1*(1), 58–70. https://doi.org/10.1108/JBSED-02-2021-0017
47. Seyadi, A., & Elali, W. (2021). The impact of strategic agility on the SMEs competitive capabilities and innovation in the kingdom of bahrain. *TechManagement and Innovation Journal, 1*(1), 63–75.
48. Deghash, A. (2019). Balanced scorecard application and its challenges. *International Journal of Business Ethics and Governance, 2*(1), 33–58. https://doi.org/10.51325/ijbeg.v2i1.41
49. Al kurdi, O. (2021). A critical comparative review of emergency and disaster management in the Arab world. *Journal of Business and Socio-economic Development, 1*(1), 25–36. https://doi.org/10.1108/JBSED-02-2021-0021
50. Al Romaihi, N. (2021). The relationship between IT governance and firm performance: A eview of the literature. *TechManagement and Innovation Journal, 1*(1), 76–96.

Index

P. Siarry et al. (eds.), *The Fusion of Internet of Things, Artificial Intelligence, and Cloud Computing in Health Care*, Internet of Things,
https://doi.org/10.1007/978-3-030-75220-0

The manufacturer's authorised representative in the EU is Springer Nature Customer Service Centre GmbH, Europaplatz 3, 69115 Heidelberg, Germany. If you have any concerns regarding our products, please contact ProductSafety@springernature.com

Printed and bound by CPI Group (UK) Ltd, Croydon, CR0 4YY
30/09/2026
02225694-0008